The Norovirus

The Norovirus
Features, Detection, and Prevention of Foodborne Disease

Chief Editor

Paul K.S. Chan

Chairman and Professor (Clinical)
Department of Microbiology, Faculty of Medicine
The Chinese University of Hong Kong, Hong Kong, China

Associate Editor

Hoi Shan Kwan

Professor
School of Life Sciences
The Chinese University of Hong Kong, Hong Kong, China

Assistant Editor

Martin C.W. Chan

Research Assistant Professor
Department of Microbiology, Faculty of Medicine
The Chinese University of Hong Kong, Hong Kong, China

ELSEVIER

AMSTERDAM • BOSTON • HEIDELBERG • LONDON
NEW YORK • OXFORD • PARIS • SAN DIEGO
SAN FRANCISCO • SINGAPORE • SYDNEY • TOKYO

Academic Press is an imprint of Elsevier

Academic Press is an imprint of Elsevier
125 London Wall, London EC2Y 5AS, United Kingdom
525 B Street, Suite 1800, San Diego, CA 92101-4495, United States
50 Hampshire Street, 5th Floor, Cambridge, MA 02139, United States
The Boulevard, Langford Lane, Kidlington, Oxford OX5 1GB, United Kingdom

Notices
Knowledge and best practice in this field are constantly changing. As new research and experience broaden our
understanding, changes in research methods, professional practices, or medical treatment may become necessary.

Practitioners and researchers must always rely on their own experience and knowledge in evaluating and using any
information, methods, compounds, or experiments described herein. In using such information or methods they should be
mindful of their own safety and the safety of others, including parties for whom they have a professional responsibility.

To the fullest extent of the law, neither the Publisher nor the authors, contributors, or editors, assume any liability for
any injury and/or damage to persons or property as a matter of products liability, negligence or otherwise, or from any
use or operation of any methods, products, instructions, or ideas contained in the material herein.

British Library Cataloguing-in-Publication Data
A catalogue record for this book is available from the British Library

Library of Congress Cataloging-in-Publication Data
A catalog record for this book is available from the Library of Congress

ISBN: 978-0-12-804177-2

For Information on all Academic Press publications
visit our website at https://www.elsevier.com

 Working together
to grow libraries in
developing countries

www.elsevier.com • www.bookaid.org

Publisher: Nikki Levy
Acquisition Editor: Patricia Osborn
Editorial Project Manager: Jaclyn Truesdell
Production Project Manager: Caroline Johnson
Designer: Victoria Pearson

Typeset by MPS Limited, Chennai, India

Contents

PART III PATHOGEN AND THE HOST

List of Contributors

Giuseppe Arcangeli
Istituto Zooprofilattico Sperimentale delle Venezie, V.le Università, Legnaro, Padova, Italy

Robert L. Atmar
Baylor College of Medicine, Houston, TX, United States

Judith Breuer
University College London, London, United Kingdom

Julianne R. Brown
Great Ormond Street Hospital for Children NHS Foundation Trust, London, United Kingdom

Martin C.W. Chan
The Chinese University of Hong Kong, Hong Kong, China

Paul K.S. Chan
The Chinese University of Hong Kong, Hong Kong, China

Mary K. Estes
Baylor College of Medicine, Houston, TX, United States

Aron J. Hall
Centers for Disease Control and Prevention, Atlanta, GA, United States

Zhong Huang
Institute Pasteur of Shanghai, Huangpu, Shanghai, China

Pattara Khamrin
Nihon University School of Medicine, Tokyo, Japan; Chiang Mai University, Chiang Mai, Thailand

Evelyn Siew-Chuan Koay
National University Health System, Singapore

Bonita E. Lee
University of Alberta, Edmonton, Alberta, Canada

Hong Kai Lee
National University Health System, Singapore

Way-Seah Lee
University of Malaya, Kuala Lumpur, Malaysia

Qingwei Liu
Institute Pasteur of Shanghai, Huangpu, Shanghai, China

Edmond A.S. Nelson
The Chinese University of Hong Kong, Hong Kong, China

Mamoru Noda
National Institute of Health Sciences, Tokyo, Japan

Shoko Okitsu
Nihon University School of Medicine, Tokyo, Japan; The University of Tokyo, Tokyo, Japan

Minesh P. Shah
Centers for Disease Control and Prevention, Atlanta, GA, United States

Xiaoli Pang
University of Alberta, Edmonton, Alberta, Canada

Sasirekha Ramani
Baylor College of Medicine, Houston, TX, United States

Hiroyuki Saito
Akita Prefectural Research Center for Public Health and Environment, Akita, Japan

Hoi Shan Kwan
The Chinese University of Hong Kong, Hong Kong, China

Tomoyuki Tanaka
Hidaka General Hospital, Gobo, Japan

Calogero Terregino
Istituto Zooprofilattico Sperimentale delle Venezie, V.le Università, Legnaro, Padova, Italy

Aksara Thongprachum
Nihon University School of Medicine, Tokyo, Japan; The University of Tokyo, Tokyo, Japan

Miho Toho
Fukui Prefectural Institute of Public Health and Environmental Science, Fukui, Japan

Hiroshi Ushijima
Nihon University School of Medicine, Tokyo, Japan; The University of Tokyo, Tokyo, Japan

Xiaoli Wang
Institute Pasteur of Shanghai, Huangpu, Shanghai, China

About the Editors

CHIEF EDITOR
PAUL K.S. CHAN, DEPARTMENT OF MICROBIOLOGY, THE CHINESE UNIVERSITY OF HONG KONG, HONG KONG, CHINA

Paul K.S. Chan, MBBS, MSc (Virology), MD, FRCPath, FHKCPath, FHKAM, is Chairman and Clinical Professor of the Department of Microbiology and Deputy Director of Stanley Ho Centre for Emerging Infectious Diseases, Faculty of Medicine, The Chinese University of Hong Kong. He is also Consultant in Microbiology for the New Territories East Cluster Hospitals of Hong Kong Hospital Authority. He graduated from University of Hong Kong in 1988 with a Bachelor of Medicine and Bachelor of Surgery. He obtained his Master of Science in Virology from London School of Hygiene and Tropical Medicine in 1995, and he obtained his Doctor of Medicine from The Chinese University of Hong Kong in 2003. He received fellowships from Royal College of Pathologists and Hong Kong College of Pathologists. He is a leading expert on clinical virology, especially on diagnosis, pathogenesis, and epidemiology. Based on original studies, he has published more than 300 articles in international peer-reviewed medical journals. In addition to academic achievements, he has made major contributions to government, professional bodies, and the community. For instance, since 2004, he has served on the Scientific Committee on Emerging and Zoonotic Diseases of the Centre for Health Protection of Hong Kong Government, providing advice on the control of infectious disease outbreaks. Since 2009, he has been a member of the Advisory Council on Food and Environmental Hygiene of Hong Kong Government, providing imperative advice on food safety. His team is monitoring the epidemiology and strain variation of norovirus in Hong Kong.

ASSOCIATE EDITOR
HOI SHAN KWAN, PROFESSOR, SCHOOL OF LIFE SCIENCES, THE CHINESE UNIVERSITY OF HONG KONG, HONG KONG, CHINA

Professor Hoi Shan Kwan has been teaching at The Chinese University of Hong Kong since 1984. He is the director of Food Research Centre (CUHK), professor of the School of Life Sciences (CUHK), and honorary professor of the School of Chinese Medicine (CUHK). He was awarded the Bronze Bauhinia Star for his meritorious public and community service, particularly his contribution to promoting food safety and quality assurance. He served as the Chairman of the Expert Committee for Food Safety of Food and Environmental Hygiene Department and as the Chairman of the Accreditation Advisory Board of Hong Kong Accreditation Service. He is currently a member of the Chinese Medicines Board of the Chinese Medicine Council of Hong Kong, the Chinese Medicine Development Committee, the Council for Testing and Certification of Innovation and Technology Commission, the Committee on Reduction of Salt and Sugar in Food, and the Scientific Committee on Enteric and Infections and Foodborne Diseases of the Centre for Health Protection. His research interests include molecular biotechnology, genetics and genomics of enteric bacteria, edible and medicinal fungi, medicinal plants, and marine animals. His funding sources include the Department of Health, Industrial Support Fund, Research Grants Council (RGC) Earmarked Grants, The Hong Kong Jockey Club Charities Trust, Research Fund for the Control of Infectious Diseases, and Research Grants Council (RGC) Central Allocation Vote. He has published more than 200 refereed papers and abstracts in international journals and conferences.

ASSISTANT EDITOR

MARTIN C.W. CHAN, DEPARTMENT OF MICROBIOLOGY, FACULTY OF MEDICINE, THE CHINESE UNIVERSITY OF HONG KONG, HONG KONG, CHINA

Martin C.W. Chan is a research assistant professor in the Department of Microbiology at the Faculty of Medicine of The Chinese University of Hong Kong. He has been working on noroviruses since 2004. His research interests include studies of the molecular epidemiology of foodborne viruses such as noroviruses and hepatitis E virus, the biological importance of gut virome, and the discovery of novel viruses.

Introduction: Noroviruses at a Glance

HISTORY
WINTER VOMITING DISEASE

The illness induced by noroviruses was recognized long before the pathogen was identified. A paper titled, "Hyperemesis Hiemis or the Winter Vomiting Disease," written by pediatrician J. Zahorsky, was published in 1929 and highlighted two salient features of the infection (Zahorsky, 1929). First, infected subjects often presented with prominent "vomiting" along with other symptoms of acute gastroenteritis, including diarrhea and mild fever. This characteristic was reproduced in subsequent outbreaks and experimental inoculation to humans. Today, "vomiting" remains a useful sign to recognize norovirus outbreak. Second, Zahorsky observed a seasonal predilection with winter predominance of those cases. This wintertime phenomenon was reiterated by a recent meta-analysis, at least for the temperate region for which most data were available (Ahmed et al., 2013). Of note, outbreaks during summertime have also been reported (Magill-Collins et al., 2015; Di Bartolo et al., 2015; Solano et al., 2014).

NORWALK AGENT

Human norovirus was previously known as Norwalk virus to signify the place where outbreaks led to identification of the virus. In October 1968, two epidemics of winter vomiting disease occurred in an elementary school in Norwalk, Ohio (Adler and Zickl, 1969). The outbreak demonstrated a few key epidemiological features of norovirus infection. It was explosive, with a high attack rate involving 50% of the students and teachers in the first wave and further affected 32% of family contacts in the second wave. The incubation period was approximately 48 hours, with a short illness duration of 12−24 hours. Nausea and vomiting were the predominant symptoms, occurred in greater than 80% of cases, whereas diarrhea occurred in 44% and fever or chills in 37%. Although the pathogen could not be identified, the infectious nature of the outbreak was proven by reproduction of symptoms in healthy adults who had received oral administration of filtrates prepared from rectal swabs taken from affected subjects (Dolin et al., 1971).

THE 27-NM VIRION

The success in human transmission study using bacteria-free filtrate of rectal swab specimens collected from outbreaks in Norwalk and other locations pinpointed a viral origin of acute gastroenteritis (Reimann et al., 1945; Gordon et al., 1947; Kojima et al., 1948; Dolin et al., 1971; Clarke et al., 1972). However, attempts to isolate the virus using standard tissue culture as well as organ culture failed to yield an etiological agent for those outbreaks (Blacklow et al., 1972). Today, isolation of noroviruses remains a difficult challenge. In 1972, Kapikian examined the stool filtrate derived from a volunteer who developed illness after oral administration of the Norwalk agent (Kapikian et al., 1972). The stool filtrate was incubated with convalescent serum of a volunteer for

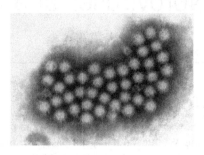

FIGURE I.1

An aggregate of noroviruses observed by negative staining of a stool sample collected from a patient with acute gastroenteritis.

examination by immune electron microscopy. Glistening aggregates of nonenveloped, antibody-coated, 27-nm virus-like particles (VLPs) resembling rhinoviruses were visualized. The etiological association of the 27-nm VLPs with disease was further demonstrated by the serological response among volunteers after challenged with Norwalk virus stool filtrate (Kapikian, 2000; Kapikian et al., 1972). Electron microscopy was the mainstay of laboratory diagnosis for norovirus infection until recently, when it was replaced by molecular techniques (Fig. I.1).

CLASSIFICATION AND STRUCTURE

Noroviruses are classified under the family *Caliciviridae*, which is composed of the following five genera of nonenveloped, positive-sense, single-stranded RNA viruses: *Norovirus*, *Sapovirus*, *Lagovirus*, *Nebovirus*, and *Vesivirus* (Green, 2013). There are two proposed genera pending consideration by the International Committee on Taxonomy of Viruses: *Recovirus* in rhesus monkeys (Farkas et al., 2008) and *Valovirus* in pigs (L'Homme et al., 2009). The human norovirus genome is approximately 7.6 kb in length, with three open reading frames (ORFs) encoding eight proteins. ORF1 encodes six nonstructural proteins. ORF2 and ORF3 encode structural viral protein 1 (VP1) and VP2, respectively. Noroviruses are genetically very diverse. Based on the sequence variation of VP1, noroviruses are separated into seven genogroups (GI−VII) and more than 40 genotypes (Donaldson et al., 2010; Zheng et al., 2006; Vinjé, 2015). Recently, virome study in bats identified several novel norovirus sequences, putatively representing an eighth genogroup (Wu et al., 2015). Among the seven genogroups, GI and GII infect humans; human infections by GIV have been documented but appear to be rare (Eden et al., 2012; Ao et al., 2014). GII viruses, specifically GII.4 variants, account for the majority of recent outbreaks worldwide. In the past two decades, at least six pandemic variants of GII.4 have emerged (Pringle et al., 2015). The emergence of novel GII.4 variants is usually, but not always, accompanied by a surge in the number of infected cases (Lopman et al., 2004a; van Beek et al., 2013). The protruding 2 (P2) domain of VP1 is the most exposed portion of norovirus virion, which is presumably also a major point of contact with neutralizing antibodies. Mutations at the P2 domain can affect the antigenic property and result in the emergence of an epidemic (Lindesmith et al., 2011; Bull et al., 2010; Shanker et al., 2011; Chan et al., 2015a).

CLINICAL FEATURES
HEALTHY INDIVIDUALS

With the increase in accessibility to sensitive molecular assays, the clinical spectrum of norovirus infection has been much better defined. At the same time, asymptomatic infection represented by the presence of viral RNA in stool is recognized to be not uncommon. The reported asymptomatic carriage rates among children range from 3% to 50%, and asymptomatic infection is not limited to areas with poor hygiene (Qi et al., 2015; Garcia et al., 2006; Marques Mendanha de Oliveira et al., 2014; Huynen et al., 2013; Frange et al., 2012). Asymptomatic infection has also been detected in adults, including food handlers, who can be a potential source of food contamination and further spread (Yu et al., 2011).

Norovirus infection affects all age groups and typically presents as acute gastroenteritis with a short incubation period of 1 or 2 days, as well as a short duration of illness of 1 or 2 days. In most healthy individuals, symptoms are mild and self-limiting. The clinical manifestations recorded in one volunteer experiment were fever (45%), diarrhea (81%), vomiting (65%), abdominal discomfort (68%), anorexia (90%), headache (81%), and myalgia (58%) (Wyatt et al., 1974). At the extremes of age, norovirus infection can be severe enough to necessitate hospitalization, and life-threatening dehydration can occur (Mattner et al., 2006; Franck et al., 2014).

IMMUNOCOMPROMISED INDIVIDUALS

Norovirus infections in immunocompromised hosts are often prolonged, more severe, and persist for long durations. A survey conducted in a pediatric hematopoietic stem cell transplant center revealed a prolong shedding of viruses for 60–380 days (median, 150 days), which requires lengthened enteral and parental nutritional support. The resolution of infection correlated with the time to $CD3^+$ T-cell recovery (Saif et al., 2011). Similar prolonged symptoms and viral shedding have also been reported from solid organ transplant patients (Coste et al., 2013) and HIV-infected subjects (Wingfield et al., 2010). In general, controlling the underlying immunosuppression brings resolution of symptoms and stops virus excretion.

TRANSMISSION AND OUTBREAKS

Kaplan's criteria, which are based on the characteristic clinical and epidemiological features, remain a useful tool to identify norovirus outbreak today, especially in circumstances in which rapid diagnostic test or specimen is not available (Table I.1) (Kaplan et al., 1982). Because humans are the only natural host of noroviruses, outbreaks always originate from either direct human-to-human transmission or contamination of the environment or vehicles by infected persons.

The fecal–oral route is the main mode of transmission. Infected individuals shed a large amount of virions in stool, with viral RNA copies as high as 10^4-10^{12} per gram of feces (Chan et al., 2006; Pang et al., 2004; Atmar et al., 2008; Aoki et al., 2010). It has been shown that the magnitude of viral shedding correlated with clinical manifestations and with the infected genotype (Lee et al., 2007; Tu et al., 2008; Kirby et al., 2014; Corcoran et al., 2014; Chan et al., 2015b).

Table I.1 Kaplan's Criteria for Norovirus-Associated Outbreak of Gastroenteritis	
Criterion	**Description**
1	Vomiting in $\geq 50\%$ of cases
2	Mean or median incubation period of 24–48 h
3	Mean or median duration of illness of 12–60 h
4	Stool culture negative for bacterial pathogens

When laboratory confirmation is not possible, the Kaplan's criteria can be used to assess whether the outbreak was likely caused by norovirus. When all four criteria are present, it is very likely that the outbreak was caused by norovirus. However, approximately 30% of norovirus outbreaks do not meet these criteria. Therefore, when these criteria are not met, the possibility of norovirus causing the outbreak is lower but still cannot be excluded.

The characteristic symptom of vomiting, and sometimes even projectile vomiting, can generate aerosolized virions that can contaminate much wider and often unnoticed areas and also objects, making the control of outbreak more difficult (Kirking et al., 2010).

Contaminated surfaces (i.e., fomites) often play an important role in propagating the infection. The extreme contagious nature of noroviruses is related to their nonenveloped virion structure, which enhances resistance to disinfection and improves survival in the environment. It has been shown that noroviruses can survive on stainless-steel surfaces for weeks at ambient temperatures (Liu et al., 2008). In general, stronger disinfectants such as hypochlorite of at least 5000 ppm (i.e., domestic bleach in 10% solution) are required to clean contaminated surfaces (Barker et al., 2004). Of note, alcohol-based hand rub, which has been promoted for preventing transmission of infections, has limited effectiveness in killing noroviruses (Said et al., 2008).

Common settings for norovirus outbreak are closed spaces in which people share common facilities, such as hospitals, nursing homes, schools, and especially public restrooms. In these settings, exposed people of all age groups can be affected (Petriqnani et al., 2015; Dancer, 2014; Iturriza-Gomara and Lopman, 2014). These closed-space outbreaks are often explosive and lead to disruption of service because closure of the facility is usually necessary to stop further propagation. Outbreaks on cruise ships are well documented and publicized. More than 95% of cruise ship acute gastroenteritis outbreaks are caused by noroviruses. A study conducted in 2005–08 including 56 large cruise ships showed that only 37% of the surfaces that had a high likelihood of being contaminated with enteric pathogens during toileting activities were cleaned at least once daily. Of note, only 35% of restroom exit door knobs or pulls were cleaned daily. Washed hands can therefore become contaminated again by touching these fomites (Carling et al., 2009). Furthermore, only 30% of baby changing tables were cleaned on a daily basis. Such suboptimal cleansing frequency probably also occurs in other settings.

Water and food are important vehicles to disseminate noroviruses, particularly in the community. Outbreaks linked to direct consumption of contaminated water, commercial ice, and exposure during swimming and other recreational activities have been documented (Cannon et al., 1991; Koopman et al., 1982). Shellfish, oysters, and other bivalves grown in contaminated water are common sources of foodborne outbreaks in the community (Loury et al., 2015; Le Guyader et al., 2000). In a raw oyster-associated outbreak reported from Shanghai, China, multiple strains of caliciviruses with 15 strains of sapoviruses, 14 strains of norovirus GI, and 17 stains of norovirus GII were found from 25 specimens. Of these, 20% and 48% were triple and double infections, respectively (Wang et al., 2015).

Vegetables and fruits are also vulnerable to contamination either at the source of production or due to hygiene breaches during the preparation process. In the European Union, there was a 4.5-fold increase in consumption of berries from 1988 to 2005 due to an increase in popularity of fruit-based products such as smoothies, ice creams, and yogurts (Commission of the European Communities, 2006). Berry production is a labor-intensive process that is vulnerable to contamination by infected food handlers, especially asymptomatic ones. A review on outbreaks associated with frozen berries in the European Union reported from 1983 to 2013 showed that norovirus was the most common pathogen implicated in 27 events in more than 15,000 cases (Tavoschi et al., 2015).

BURDEN

Acute gastroenteritis accounts for the second greatest burden of all infectious diseases worldwide (Murray et al., 2012; Lozano et al., 2012). The World Health Organization (WHO) estimates that norovirus and *Campylobacter* spp. are the most common etiological agents causing foodborne illness worldwide (WHO, 2015). In the 2010 WHO Estimates, norovirus is one of the leading causes of death in diarrheal diseases in all six WHO regions except Europe, and it ranks fourth among 22 foodborne pathogens in terms of disability-adjusted life-years globally (Pires et al., 2015; Kirk et al., 2015). Based on an analysis of 175 published studies covering 187,336 cases of acute gastroenteritis, it was estimated that norovirus associated with 18% (95% CI: 17−20%) of all diarrhea cases worldwide affecting all age groups (Ahmed et al., 2014). The estimated prevalence of norovirus infection tended to be higher in the community (24%) and outpatients (20%) compared to inpatients (17%), reflecting the generally mild nature of norovirus-associated gastroenteritis. Norovirus is estimated to cause approximately 200,000 deaths annually worldwide, with approximately 70,000 young children in developing countries. All ages are affected, with the highest incidence in children. Severe outcomes are mainly seen in young children and elderly. Among the 1877 norovirus outbreaks identified in England and Wales in 1992−2000, 40% occurred in hospitals and a similar fraction (39%) was detected in residential care facilities (Lopman et al., 2003). A survey involving 386 outbreaks in 289 US hospitals showed that norovirus was the most frequent cause of hospital-acquired infection, accounting for 18% of outbreaks and greater than 65% of hospital unit closures (Rhinehart et al., 2012).

The infection control measures necessary to stop norovirus outbreak often lead to major disruption of health service, resulting in substantial economic loss. For instance, an outbreak in a Swiss hospital reported a cost of $40,675 for additional diagnostic materials, health care, revenue loss, and sick leave (Zingg et al., 2005). In the United Kingdom, nosocomial outbreaks of acute gastroenteritis cost approximately $184 million annually (Lopman et al., 2004b).

VIRUS DETECTION

Prompt and accurate detection of noroviruses is of paramount importance to identify the etiological agent of suspected cases or contaminated vehicles and to interrupt virus transmission in both health care and community settings. Before the molecular era, electron microscopy and enzyme immunoassay (EIA) were used for norovirus detection (Vinjé, 2015). However, these techniques are of low throughput and have suboptimal sensitivity. The sensitivity of EIAs, for example, ranges from 32%

to 92% (Robilotti et al., 2015). Currently, there is only one commercial EIA cleared for norovirus diagnosis by the US Food and Drug Administration (CDC, 2014). Today, broadly reactive real-time reverse transcription—polymerase chain reaction (RT-PCR) assays for norovirus RNA detection are available and commonly used. They are also the de facto gold standard for evaluating the performance of different virus detection platforms (Kojima et al., 2002; Kageyama et al., 2003; Vinjé, 2015; Pang and Lee, 2015; Farkas et al., 2015). High-throughput multiplex nucleic acid amplification test (NAAT)-based assays to detect a panel of diarrheagenic viruses and bacteria have been recently introduced to the market (Navidad et al., 2013; Khare et al., 2014). With technological advances and the reduced cost of massively parallel sequencing, virus-targeted whole genome sequencing is now feasible in a proof-of-concept study and may play a role in the management of norovirus outbreaks in the future (Bavelaar et al., 2015).

VACCINE DEVELOPMENT

Given the public health burden of foodborne norovirus infections and the economic cost associated with containment of outbreaks, service interruption in health care facilities, and treatment of disease, there is a strong demand for a norovirus vaccine (Debbink et al., 2014; Aliabadi et al., 2015). In a small-scale, randomized, double-blind, placebo-controlled, multicenter trial, a norovirus virus like particle (VLP) vaccine was shown to offer protection against Norwalk virus (GI.1) infection (Atmar et al., 2011). Because norovirus is genetically very diverse, a multivalent vaccine may prove more useful in real-world settings than a monovalent vaccine. Human volunteer challenge studies provide preliminary evidence that a bivalent norovirus VLP vaccine that includes GII.4 could trigger immune response and may alleviate gastroenteritis symptoms (Bernstein et al., 2015; Treanor et al., 2014). The smaller-sized norovirus P particle, which is composed of only the P domain of VP1, is immunogenic and serves as an attractive alternative to VLP for the manufacture of norovirus vaccine (Tan et al., 2011; Xia et al., 2011). One major hurdle in developing norovirus vaccine is the lack of a robust in vitro cell culture model for human noroviruses. Recently, it has been reported that human noroviruses infect and replicate in B cells, but this finding has not yet been reproduced in other laboratories (Jones et al., 2014, 2015). Without a cell culture system, identification of broadly neutralizing epitopes and antibodies against human norovirus remains challenging.

CONCLUSIONS AND PERSPECTIVES

Substantial progress has been made in the past few decades to better our understanding of the biology, epidemiology, and clinical picture of noroviruses. Challenges remain and knowledge gaps need to be filled. Asymptomatic norovirus shedding is commonly observed in healthy individuals. The role of asymptomatic norovirus shedding in outbreak settings needs to be clarified. Does norovirus infection mediate humans' gut microbiome and influence other systemic chronic diseases? Several vaccines are in the pipeline and undergoing clinical trials. Given the very low mortality of norovirus gastroenteritis, it is a consensus that norovirus vaccination may need to target specific populations such as food handlers and health care professionals, who are prone to disseminating noroviruses, as well as young children and the elderly, who are at risk of more severe presentation and adverse outcome. Vaccine efficacy in these groups of people needs to be evaluated. Novel pandemic norovirus GII.4 variants emerge every 2–4 years. What is the reservoir? Because human noroviruses have no known hosts other than humans, it is speculated that unchecked norovirus evolution in infected immunocompromised patients or malnourished individuals may seed the next pandemic strain. If this is true, it means that the emergence of novel norovirus strains is stochastic and unpredictable. This poses a significant challenge with regard to vaccine formulation and design. To answer questions, we need better tools. Recent successful cultivation of human noroviruses in B cells is a triumph in the field. However, this victory definitely invites more questions than it answers. How does norovirus B-cell infection lead to vomiting and diarrhea? It seems we are just beginning to understanding noroviruses.

Paul K.S. Chan, Hoi Shan Kwan and Martin C.W. Chan

The Chinese University of Hong Kong, Hong Kong, China

REFERENCES

Adler, J.L., Zickl, R., 1969. Winter vomiting disease. J. Infect. Dis. 119 (6), 668–673.

Ahmed, S.M., Lopman, B.A., Levy, K., 2013. A systematic review and meta-analysis of the global seasonality of norovirus. PLos ONE 8 (10), e75922.

Ahmed, S.M., Hall, A.J., Robinson, A.E., Verhoef, L., Premkumar, P., Parashar, U.D., et al., 2014. Global prevalence of norovirus in cases of gastroenteritis: a systematic review and meta-analysis. Lancet Infect. Dis. 14 (8), 725–730.

Aliabadi, N., Lopman, B.A., Parashar, U.D., Hall, A.J., 2015. Progress toward norovirus vaccines: considerations for further development and implementation in potential target populations. Expert. Rev. Vaccines 14 (9), 1241–1253.

Ao, Y.Y., Yu, J.M., Li, L.L., Jin, M., Duan, Z.J., 2014. Detection of human norovirus GIV. 1 in China: a case report. J. Clin. Virol. 61 (2), 298–301.

Aoki, Y., Suto, A., Mizuta, K., Ahiko, T., Osaka, K., Matsuzaki, Y., 2010. Duration of norovirus excretion and the longitudinal course of viral load in norovirus-infected elderly patients. J. Hosp. Infect. 75 (1), 42–46.

Atmar, R.L., Bernstein, D.I., Harro, C.D., Al-Ibrahim, M.S., Chen, W.H., Ferreira, J., et al., 2011. Norovirus vaccine against experimental human Norwalk virus illness. New Engl. J. Med. 365 (23), 2178–2187.

Atmar, R.L., Opekun, A.R., Gilger, M.A., Estes, M.K., Crawford, S.E., Neill, F.H., et al., 2008. Norwalk virus shedding after experimental human infection. Emerg. Infect. Dis. 14 (10), 1553–1557.

Barker, J., Vipond, I.B., Bloomfield, S.F., 2004. Effects of cleaning and disinfection in reducing the spread of norovirus contamination via environmental surfaces. J. Hosp. Infect. 58 (1), 42–49.

Bavelaar, H.H., Rahamat-Langendoen, J., Niesters, H.G., Zoll, J., Melchers, W.J., 2015. Whole genome sequencing of fecal samples as a tool for the diagnosis and genetic characterization of norovirus. J. Clin. Virol. 72, 122–125.

Bernstein, D.I., Atmar, R.L., Lyon, G.M., Treanor, J.J., Chen, W.H., Jiang, X., et al., 2015. Norovirus vaccine against experimental human GII.4 virus illness: a challenge study in healthy adults. J. Infect. Dis. 211 (6), 870–878.

Blacklow, N.R., Dolin, R., Fedson, D.S., et al., 1972. Acute infectious nonbacterial gastroenteritis: etiology and pathogenesis. A combined clinical staff conference at the Clinical Center of the National Institutes of Health. Ann. Intern. Med. 76, 993–1008.

Bull, R.A., Eden, J.S., Rawlinson, W.D., White, P.A., 2010. Rapid evolution of pandemic noroviruses of the GII.4 lineage. PLoS Pathog. 6 (3), e1000831.

Cannon, R.O., Poliner, J.R., Hirschhorn, R.B., Rodeheaver, D.C., Silverman, P.R., Brown, E.A., et al., 1991. A multistate outbreak of Norwalk virus gastroenteritis associated with consumption of commercial ice. J. Infect. Dis. 164, 860–863.

Carling, P.C., Bruno-Murtha, L.A., Griffiths, J.K., 2009. Cruise ship environmental hygiene and the risk of norovirus infection outbreaks: an objective assessment of 56 vessels over 3 years. Clin. Infect. Dis. 49 (9), 1312–1317.

Centers for Disease Control and Prevention, 2014. Norovirus-diagnostic methods. Last updated: 2014 May. Available from: <http://www.cdc.gov/norovirus/lab-testing/diagnostic.html>.

Chan, M.C., Lee, N., Hung, T.N., Kwok, K., Cheung, K., Tin, E.K., et al., 2015a. Rapid emergence and predominance of a broadly recognizing and fast-evolving norovirus GII. 17 variant in late 2014. Nat. Commun. 6, 10061.

Chan, M.C., Leung, T.F., Chung, T.W., Kwok, A.K., Nelson, E.A., Lee, N., et al., 2015b. Virus genotype distribution and virus burden in children and adults hospitalized for norovirus gastroenteritis, 2012–2014, Hong Kong. Sci. Rep. 5, 11507.

Chan, M.C., Sung, J.J., Lam, R.K., Chan, P.K., Lee, N.L., Lai, R.W., et al., 2006. Fecal viral load and norovirus-associated gastroenteritis. Emerg. Infect. Dis. 12 (8), 1278–1280.

Clarke, S.K.R., Cook, G.T., Egglestone, S.I., et al., 1972. A virus from epidemic vomiting disease. Br. Med. J. 3, 86–89.

Commission of the European Communities, 2006. Commission staff working document-Annex to the report from the commission to the council and the European Parliament on the situation of the sector of soft fruits and cherries intended for processing: review of the sector of soft fruits and cherries intended for processing in the EU. Brussels: Commission of the European Communities. Available from: <http://ec.europa.eu/agriculture/publi/reports/fruitveg/softfruit/workdoc_en.pdf>.

Corcoran, M.S., van Well, G.T., van Loo, I.H., 2014. Diagnosis of viral gastroenteritis in children: interpretation of real-time PCR results and relation to clinical symptoms. Eur. J. Clin. Microbiol. Infect. Dis. 33 (10), 1663–1673.

Coste, J.F., Vuiblet, V., Moustapha, B., Bouin, A., Lavaud, S., Toupance, O., et al., 2013. Microbiological diagnosis of severe diarrhea in kidney transplant recipients by use of multiplex PCR assays. J. Clin. Microbiol. 51 (6), 1841–1849.

Dancer, S.J., 2014. Controlling hospital-acquired infection: focus on the roles of the environment and new technologies for decontamination. Clin. Microbiol. Rev. 27 (4), 665–690.

Debbink, K., Lindesmith, L.C., Baric, R.S., 2014. The state of norovirus vaccines. Clin. Infect. Dis. 58 (12), 1746–1752.

Di Bartolo, I., Pavoni, E., Tofani, S., Consoli, M., Galuppini, E., Losio, M.N., et al., 2015. Waterborne norovirus outbreak during a summer excursion in Northern Italy. New Microbiol. 38 (1), 109–112.

Dolin, R., Blacklow, N.R., DuPont, H., Formal, S., Buscho, R.F., Kasel, J.A., et al., 1971. Transmission of acute infectious nonbacterial gastroenteritis to volunteers by oral administration of stool filtrates. J. Infect. Dis. 123 (3), 307–312.

Donaldson, E.F., Lindesmith, L.C., Lobue, A.D., Baric, R.S., 2010. Viral shape-shifting: norovirus evasion of the human immune system. Nat. Rev. Microbiol. 8 (3), 231–241.

Eden, J.S., Lim, K.L., White, P.A., 2012. Complete genome of the human norovirus GIV. 1 strain Lake Macquarie virus. J. Virol. 86 (18), 10251–10252.

Farkas, T., Sestak, K., Wei, C., Jiang, X., 2008. Characterization of rhesus monkey calicivirus representing a new genus of Caliciviridae. J. Virol. 82 (11), 5408–5416.

Farkas, T., Singh, A., Le Guyader, F.S., La Rosa, G., Saif, L., McNeal, M., 2015. Multiplex real-time RT-PCR for the simultaneous detection and quantification of GI, GII and GIV noroviruses. J. Virol. Methods 223, 109–114.

Franck, K.T., Fonager, J., Ersbøll, A.K., Böttiger, B., 2014. Norovirus epidemiology in community and health care settings and association with patient age, Denmark. Emerg. Infect. Dis. 20 (7), 1123–1131.

Frange, P., Touzot, F., Debre, M., Heritier, S., Leruez-Ville, M., Cros, G., et al., 2012. Prevalence and clinical impact of norovirus fecal shedding in children with inherited immune deficiencies. J. Infect. Dis. 206 (8), 1269–1274.

Garcia, C., DuPont, H.L., Long, K.Z., Santos, J.I., Ko, G., 2006. Asymptomatic norovirus infection in Mexican children. J. Clin. Microbiol. 44 (8), 2997–3000.

Gordon, I., Ingraham, H.S., Korns, R.F., 1947. Transmission of epidemic gastroenteritis to human volunteers by oral administration of fecal filtrates. J. Exp. Med. 86 (5), 409–422.

Green, K.Y., 2013. Caliciviridae: the noroviruses. In: sixth ed Knipe, D.M., Howley, P.M., Cohen, J.I., Griffin, D.E., Lamb, R.A., Martin, M.A., Racaniello, V.R., Roizman, B. (Eds.), Fields Virology, vol. 1. Lippincott Williams & Wilkins, Philadelphia, PA.

Huynen, P., Mauroy, A., Martin, C., Savadogo, L.G., Boreux, R., Thiry, E., et al., 2013. Molecular epidemiology of norovirus infections in symptomatic and asymptomatic children from Bobo Dioulasso, Burkina Faso. J. Clin. Virol. 58 (3), 515–521.

Iturriza-Gomara, M., Lopman, B., 2014. Norovirus in healthcare settings. Curr. Opin. Infect. Dis. 27 (5), 437–443.

Jones, M.K., Grau, K.R., Costantini, V., Kolawole, A.O., de Graaf, M., Freiden, P., et al., 2015. Human norovirus culture in B cells. Nat. Protoc. 10 (12), 1939–1947.

Jones, M.K., Watanabe, M., Zhu, S., Graves, C.L., Keyes, L.R., Grau, K.R., et al., 2014. Enteric bacteria promote human and mouse norovirus infection of B cells. Science 346 (6210), 755–759.

Kageyama, T., Kojima, S., Shinohara, M., Uchida, K., Fukushi, S., Hoshino, F.B., et al., 2003. Broadly reactive and highly sensitive assay for Norwalk-like viruses based on real-time quantitative reverse transcription-PCR. J. Clin. Microbiol. 41 (4), 1548–1557.

Kapikian, A.Z., Wyatt, R.G., Dolin, R., Thornhill, T.S., Kalica, A.R., Chanock, R.M., 1972. Visualization by immune electron microscopy of a 27 nm particle associated with acute infectious nonbacterial gastroenteritis. J. Virol. 10 (5), 1075–1081.

Kapikian, A.Z., 2000. The discovery of the 27-nm Norwalk virus: an historic perspective. J. Infect. Dis. 181 (Suppl. 2), S295–S302.

Kaplan, J.E., Feldman, R., Campbell, D.S., Lookabaugh, C., Gary, G.W., 1982. The frequency of a Norwalk-like pattern of illness in outbreaks of acute gastroenteritis. Am. J. Public Health 72 (12), 1329–1332.

Khare, R., Espy, M.J., Cebellinski, E., Boxrud, D., Sloan, L.M., Cunningham, S.A., et al., 2014. Comparative evaluation of two commercial multiplex panels for detection of gastrointestinal pathogens by use of clinical stool specimens. J. Clin. Microbiol. 52 (10), 3667–3673.

Kirby, A.E., Shi, J., Montes, J., Lichtenstein, M., Moe, C.L., 2014. Disease course and viral shedding in experimental Norwalk virus and Snow Mountain virus infection. J. Med. Virol. 86 (12), 2055–2064.

Kirk, M.D., Pires, S.M., Black, R.E., Caipo, M., Crump, J.A., Devleesschauwer, B., et al., 2015. World Health Organization estimates of the global and regional disease burden of 22 foodborne bacterial, protozoal, and viral diseases, 2010: a data synthesis. PLoS Med. 12 (12), e1001921.

Kirking, H.L., Cortes, J., Burrer, S., Hall, A.J., Cohen, N.J., Lipman, H., et al., 2010. Likely transmission of norovirus on an airplane, October 2008. Clin. Infect. Dis. 50 (9), 1216–1221.

Kojima, S., Fukumi, H., Kusama, H., et al., 1948. Studies on the causative agent of the infectious diarrhea. Records of the experiments on human volunteers. Jpn. Med. J. 1, 467–476.

Kojima, S., Kageyama, T., Fukushi, S., Hoshino, F.B., Shinohara, M., Uchida, K., et al., 2002. Genogroup-specific PCR primers for detection of Norwalk-like viruses. J. Virol. Methods 100 (1−2), 107−114.

Koopman, J.S., Eckert, E.A., Greenberg, H.B., Strohm, B.C., Isaacson, R.E., Monto, A.S., 1982. Norwalk virus enteric illness acquired by swimming exposure. Am. J. Epidemiol. 115 (2), 173−177.

L'Homme, Y., Sansregret, R., Plante-Fortier, E., Lamontagne, A.M., Ouardani, M., Lacroix, G., et al., 2009. Genomic characterization of swine caliciviruses representing a new genus of Caliciviridae. Virus Genes 39 (1), 66−75.

Le Guyader, F., Haugarreau, L., Miossec, L., Dubois, E., Pommepuy, M., 2000. Three-year study to assess human enteric viruses in shellfish. Appl. Environ. Microb. 66 (8), 3241−3248.

Lee, N., Chan, M.C., Wong, B., Choi, K.W., Sin, W., Lui, G., et al., 2007. Fecal viral concentration and diarrhea in norovirus gastroenteritis. Emerg. Infect. Dis. 13 (9), 1399−1401.

Lindesmith, L.C., Donaldson, E.F., Baric, R.S., 2011. Norovirus GII.4 strain antigenic variation. J. Virol. 85 (1), 231−242. Available from: <http://dx.doi.org/10.1128/JVI>.

Liu, P., Wong, E., Moe, C.L. (2008) Survival of norovirus, ms2 coliphage, and E. coli on surfaces and in solution [abstract K-4142]. In: Program and Abstracts of the 46th Annual Meeting of the Infectious Diseases Society of America, San Diego, CA.

Lopman, B., Vennema, H., Kohli, E., Pothier, P., Sanchez, A., Negredo, A., et al., 2004a. Increase in viral gastroenteritis outbreaks in Europe and epidemic spread of new norovirus variant. Lancet 363 (9410), 682−688.

Lopman, B.A., Adak, G.K., Reacher, M.H., Brown, D.W., 2003. Two epidemiologic patterns of norovirus outbreaks: surveillance in England and Wales, 1992−2000. Emerg. Infect. Dis. 9 (1), 71−77.

Lopman, B.A., Reacher, M.H., Vipond, I.B., et al., 2004b. Epidemiology and cost of nosocomial gastroenteritis, Avon, England, 2002−2003. Emerg. Infect. Dis. 10 (10), 1827−1834.

Loury, P., Le Guyader, F.S., Le Saux, J.C., Ambert-Balay, K., Parrot, P., Hubert, B., 2015. A norovirus oyster-related outbreak in a nursing home in France, January 2012. Epidemiol. Infect. 143 (12), 2486−2493.

Lozano, R., Naghavi, M., Foreman, K., et al., 2012. Global and regional mortality from 235 causes of death for 20 age groups in 1990 and 2010: a systematic analysis for the Global Burden of Disease Study 2010. Lancet 380 (9859), 2095−2128.

Magill-Collins, A., Gaither, M., Gerba, C.P., Kitajima, M., Iker, B.C., Stoehr, J.D., 2015. Norovirus outbreaks among Colorado River rafters in the Grand Canyon, Summer 2012. Wilderness Environ. Med. 26 (3), 312−318.

Marques Mendanha de Oliveira, D., Souza, M., Souza Fiaccadori, F., Cesar Pereira Santos, H., das Dores de Paula Cardoso, D., 2014. Monitoring of calicivirus among day-care children: evidence of asymptomatic viral excretion and first report of GI.7 norovirus and GI.3 sapovirus in Brazil. J. Med. Virol. 86 (9), 1569−1575.

Mattner, F., Sohr, D., Heim, A., Gastmeier, P., Vennema, H., Koopmans, M., 2006. Risk groups for clinical complications of norovirus infections: and outbreak investigation. Clin. Microbiol. Infect. 12 (1), 69−74.

Murray, C.J., Vos, T., Lozano, R., et al., 2012. Disability-adjusted life years (DALYs) for 291 diseases and injuries in 21 regions, 1990−2010: a systematic analysis for the Global Burden of Disease Study 2010. Lancet 380, 2197−2223.

Navidad, J.F., Griswold, D.J., Gradus, M.S., Bhattacharyya, S., 2013. Evaluation of Luminex xTAG gastrointestinal pathogen analyte-specific reagents for high-throughput, simultaneous detection of bacteria, viruses, and parasites of clinical and public health importance. J. Clin. Microbiol. 51 (9), 3018−3024.

Pang, X., Lee, B.E., 2015. Laboratory diagnosis of noroviruses: present and future. Clin. Lab. Med. 35 (2), 345−362.

Pang, X., Lee, B., Chui, L., Preiksaitis, J.K., Monroe, S.S., 2004. Evaluation and validation for real-time reverse transcription-pcr assay using the LightCycler system for detection and quantitation of norovirus. J. Clin. Microbiol. 42 (10), 4679−4685.

Petriqnani, M., van Beek, J., Borsboom, G., Richardus, J.H., Koopmans, M., 2015. Norovirus introduction routes into nursing homes and risk factors for spread: a systematic review and meta-analysis of observational studies. J. Hosp. Infect. 89 (3), 163−178.

Pires, S.M., Fischer-Walker, C.L., Lanata, C.F., Devleesschauwer, B., Hall, A.J., Kirk, M.D., et al., 2015. Aetiology-specific estimates of the global and regional incidence and mortality of diarrhoeal diseases commonly transmitted through food. PLoS ONE 10 (12), e0142927.

Pringle, K., Lopman, B., Vega, E., Vinjé, J., Parashar, U.D., Hall, A.J., 2015. Noroviruses: epidemiology, immunity and prospects for prevention. Future Microbiol. 10 (1), 53−67.

Qi, R., Ye, C., Chen, C., Yao, P., Hu, F., Lin, Q., 2015. Norovirus prevention and the prevalence of asymptomatic norovirus infection in kindergartens and primary schools in Changzhou, China: status of the knowledge, attitudes, behaviors, and requirements. Am. J. Infect. Control. 43 (8), 833−838.

Reimann, H.A., Prince, A.H., Hodges, J.H., 1945. The cause of epidemic diarrhea, nausea and vomiting (viral dysentery?). Proc. Soc. Exp. Biol. Med. 59 (9), 8−9.

Rhinehart, E., Walker, S., Murphy, D., O'Reilly, K., Leeman, P., 2012. Frequency of outbreak investigations in US hospitals: results of a national survey of infection preventionists. Am. J. Infect. Contr. 40 (1), 2−8.

Robilotti, E., Deresinski, S., Pinsky, B.A., 2015. Norovirus. Clin. Microbiol. Rev. 28 (1), 134−164.

Said, M.A., Perl, T.M., Sears, C.L., 2008. Gastrointestinal flu: norovirus in healthcare and long-term care facilities. Clin. Infect. Dis. 47 (9), 1202−1208.

Saif, M.A., Bonney, D.K., Bigger, B., Forsythe, L., Williams, N., Page, J., et al., 2011. Chronic norovirus infection in pediatric hematopoietic stem cell transplant recipients: a cause of prolonged intestinal failure requiring intensive nutritional support. Pediatr. Transplant.. 15 (5), 505−509.

Shanker, S., Choi, J.M., Sankaran, B., Atmar, R.L., Estes, M.K., Prasad, B.V., 2011. Structural analysis of histo-blood group antigen binding specificity in a norovirus GII.4 epidemic variant: implications for epochal evolution. J. Virol. 85 (17), 8635−8645.

Solano, R., Alseda, M., Godoy, P., Sanz, M., Bartolomé, R., Manzanares-Laya, S., et al., 2014. Working Group for the Study of Acute Gastroenteritis in Catalonia. Person-to-person transmission of norovirus resulting in an outbreak of acute gastroenteritis at a summer camp. Eur. J. Gastroenterol. Hepatol. 26 (10), 1160−1166.

Tan, M., Huang, P., Xia, M., Fang, P.A., Zhong, W., McNeal, M., et al., 2011. Norovirus P particle, a novel platform for vaccine development and antibody production. J. Virol. 85 (2), 753−764.

Tavoschi, L., Severi, E., Niskanen, T., Boelaert, F., Rizzi, V., Liebana, E., et al., 2015. Food-borne diseases associated with frozen berries consumption: a historical perspective, European Union, 1983 to 2013. Euro. Surveill. 20 (29), 21193.

Treanor, J.J., Atmar, R.L., Frey, S.E., Gormley, R., Chen, W.H., Ferreira, J., et al., 2014. A novel intramuscular bivalent norovirus virus-like particle vaccine candidate-reactogenicity, safety, and immunogenicity in a phase 1 trial in healthy adults. J. Infect. Dis. 210 (11), 1769−1771.

Tu, E.T., Bull, R.A., Kim, M.J., McIver, C.J., Heron, L., Rawlinson, W.D., et al., 2008. Norovirus excretion in an aged-care setting. J. Clin. Microbiol. 46 (6), 2119−2121.

van Beek, J., Ambert-Balay, K., Botteldoorn, N., Eden, J.S., Fonager, J., Hewitt, J., et al., 2013. Incubations for worldwide increased norovirus activity associated with emergence of a new variant of genotype II.4, late 2012. Euro. Surveill. 18 (1), 8−9.

Vinjé, J., 2015. Advances in laboratory methods for detection and typing of norovirus. J. Clin. Microbiol. 53 (2), 373−381.

Wang, Y., Zhang, J., Shen, Z., 2015. The impact of calicivirus mixed infection in an oyster-associated outbreak during a food festival. J. Clin. Virol. 73, 55−63.

Wingfield, T., Gallimore, C.I., Xerry, J., Gray, J.J., Klapper, P., Guiver, M., et al., 2010. Chronic norovirus infection in an HIV-positive patient with persistent diarrhea: a novel cause. J. Clin. Virol. 49 (3), 219−222.

World Health Organization. (2015) WHO estimates of the global burden of foodborne diseases. Available from: <http://www.who.int/foodsafety/areas_work/foodborne-diseases/ferg/en/>.

Wu, Z., Yang, L., Ren, X., He, G., Zhang, J., Yang, J., et al., 2015. Deciphering the bat virome catalog to better understand the ecological diversity of bat viruses and the bat origin of emerging infectious diseases. ISME J. 10 (3), 609−620.

Wyatt, R.G., Dolin, R., Blacklow, N.R., DuPont, H.L., Buscho, R.F., Thornhill, T.S., et al., 1974. Comparison of three agents of acute infectious nonbacterial gastroenteritis by cross-challenge in volunteers. J. Infect. Dis. 129 (6), 709−714.

Xia, M., Tan, M., Wei, C., Zhong, W., Wang, L., McNeal, M., et al., 2011. A candidate dual vaccine against influenza and noroviruses. Vaccine 29 (44), 7670−7677.

Yu, J.H., Kim, N.Y., Lee, E.J., Jeon, I.S., 2011. Norovirus infections in asymptomatic food handlers in elementary schools without norovirus outbreaks in some regions of Incheon, Korea. J. Korean Med. Sci. 26 (6), 734−739.

Zahorsky, J., 1929. Hyperemesis hiemis or the winter vomiting disease. Arch. Pediar. 46, 391−395.

Zheng, D.P., Ando, T., Fankhauser, R.L., Beard, R.S., Glass, R.I., Monroe, S.S., 2006. Norovirus classification and proposed strain nomenclature. Virology 346 (2), 312−323.

Zingg, W., Colombo, C., Jucker, T., Bossart, W., Ruef, C., 2005. Impact of an outbreak of norovirus infection on hospital resources. Infect. Control. Hosp. Epidemiol. 26 (3), 263−267.

HEALTH IMPACT

GLOBAL DISEASE BURDEN OF FOODBORNE ILLNESSES ASSOCIATED WITH NOROVIRUS

Minesh P. Shah and Aron J. Hall

Centers for Disease Control and Prevention, Atlanta, GA, United States

1.1 BACKGROUND

Noroviruses are a genetically diverse group of viruses in the *Caliciviridae* family that cause the clinical syndrome of acute gastroenteritis. The first norovirus was described when a viral particle was observed by electron microscopy in a stool sample derived from a 1968 outbreak in Norwalk, Ohio, leading to the initial name of Norwalk virus (Kapikian et al., 1972). Norwalk virus was the first virus shown to cause gastroenteritis. Since then, other "Norwalk-like viruses" have been discovered; currently, noroviruses are classified into genogroups GI−GVII (Vinjé, 2015). Genogroups GI, GII, and, to a lesser extent, GIV are known to cause human disease. According to several estimates using different methodologies detailed in this chapter, norovirus is the leading infectious cause of both sporadic (or endemic) cases and reported outbreaks of foodborne illness in the world (Havelaar et al., 2015; Pires et al., 2015; Kirk et al., 2015; Ahmed et al., 2014; Hall et al., 2014; Thomas et al., 2013; Havelaar et al., 2012; Thongprachum et al., 2016).

Norovirus infections cause acute gastroenteritis, presenting as acute-onset vomiting and/or diarrhea. Vomiting-only and diarrhea-only illness can occur with varying estimates of frequency, depending on the population and transmission mode studied (Gotz et al., 2001; Rockx et al., 2002; Arness et al., 2000; Lopman et al., 2004; Wikswo et al., 2013). When present, diarrhea is typically watery, nonbloody, and may be accompanied by abdominal cramps, nausea, and fever. Asymptomatic norovirus infection can be identified through stool shedding of norovirus in patients without gastroenteritis, and it has been found in 3−10% of children and adults in both lower- and higher-income countries (Ahmed et al., 2014).

The incubation period lasts 12−48 hours, and the clinical syndrome is typically 12−72 hours. Although most infections will result in full recovery (Rockx et al., 2002), severe outcomes such as hospitalization and death do occur, particularly among children younger than age 5 years, adults older than age 65 years, and immunocompromised hosts (Hall et al., 2013b; O'Brien et al., 2016; de Wit et al., 2001b; Bok and Green, 2012). In higher-income countries, norovirus infections are responsible for 10−20% of gastroenteritis hospitalizations and deaths among older adults, with long-term care facilities experiencing frequent norovirus outbreaks (Lindsay et al., 2015). In lower-income countries, there is a younger age distribution, with most norovirus infections in children occurring between 6 and 23 months of age (Shioda et al., 2015).

The Norovirus. DOI: http://dx.doi.org/10.1016/B978-0-12-804177-2.00001-4

Several traits contribute to the high incidence of norovirus infection. They are highly infectious, with estimates of infectious dose ranging from 18 to 2800 particles (Teunis et al., 2008; Atmar et al., 2014). There is a prolific period of viral shedding, which may begin before symptom onset, peaks 4 days after exposure, and may persist for several weeks after resolution of symptoms (Aoki et al., 2010). Noroviruses are stable in the environment, remaining infectious in experimentally spiked groundwater samples for more than 60 days and detectable for more than 3 years (Seitz et al., 2011). Although initial studies suggested that noroviruses produced immunity for approximately 6–24 months (Parrino et al., 1977), recent modeling studies suggest immunity lasts longer—from 4 to 9 years (Simmons et al., 2013). Regardless of the duration of immunity, reinfection with norovirus is common (Saito et al., 2014; Lopman et al., 2015). Host susceptibility to infection is influenced by genetic profiles; notably, individuals with nonfunctional *FUT2* genes exhibit innate resistance to norovirus infections (Kambhampati et al., 2016).

1.2 DETERMINING THE DISEASE BURDEN OF FOODBORNE NOROVIRUS

In 2007, the World Health Organization (WHO) established the Foodborne Disease Burden Epidemiology Reference Group (FERG) to create a systematic approach to estimate the global burden of all foodborne diseases. FERG assessed a comprehensive list of hazards that cause foodborne disease, including enteric pathogens (including norovirus), invasive infectious agents (e.g., hepatitis A), helminths (e.g., ascaris), and chemicals and toxins (e.g., aflatoxin) (Kuchenmuller et al., 2009). The methodology employed by FERG provides a useful framework for understanding the various inputs necessary for generating such disease burden estimates (Kuchenmuller et al., 2013; Devleesschauwer et al., 2015). This chapter utilizes that framework to highlight the various data sources and estimates available, as well as remaining gaps. This approach involves the following steps:

1. Estimate the global incidence of all-cause diarrheal disease.
2. Estimate the proportion of total diarrheal disease caused by noroviruses.
3. Adjust the norovirus diarrhea estimate for vomiting-only cases of norovirus.
4. Estimate the fraction of all norovirus cases that are foodborne.
5. Apply the foodborne fraction to various measures of norovirus disease burden, including incidence of cases, hospitalizations, deaths, and disability-adjusted life years (DALYs).

For each of the previous steps, there are a variety of methodological approaches and challenges that are reviewed herein.

1.2.1 GLOBAL INCIDENCE OF DIARRHEAL DISEASES

In 1990, WHO and World Bank launched the Global Burden of Disease (GBD) study to comprehensively and systematically measure the state of health in the world (Murray and Lopez, 1996). The first GBD study estimated that diarrheal diseases were responsible for almost 3 million deaths in adults and children annually, accounting for the second highest age-adjusted death rate of all infectious etiologies (Murray and Lopez, 1997a,b). Since that time, advances in health, sanitation, and hygiene have led to a modest 7% decrease in diarrheal illnesses but a dramatic 50% reduction in diarrheal deaths by 2013, according to the most recent GBD update (GBD 2013 Mortality and

Causes of Death Collaborators, 2015; Vos et al., 2015). Despite this reduction in mortality, diarrheal diseases remain the fourth-leading infectious cause of death in all ages and the second-leading infectious cause of death in children worldwide (GBD 2013 Mortality and Causes of Death Collaborators, 2015; Liu et al., 2015). Developing countries bear the greatest burden of deaths from diarrhea, encompassing nearly 90% of global diarrheal deaths and a mortality rate almost 90 times that of developed nations (Global Burden of Disease Pediatrics, 2016).

In addition to the GBD studies, systematic literature reviews have found a modest decline in global diarrhea incidence in both children and adults, and specifically for children younger than 5 years of age in low- and middle-income countries (Walker et al., 2013; Walker and Black, 2010; Fischer Walker et al., 2012). Globally, children younger than 5 years of age experience 2.7 (95% confidence interval (CI), 2.1−3.2) episodes of diarrhea per year, with a regional range of 2.2 (95% CI, 1.3−2.5) in the Western Pacific to 3.3 (95%, CI, 2.1−5.0) in Africa (Walker et al., 2013). In 2001, WHO and UNICEF launched the Child Health Epidemiology Reference Group (CHERG), a second major disease burden study, this one focused on children younger than age 5 years (Liu et al., 2012). For 2013, CHERG estimated approximately 560,000 diarrheal deaths in children younger than age 5 years, the third leading cause of childhood death after birth complications and pneumonia (Liu et al., 2015).

Both GBD and CHERG estimates, summarized in Table 1.1, use similar methodology, extracting information from country-specific vital registration data when available, supplemented with verbal autopsy studies. However, there are differences in each group's approach to estimating cause-specific mortality. To account for countries with limited vital registration data, GBD grouped countries into regions and super-regions, using data from neighboring countries with similar attributes to fill in data gaps. CHERG identified thresholds to categorize countries into high- and low-mortality and high- and low-quality vital registration data groups. Despite these differences in data sources, as well as differences in data processing approaches, the resulting estimates of diarrhea mortality among children were very similar between these two studies (Kovacs et al., 2015).

1.2.2 ATTRIBUTABLE PROPORTION OF DIARRHEAL DISEASE TO NOROVIRUS

Perhaps the most challenging aspect of estimating the global burden of norovirus disease is determining the proportion of all diarrheal disease that is due to norovirus. Because norovirus causes a relatively nonspecific clinical syndrome, laboratory confirmation is necessary to distinguish norovirus from other etiologic agents of gastroenteritis. Current diagnostics rely on molecular methods that are largely restricted to public health and research laboratories in higher-income countries and also are highly sensitive and thus do not distinguish symptomatic from asymptomatic infections. Health care utilization and laboratory testing for gastroenteritis vary greatly by population, further complicating efforts to extrapolate from site-specific studies (Yen and Hall, 2013).

The ideal strategy to estimate norovirus burden is active population-based surveillance, which involves systematic sampling of all age cases within a known catchment area, allowing for the calculation of incidence rates of disease. This approach is not widely practiced given the expense and required labor. Examples of active surveillance include the Sensor Study in the Netherlands and the studies of Infectious Intestinal Disease (IID) in the United Kingdom (de Wit et al., 2001b; Tam et al., 2012b). The IID study is illustrative of the underestimation of community norovirus disease when data sources are limited to health care provider or national reporting surveillance methods.

Table 1.1 Worldwide Diarrheal Illnesses and Deaths Estimated by Global Burden of Disease (GBD) and Child Health Epidemiology Reference Group (CHERG) Studies, 2013[a]

Study (Organization)	Diarrheal Illnesses (×1000), All Ages	Diarrheal Illnesses (×1000), Children <5 Years Old	Diarrheal Deaths, All Ages	Diarrheal Deaths, Children <5 Years Old	References
GBD (Institute for Health Metrics Evaluation)	2,711,253 (2,666,452–2,761,161)		1,264,100 (1,151,200–1,383,200)	519,700 (434,900–598,300)	Global (2015), Vos et al. (2015)
CHERG (WHO/UNICEF)				578,000 (448,000–750,000)	Liu et al. (2015)
Systematic literature reviews (JHU/WHO)	2,839,358	1,731,300 (1,375,700–2,032,800)		711,800 (491,100–1,049,300)	Walker et al. (2013), Walker and Black (2010)

JHU, Johns Hopkins University.
[a]Diarrheal illnesses and deaths presented as point estimates (95% CI).

In the United Kingdom, the incidence rate of norovirus was almost 23 times higher in community-based surveillance compared to general practice, and it was almost 300 times higher compared to cases reported to national surveillance (Tam et al., 2012b).

An alternative to active surveillance is passive laboratory-confirmed surveillance, which involves sampling of routinely submitted stools. In one example, random samples of fecal specimens submitted for routine clinical studies (bacterial culture) were subsequently tested for norovirus. The samples were derived from a known population catchment based on health maintenance organization (HMO) membership, allowing for norovirus incidence calculations (Hall et al., 2011).

A challenge in interpreting studies of norovirus detection in stool samples is knowing when the detected virus is indicative of a disease-causing infection. In the original IID study in the United Kingdom, norovirus was found in 16% of controls compared to 36% of cases when samples were retested using real-time reverse transcriptase—polymerase chain reaction (Amar et al., 2007). An active surveillance study of children younger than 5 years of age with medically attended gastroenteritis in the United States found norovirus in 4% of controls compared to 21% in cases with gastroenteritis (Payne et al., 2013). The Etiology, Risk Factors, and Interactions of Enteric Infection and Malnutrition and the Consequences for Child Health and Development (MAL-ED) study is a birth cohort study that performed routine stool testing in children younger than age 2 years in eight developing countries. Across all sites, norovirus was found in 19% of asymptomatic stool samples compared to 23.5% of diarrheal stool samples (Rouhani et al., 2016). A meta-analysis of 20 studies that included data for both cases of acute gastroenteritis and a healthy control group found that norovirus was detected in 7% (95% CI, 3−10%) of controls compared to 20% (95% CI, 16−24%) of cases (Ahmed et al., 2014). Differences in case and control inclusion criteria, norovirus testing methodology, and study design and setting can at least partly explain the variation in norovirus detection in healthy controls, although differences in frequency of exposure and force of infection may also play a role (Lopman et al., 2014).

The presence of norovirus in asymptomatic stool specimens does not necessarily diminish the role of norovirus in causing illness because high levels of asymptomatic infection may be a result of frequent exposure. The challenge in interpreting asymptomatic norovirus infection is illustrated when comparing the disparate conclusions reached by two large studies aiming to identify the etiology of diarrhea in developing countries—the previously mentioned MAL-ED study and the Global Enteric Multicenter Study (GEMS), which enrolled children younger than 5 years of age in four African and three Asian sites (Rouhani et al., 2016; Kotloff et al., 2013). MAL-ED is a birth cohort study that performed routine testing in children in the community, whereas GEMS is a case−control study of severe disease presenting to health facilities. For diagnostic testing, GEMS used conventional PCR, whereas MAL-ED used more sensitive real-time assays. With these design differences in mind, MAL-ED found that 89% of children experienced at least one norovirus infection before age 24 months, with severity of norovirus-associated diarrhea similar to the severity of diarrhea from all other pathogens (Rouhani et al., 2016). Conversely, the GEMS study found that norovirus was a significant cause of diarrhea in only two of its sites, and norovirus was not considered a top-five pathogen in any age group (Kotloff et al., 2013).

A key limitation with both active and passive surveillance studies is that they are only performed in a single or handful of sites and thus generalizability to broader populations is a concern. A potential alternative for estimating norovirus illness is national or nationally representative databases that rely on medical diagnosis codes, such as the International Classification of Disease (ICD).

However, specific coding for norovirus is rarely done due to the limited availability of direct testing for norovirus among sporadic illnesses (Payne et al., 2013). To overcome this limitation, modeling studies have been done to indirectly estimate the proportion of acute gastroenteritis caused by norovirus. The general approach is to use time-series regression modeling to estimate the proportion of cause-unspecified acute gastroenteritis that can be attributed to norovirus based on the observed incidence and seasonality of cases attributed to other specific causes. This approach has been used to estimate norovirus deaths among elderly populations in England and Wales (Harris et al., 2008), as well as deaths, hospitalizations, and ambulatory visits across the age spectrum in the United States (Lopman et al., 2011; Hall et al., 2012; Gastanaduy et al., 2013). Country-specific studies of acute gastroenteritis with estimated norovirus incidence are summarized in Table 1.2.

In 2014, a systematic review and meta-analysis assessed the role of norovirus as a cause of endemic acute gastroenteritis worldwide (Ahmed et al., 2014). The review included 175 published articles with a combined total of 187,336 patients with acute gastroenteritis, and it estimated norovirus to be present in 18% (95% CI, 17−20%) of all cases. The review noted a higher norovirus prevalence in community (24%; 95% CI, 18−30%) and outpatient (20%; 95% CI, 16−24%) settings compared with inpatient (17%; 95% CI, 15−19%) settings. Norovirus prevalence was also higher in low-mortality developing countries (19%; 95% CI, 16−22%) and developed countries (20%; 95% CI, 17−22%) compared with high-mortality developing countries (14%; 95% CI, 11−16%). Interestingly, patient age was not associated with norovirus prevalence. This review was an update from a 2008 review using similar methods, which calculated a pooled proportion of 12% norovirus prevalence based on a much smaller count of 31 publications of endemic norovirus (Patel et al., 2008).

1.2.3 ADJUSTMENT FOR VOMITING-ONLY PRESENTATIONS OF NOROVIRUS

Unlike many other common etiologies of acute gastroenteritis, norovirus infection often results in a vomiting-only presentation. As such, the preceding methods of estimating norovirus disease by applying the attributable proportion of norovirus to all diarrheal illnesses underestimate the true burden of norovirus. Data on vomiting-only presentations in norovirus disease are available from norovirus challenge studies; outbreak analyses; and surveillance studies from community, outpatient, inpatient, and emergency department settings. A meta-analysis of 21 such studies found that vomiting-only illnesses constituted 0−45% of all norovirus disease, with a pooled proportion of 17% (95% CI, 13−22%) (Shioda, personal communication). This estimate is similar to the 19% value used by FERG (Kirk et al., 2015). From this proportion, a vomiting-inflation factor (VIF) can be calculated as follows:

$$1/(1 - \text{proportion of vomiting-only norovirus illnesses}) = 1/(1 - 0.17) = 1.2$$

This VIF can then be multiplied by the estimated number of norovirus diarrhea cases to yield an overall estimate of norovirus disease.

1.2.4 ESTIMATING THE FOODBORNE FRACTION OF ALL NOROVIRUS DISEASE

Noroviruses can be transmitted through a variety of modes, including foodborne, person-to-person, waterborne, and environmental contamination. Although person-to-person is likely the most common transmission mode for norovirus (Hall et al., 2013a), norovirus disease occurs with such great

Table 1.2 Selected Studies of Acute Gastroenteritis by Country, With Estimates of Norovirus Disease[a]

Methodologic Approach	Countries	Years	Ages	Setting	No. of Specimens Tested	Norovirus Positive	Norovirus Incidence Rate	References
Active, population-based surveillance	United Kingdom	2008–2009	All	Community	782	16.5% (14–19.3)	47.0/1000 py (39.1–56.5)	Tam et al. (2012a,b)
Active, population-based surveillance	United Kingdom	2008–2009	All	General practice	108	12.4% (10.2–14.7)	2.07/1000 py (1.44–2.99)	Tam et al. (2012a,b)
Active, population-based surveillance	The Netherlands	1998–1999	All	Community	709	16%	31.1/1000 py	de Wit et al. (2001b)
Active, population-based surveillance	The Netherlands	1998–1999	All	General practice	854	5%		de Wit et al. (2001a)
Active, population-based surveillance	United States	2008–2010	<5 years	Hospital and emergency department	1295	21%	26.0–36.8/1000 py	Payne et al. (2013)
Active, population-based surveillance (birth cohort)	Bangladesh, India, Nepal, Pakistan, South Africa, Tanzania, Brazil, Peru	2009–2012	<2 years	Community	770	23.5%	1.87–13.43/100 child-months (depending on genotype and country)	Rouhani et al. (2016)
Active, population-based surveillance (birth cohort)	Ecuador		<3 years	Community	438	18%		Lopman et al. (2015)
Active, population-	France	1998–2000	All	Community	161	19.2%		Chikhi-Brachet et al. (2002)

(Continued)

Table 1.2 Selected Studies of Acute Gastroenteritis by Country, With Estimates of Norovirus Disease[a] *Continued*

Methodologic Approach	Countries	Years	Ages	Setting	No. of Specimens Tested	Norovirus Positive	Norovirus Incidence Rate	References
based surveillance								
Passive surveillance	United States (Georgia)	2004–2005	All	Community	572	16%	65/1000 py (37–120)	Hall et al. (2011)
Passive surveillance	United States (Georgia)	2004–2005	All	Outpatient	572	12%	6.4/1000 py (3.6–12)	Hall et al. (2011)
Indirect attribution from regression modeling	United States	1996–2007	All	Hospitals	N/A	13%, 0–4 years; 8%, >65 years	24/100,000	Lopman et al. (2011)
Indirect attribution	United States	1999–2007	All	Deaths	N/A	7.1%, all ages; 4.5%, 0–4 years; 7.7%, >65 years	2.7 deaths/ 1,000,000	Hall et al. (2012)
Indirect attribution	United States	2001–2009	All	Outpatient and emergency department	N/A	13%	13.5/10,000 (outpatient) 57.2/10,000 (emergency department)	Gastanaduy et al. (2013)
Indirect attribution	Australia	2010	All	Community	N/A	10%		Kirk et al. (2014)

N/A, *not applicable; py, person-years.*
[a]*Norovirus positive percentages and incidence rates presented as point estimates (95% CI).*

frequency that it remains the leading etiology of foodborne disease outbreaks (Pires et al., 2015; Hall et al., 2014). Norovirus contamination of food is most commonly attributed to infectious food workers (70% in a review of US outbreaks) (Hall et al., 2014). When specific food items have been identified during norovirus outbreaks, greater than 90% were contaminated during preparation, and 75% were foods eaten raw (Hall et al., 2014).

The foodborne fraction of norovirus disease has previously been estimated from epidemiologic investigations of outbreaks, but these analyses are limited to a small number of countries and may not be representative of endemic (nonoutbreak) disease. An extension of outbreak surveillance analysis involves using laboratory-confirmed disease to identify the foodborne fraction of specific norovirus genotypes, which assumes that individual genotypes have different tendencies for foodborne transmission. A review of laboratory surveillance data from the United States, Europe, and New Zealand, as well as a systematic literature review of outbreak reports from other countries, estimated a foodborne fraction of 14% for all norovirus genotypes, with a lower foodborne fraction of 10% for the GII.4 genotype, the genotype most often implicated in both endemic disease and outbreaks (Verhoef et al., 2015). Studies estimating foodborne fraction from surveillance systems are summarized in Table 1.3.

Given the limited availability and limitations of outbreak epidemiologic and laboratory surveillance for estimating foodborne fraction, an alternative method that has been frequently used is formal expert elicitation. Expert elicitation is a process that involves identifying international experts in the specific field of interest, assessing the quality of the experts' opinions through introductory questions, and then asking each expert to provide a central estimate with uncertainty bounds. This approach was utilized by FERG to estimate the foodborne fraction of all hazards, including norovirus (Hald et al., 2016). The FERG study pooled subregional estimates using 100 experts, with the foodborne fraction of norovirus ranging from 12% to 26% by subregion (Hald et al., 2016).

1.2.5 ESTIMATING THE DISEASE BURDEN

The disease burden of an illness can be measured in several ways, such as incidence (number of cases during a time period), hospitalizations, deaths, and disability. The estimates for incidence of

Table 1.3 Estimates of Foodborne Fraction of Norovirus Disease From Outbreak Surveillance Systems

Countries	Years	Report Type	Total Norovirus Illnesses	Foodborne Fraction (%)	Reference
United States	2009–2012	Outbreak epidemiologic investigations	4318 outbreaks	23	Hall et al. (2014)
England and Wales	1995	Outbreak epidemiologic investigations	647,701 cases	11	Adak et al. (2002)
Global	2009–2012	Outbreak laboratory investigations	5393 outbreaks (89% from the United States and Europe)	14	Verhoef et al. (2015)

norovirus disease were discussed previously in this chapter. When applying these estimates to the disease burden measures noted previously, it is important to note that foodborne norovirus illness may exhibit different patterns of disease burden than nonfoodborne norovirus illness. For example, an analysis of norovirus outbreak surveillance from the United States showed that compared to non-foodborne outbreaks, foodborne outbreaks had fewer cases, lower proportions of cases who were hospitalized and who died, but higher proportions of cases with emergency department visits (Hall et al., 2014).

Direct country-specific estimates for hospitalizations and mortality by pathogen are limited, with published reports from only a small number of higher-income countries (noted in the tables in this chapter). The FERG study used these direct estimates for each country, where available, and then applied pooled estimates from these studies to 61 high-income and low-mortality countries to extrapolate hospitalizations and mortality (Pires et al., 2015). For the other 133 countries, the FERG study used data from a systematic review of community, outpatient, and inpatient studies to create WHO subregional estimates of disease burden and apply these estimates to all countries within the region.

In the 1990s, the measure of DALYs was developed to provide an aggregate of the number of years lost to acute illness, long-term disability, or early death (Murray, 1994). The DALY is calculated by summing the number of healthy years of life lost (YLL) due to premature mortality and the number of years lost due to disability (YLD) for each health state associated with that illness (DALY = YLL + YLD). The DALY measure allows for comparisons of disease burden from different types of illness and across countries of varying health and life expectancies.

Gastroenteritis results in an acute health state (vomiting and/or diarrhea), which can range in severity from mild to death. Gastroenteritis can also result in chronic health states such as stunting, Guillain–Barré syndrome, and postinfectious irritable bowel syndrome, although not all of these conditions have been associated with norovirus infection specifically (Devleesschauwer et al., 2015; Scallan et al., 2015). To calculate YLD to a specific illness or pathogen, disability weights have been calculated and revised in 2013 to represent the magnitude of health loss associated with a health state or outcome (Salomon et al., 2015). In this revision, on a scale of 0 (no disability) to 1 (completely disabled), diarrhea was assigned disability weights of 0.074 (mild), 0.188 (moderate), and 0.247 (severe). Based on how frequently norovirus results in mild, moderate, and severe gastroenteritis, a FERG-commissioned study used prior (2010) measures of disability weights and created one disability weight for norovirus infection, measured at 0.074 (Devleesschauwer et al., 2015).

The FERG estimates of foodborne disease burden provide the most comprehensive global approach to date. The FERG methodology organized countries by subregions using WHO geographic regions (http://www.who.int/about/regions/en/) and five strata of child and adult mortality as described by the GBD studies (Ezzati et al., 2002). Country-specific data on gastroenteritis incidence, norovirus proportion, foodborne fraction, and disease burden were used where available, but this was limited to seven high-income countries (United States, United Kingdom, the Netherlands, France, Australia, New Zealand, and Canada). Estimates for the other countries in high-income subregions were extrapolated from these seven countries. For low- and middle-income countries, estimates were made by subregion using available community, outpatient, and inpatient studies from neighboring countries with similar mortality profiles (Kirk et al., 2015). FERG estimates for all-cause foodborne disease, with norovirus highlighted, are summarized in Table 1.4 (Havelaar et al., 2015).

The FERG subregional estimates of disease burden are further divided by age group (children <5 years and adults and children ≥5 years) (Havelaar et al., 2015). Per capita rates of norovirus

Table 1.4 Foodborne Disease Burden Estimates From the FERG, 2010[a]			
Hazard	Foodborne Illnesses	Foodborne Deaths	Foodborne DALYs
All etiologies (11 diarrheal agents, 7 invasive infectious agents, 10 helminths, 3 chemicals/toxins)	600,652,361 (417,646,804–962,834,044)	418,608 (305,128–498,419)	32,841,428 (24,809,085–46,274,735)
All diarrheal agents (norovirus, 7 bacteria, 3 protozoa)	548,595,679 (369,976,912–888,528,014)	230,111 (160,039–322,359)	17,659,226 (12,458,675–24,516,338)
Norovirus	124,803,946 (70,311,254–251,352,877)	34,929 (15,916–79,620)	2,496,078 (1,175,658–5,511,092)
Norovirus rank among all hazards	1	4	5
[a]*Foodborne illnesses, deaths, and DALYs presented as point estimates (95% CIs).*			

foodborne illnesses and deaths by subregion can be applied to each country's population to obtain country-specific estimates of disease burden, and these are shown in Figs. 1.1 and 1.2.

The country-level estimates illustrate that foodborne norovirus disease occurs in all regions of the world, with the number of illnesses reasonably approximating country size (i.e., the most populous countries have the highest number of illnesses). The global rate of foodborne norovirus illnesses in children younger than age 5 years is estimated at 5404 (95% CI, 3062–9312) per 100,000, with an estimate three times higher in the most affected WHO subregion (9221 in high-mortality Americas) than in the least-affected subregion (2875 in low-mortality Americas). For adults and children age 5 years or older, the global rate of foodborne norovirus illnesses is estimated at 1427 (95% CI, 738–3309) per 100,000, with an estimate five times higher in the most-affected subregion (2225 in high-mortality Eastern Mediterranean) than in the least-affected subregion (431 in low-mortality Southeast Asia) (Foodborne Disease Burden Epidemiology Reference Group (FERG), 2015).

Deaths due to foodborne norovirus disease, however, are dependent on factors other than population size and thus show a greater range in rates by subregion. The global rate of foodborne norovirus deaths in children younger than age 5 years is estimated at 1 (95% CI, 0.7–3) per 100,000, with an estimate 29 times higher in the most-affected subregions (2 in high-mortality Africa and Southeast Asia) than in the least-affected subregion (0.07 in low-mortality Americas). For adults and children age 5 years or older, the global rate of foodborne norovirus deaths is estimated at 0.4 (95% CI, 0.2–1) per 100,000, with an estimate 45 times higher in the most-affected subregions (0.9 in high-mortality Africa and Southeast Asia) than in the least-affected subregion (0.02 in low-mortality Western Pacific).

1.3 CONCLUSIONS AND PERSPECTIVES

Noroviruses are the leading cause of foodborne illnesses worldwide, causing an estimated 125 million illnesses, 35,000 deaths, and 2.5 million DALYs annually. These estimates are only for the foodborne fraction of norovirus, which is estimated as 18% of all norovirus disease. Thus, the total

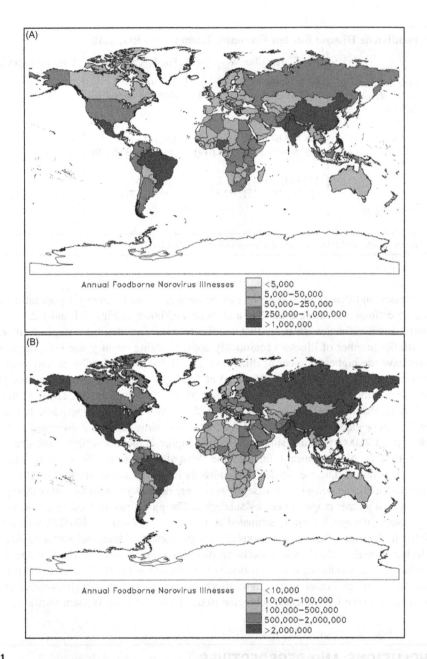

FIGURE 1.1

Global annual foodborne norovirus illnesses in (A) children aged <5 years and (B) adults and children aged ≥5 years. Country-specific estimates were calculated by applying the FERG median estimate for per capita foodborne norovirus illnesses by age group (Foodborne Disease Burden Epidemiology Reference Group (FERG), 2015) to 2014 United Nations population estimates (United Nations Department of Economic and Social Affairs, 2015).

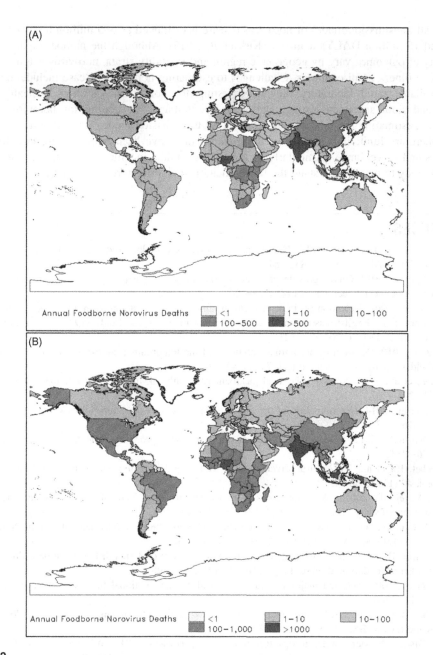

FIGURE 1.2

Global annual foodborne norovirus deaths in (A) children aged <5 years and (B) adults and children
aged ≥ 5 years. Country-specific estimates were calculated by applying the FERG median estimate for per capita
foodborne norovirus deaths by age group (Foodborne Disease Burden Epidemiology Reference Group (FERG),
2015) to 2014 population estimates (United Nations Department of Economic and Social Affairs, 2015).

burden of all transmission modes of norovirus disease is estimated as 685 million illnesses, 210,000 deaths, and 15 million DALYs annually (Kirk et al., 2015). Although the number of illnesses and the severity of outcomes vary by geographic region and mortality strata, norovirus is a major cause of foodborne illness in all countries. Challenges to estimating norovirus disease include the lack of widely available rapid laboratory diagnostic testing for norovirus, variation in health-seeking behavior and stool specimen testing, and inconsistent diagnostic coding for norovirus disease. Furthermore, estimating the foodborne fraction of all transmission modes for norovirus is challenging, and there are limitations to each of the methods that have been employed to date. Improved diagnostics and surveillance, particularly in lower- and middle-income countries, is a priority area for further study to better understand the full burden of foodborne norovirus disease.

REFERENCES

Adak, G.K., Long, S.M., O'Brien, S.J., 2002. Trends in indigenous foodborne disease and deaths, England and Wales: 1992 to 2000. Gut 51 (6), 832–841.

Ahmed, S.M., et al., 2014. Global prevalence of norovirus in cases of gastroenteritis: a systematic review and meta-analysis. Lancet Infect. Dis. 14 (8), 725–730.

Amar, C.F., et al., 2007. Detection by PCR of eight groups of enteric pathogens in 4,627 faecal samples: re-examination of the English case–control Infectious Intestinal Disease Study (1993–1996). Eur. J. Clin. Microbiol. Infect. Dis. 26 (5), 311–323.

Aoki, Y., et al., 2010. Duration of norovirus excretion and the longitudinal course of viral load in norovirus-infected elderly patients. J. Hosp. Infect. 75 (1), 42–46.

Arness, M.K., et al., 2000. Norwalk-like viral gastroenteritis outbreak in U.S. Army trainees. Emerg. Infect. Dis. 6 (2), 204–207.

Atmar, R.L., et al., 2014. Determination of the 50% human infectious dose for Norwalk virus. J. Infect. Dis. 209 (7), 1016–1022.

Bok, K., Green, K.Y., 2012. Norovirus gastroenteritis in immunocompromised patients. New Eng. J. Med. 367 (22), 2126–2132.

Chikhi-Brachet, R., et al., 2002. Virus diversity in a winter epidemic of acute diarrhea in France. J. Clin. Microbiol. 40 (11), 4266–4272.

de Wit, M.A., et al., 2001a. A comparison of gastroenteritis in a general practice-based study and a community-based study. Epidemiol. Infect. 127 (3), 389–397.

de Wit, M.A.S., et al., 2001b. Sensor, a Population-Based Cohort Study on Gastroenteritis in the Netherlands: Incidence and Etiology. Am. J. Epidemiol. 154 (7), 666–674.

Devleesschauwer, B., et al., 2015. Methodological framework for World Health Organization estimates of the global burden of foodborne disease. PLoS ONE 10 (12), e0142498.

Ezzati, M., et al., 2002. Selected major risk factors and global and regional burden of disease. Lancet 360 (9343), 1347–1360.

Fischer Walker, C.L., et al., 2012. Diarrhea incidence in low- and middle-income countries in 1990 and 2010: a systematic review. BMC Public Health 12, 220.

Foodborne Disease Burden Epidemiology Reference Group (FERG), 2015. WHO estimates of the global burden of foodborne diseases—online tool. 2015. Available from: <http://www.who.int/foodsafety/areas_work/foodborne-diseases/ferg/en/>.

Gastanaduy, P.A., et al., 2013. Burden of norovirus gastroenteritis in the ambulatory setting—United States, 2001–2009. J. Infect. Dis. 207 (7), 1058–1065.

GBD 2013 Mortality and Causes of Death Collaborators, 2013. Global, regional, and national age-sex specific all-cause and cause-specific mortality for 240 causes of death, 1990–2013: a systematic analysis for the Global Burden of Disease Study 2013. Lancet 385 (9963), 117–171.

Global Burden of Disease Pediatrics, 2016. Global and national burden of diseases and injuries among children and adolescents between 1990 and 2013: findings from the global burden of disease 2013 study. JAMA Pediatr.

Gotz, H., et al., 2001. Clinical spectrum and transmission characteristics of infection with Norwalk-like virus: findings from a large community outbreak in Sweden. Clin. Infect. Dis. 33 (5), 622–628.

Hald, T., et al., 2016. World Health Organization estimates of the relative contributions of food to the burden of disease due to selected foodborne hazards: a structured expert elicitation. PLoS ONE 11 (1), e0145839.

Hall, A.J., et al., 2011. Incidence of acute gastroenteritis and role of norovirus, Georgia, USA, 2004–2005. Emerg. Infect. Dis. 17 (8), 1381–1388.

Hall, A.J., et al., 2012. The roles of Clostridium difficile and norovirus among gastroenteritis-associated deaths in the United States, 1999–2007. Clin. Infect. Dis. 55 (2), 216–223.

Hall, A.J., et al., 2013a. Acute gastroenteritis surveillance through the national outbreak reporting system, United States. Emerg. Infect. Dis. 19 (8), 1305–1309.

Hall, A.J., et al., 2013b. Norovirus disease in the United States. Emerg. Infect. Dis. 19 (8), 1198–1205.

Hall, A.J., et al., 2014. Vital signs: foodborne norovirus outbreaks—United States, 2009–2012. MMWR Morb. Mortal Wkly. Rep. 63 (22), 491–495.

Harris, J.P., et al., 2008. Deaths from norovirus among the elderly, England and Wales. Emerg. Infect. Dis. 14 (10), 1546–1552.

Havelaar, A.H., et al., 2012. Disease burden of foodborne pathogens in the Netherlands, 2009. Int. J. Food Microbiol. 156 (3), 231–238.

Havelaar, A.H., et al., 2015. World Health Organization global estimates and regional comparisons of the burden of foodborne disease in 2010. PLoS Med. 12 (12), e1001923.

Kambhampati, A., et al., 2016. Host genetic susceptibility to enteric viruses: a systematic review and metaanalysis. Clin. Infect. Dis. 62 (1), 11–18.

Kapikian, A.Z., et al., 1972. Visualization by Immune Electron Microscopy of a 27-nm Particle Associated with Acute Infectious Nonbacterial Gastroenteritis. Journal of Virology 10 (5), 1075–1081.

Kirk, M., et al., 2014. Foodborne illness, Australia, circa 2000 and circa 2010. Emerg. Infect. Dis. 20 (11), 1857–1864.

Kirk, M.D., et al., 2015. World Health Organization estimates of the global and regional disease burden of 22 foodborne bacterial, protozoal, and viral diseases, 2010: a data synthesis. PLoS Med. 12 (12), e1001921.

Kotloff, K.L., et al., 2013. Burden and aetiology of diarrhoeal disease in infants and young children in developing countries (the Global Enteric Multicenter Study, GEMS): a prospective, case–control study. Lancet 6736.

Kovacs, S.D., et al., 2015. Deconstructing the differences: a comparison of GBD 2010 and CHERG's approach to estimating the mortality burden of diarrhea, pneumonia, and their etiologies. BMC Infect. Dis. 15 (1), 1–15.

Kuchenmuller, T., et al., 2009. Estimating the global burden of foodborne diseases—a collaborative effort. Euro. Surveill. 14, 18.

Kuchenmuller, T., et al., 2013. World Health Organization initiative to estimate the global burden of foodborne diseases. Rev. Sci. Tech. 32 (2), 459–467.

Lindsay, L., et al., 2015. A decade of norovirus disease risk among older adults in upper-middle and high income countries: a systematic review. BMC Infect. Dis. 15, 425.

Liu, L., et al., 2012. Global, regional, and national causes of child mortality: an updated systematic analysis for 2010 with time trends since 2000. Lancet 379.

Liu, L., et al., 2015. Global, regional, and national causes of child mortality in 2000–13, with projections to inform post-2015 priorities: an updated systematic analysis. The Lancet 385 (9966), 430–440.

Lopman, B.A., et al., 2004. Clinical manifestation of norovirus gastroenteritis in health care settings. Clin. Infect. Dis. 39 (3), 318–324.

Lopman, B.A., et al., 2011. Increasing rates of gastroenteritis hospital discharges in US adults and the contribution of norovirus, 1996–2007. Clin. Infect. Dis. 52 (4), 466–474.

Lopman, B., et al., 2014. Epidemiologic implications of asymptomatic reinfection: a mathematical modeling study of norovirus. Am. J. Epidemiol. 179 (4), 507–512.

Lopman, B.A., et al., 2015. Norovirus infection and disease in an Ecuadorian Birth Cohort: association of certain norovirus genotypes with host FUT2 secretor status. J. Infect. Dis. 211 (11), 1813–1821.

Murray, C.J., 1994. Quantifying the burden of disease: the technical basis for disability-adjusted life years. Bull. World Health Organization 72 (3), 429–445.

Murray, C.J.L., Lopez, A.D., 1996. The Global Burden of Disease: A Comprehensive Assessment of Mortality and Disability From Diseases, Injuries, and Risk Factors in 1990 and Projected to 2020. Harvard School of Public Health on Behalf of the World Health Organization and the World Bank, Cambridge, MA.

Murray, C.J., Lopez, A.D., 1997a. Global mortality, disability, and the contribution of risk factors: Global Burden of Disease Study. Lancet 349 (9063), 1436–1442.

Murray, C.J.L., Lopez, A.D., 1997b. Mortality by cause for eight regions of the world: Global Burden of Disease Study. The Lancet 349 (9061), 1269–1276.

O'Brien, S.J., et al., 2016. Age-specific incidence rates for norovirus in the community and presenting to primary healthcare facilities in the United Kingdom. J. Infect. Dis. 213 (Suppl. 1), S15–S18.

Parrino, T.A., et al., 1977. Clinical immunity in acute gastroenteritis caused by Norwalk agent. New Engl. J. Med. 297 (2), 86–89.

Patel, M.M., et al., 2008. Systematic literature review of role of noroviruses in sporadic gastroenteritis. Emerg. Infect. Dis. 14 (8), 1224–1231.

Payne, D.C., et al., 2013. Norovirus and medically attended gastroenteritis in U.S. children. New Engl. J. Med. 368 (12), 1121–1130.

Pires, S.M., et al., 2015. Aetiology-specific estimates of the global and regional incidence and mortality of diarrhoeal diseases commonly transmitted through Food. PLoS ONE 10 (12), e0142927.

Rockx, B., et al., 2002. Natural history of human calicivirus infection: a prospective cohort study. Clin. Infect. Dis. 35 (3), 246–253.

Rouhani, S., et al., 2016. Norovirus infection and acquired immunity in 8 countries: results from the MAL-ED study. Clin. Infect. Dis.

Saito, M., et al., 2014. Multiple norovirus infections in a birth cohort in a Peruvian Periurban community. Clin. Infect. Dis. 58 (4), 483–491.

Salomon, J.A., et al., 2015. Disability weights for the Global Burden of Disease 2013 study. Lancet Global Health 3 (11), e712–e723.

Scallan, E., et al., 2015. An assessment of the human health impact of seven leading foodborne pathogens in the United States using disability adjusted life years. Epidemiol. Infect. 143 (13), 2795–2804.

Seitz, S.R., et al., 2011. Norovirus infectivity in humans and persistence in water. Appl. Environ. Microbiol. 77 (19), 6884–6888.

Shioda, K., et al., 2015. Global age distribution of pediatric norovirus cases. Vaccine 33 (33), 4065–4068.

Simmons, K., et al., 2013. Duration of immunity to norovirus gastroenteritis. Emerg. Infect. Dis. 19 (8), 1260–1267.

Tam, C.C., et al., 2012a. Changes in causes of acute gastroenteritis in the United Kingdom over 15 years: microbiologic findings from 2 prospective, population-based studies of infectious intestinal disease. Clin. Infect. Dis. 54 (9), 1275–1286.

Tam, C.C., et al., 2012b. Longitudinal study of infectious intestinal disease in the UK (IID2 study): incidence in the community and presenting to general practice. Gut 61 (1), 69−77.

Teunis, P.F., et al., 2008. Norwalk virus: how infectious is it? J. Med. Virol. 80 (8), 1468−1476.

Thomas, M.K., et al., 2013. Estimates of the burden of foodborne illness in Canada for 30 specified pathogens and unspecified agents, circa 2006. Foodborne Pathog. Dis. 10 (7), 639−648.

Thongprachum, A., et al., 2016. Epidemiology of gastroenteritis viruses in Japan: prevalence, seasonality, and outbreak. J. Med. Virol. 88 (4), 551−570.

United Nations Department of Economic and Social Affairs, Population Division. World population prospects, the 2015 revision. 2015. Available from: <http://esa.un.org/unpd/wpp/Download/Standard/Population/>.

Verhoef, L., et al., 2015. Norovirus genotype profiles associated with foodborne transmission, 1999−2012. Emerg. Infect. Dis. 21 (4), 592−599.

Vinjé, J., 2015. Advances in laboratory methods for detection and typing of norovirus. J. Clin. Microbiol. 53 (2), 373−381.

Vos, T., et al., 2015. Global, regional, and national incidence, prevalence, and years lived with disability for 301 acute and chronic diseases and injuries in 188 countries, 1990−2013: a systematic analysis for the Global Burden of Disease Study 2013. Lancet 386 (9995), 743−800.

Walker, C.L., Black, R.E., 2010. Diarrhoea morbidity and mortality in older children, adolescents, and adults. Epidemiol. Infect. 138 (9), 1215−1226.

Walker, C.L., et al., 2013. Global burden of childhood pneumonia and diarrhoea. Lancet 381 (9875), 1405−1416.

Wikswo, M.E., et al., 2013. Clinical profile of children with norovirus disease in rotavirus vaccine era. Emerg. Infect. Dis. 19 (10), 1691−1693.

Yen, C., Hall, A.J., 2013. Editorial commentary: challenges to estimating norovirus disease burden. J. Pediatric Infect. Dis. Soc. 2 (1), 61−62.

OVERVIEW OF NOROVIRUS AS A FOODBORNE PATHOGEN

2

Hoi Shan Kwan, Paul K.S. Chan and Martin C.W. Chan

The Chinese University of Hong Kong, Hong Kong, China

2.1 GLOBAL BURDEN OF NOROVIRUS INFECTIONS

Food safety is a major public health concern throughout the world. In 2015, the World Health Organization (WHO) published the first-ever estimates of the global and regional burden of foodborne diseases (WHO, 2015a). The WHO report estimated that eating contaminated food causes almost 1 in 10 people to become ill every year and 420,000 deaths. The tremendous burden of foodborne diseases shows that food safety is an important issue for the world, particularly Africa, Southeast Asia, and the Americas. It is clear that foodborne diseases affect people of all ages, particularly children younger than age 5 years and people in low-income countries. Children younger than age 5 years are at particularly high risk, with 125,000 children dying from foodborne diseases every year. WHO African and Southeast Asia regions have the highest burden of foodborne diseases. Another WHO report provides an online tool for researchers to study foodborne diseases and policymakers to set up and implement strategies to improve food safety (WHO, 2015b). In this WHO report, noroviruses were chosen as the only diarrheal virus in the estimation, indicating the importance of these viruses in foodborne diseases worldwide. Indeed, noroviruses are among the leading causes of foodborne diarrheal diseases in eastern Mediterranean countries, the Americas, and Southeast Asia. For example, annually in eastern Mediterranean countries, norovirus causes 15 million of a total of 23 million foodborne illnesses (WHO, 2015a).

Norovirus was first identified microscopically in Norwalk, Ohio, in 1972 from a foodborne disease outbreak. It was named Norwalk virus and later included more isolates, which were called Norwalk-like viruses and are now termed noroviruses. It has yet to be cultured. It belongs to a group referred to as SRSV for "small round structured viruses" of the family Caliciviridae. It has been estimated that each year, noroviruses are responsible for 64,000 diarrheal episodes requiring hospitalization, 900,000 clinic visits among children in industrialized nations, and 200,000 deaths of children younger than age 5 years in the developing world (Patel et al., 2008). WHO (2015b) estimated that noroviruses caused 125 million diarrheal illnesses and 35,000 deaths in 2010 globally. The burden of noroviruses is approximately 23% of a total of 550 million cases of foodborne diarrhea disease and chemical intoxication (Fig. 2.1) (WHO, 2015b). Indeed, Hall and colleagues from the Centers for Disease Control and Prevention (CDC) performed a meta-analysis that estimated noroviruses cause 570−800 deaths, 56,000−71,000 hospitalizations, 400,000 emergency visits, 1.7−1.9 million outpatient visits, and 19−21 million total illnesses per year in the

The Norovirus. DOI: http://dx.doi.org/10.1016/B978-0-12-804177-2.00002-6

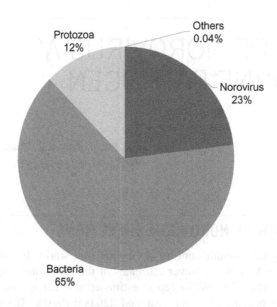

FIGURE 2.1

Proportions of foodborne illnesses with different etiologies in the world, 2010. Global foodborne diarrheal diseases and chemical intoxication. Total count: 541,609,603.

From: World Health Organization (WHO), 2015b. WHO estimates of the global burden of foodborne diseases. Available from: <https://extranet.who.int/sree/Reports?op = vs&path = /WHO_HQ_Reports/G36/PROD/EXT/FoodborneDiseaseBurden>.

United States alone (Hall et al., 2012). The proportion of noroviruses among foodborne illnesses in the United States is approximately 32%, which represents the same share as all bacterial foodborne diseases combined (Fig. 2.2) (CDC, 2013). A recent analysis suggested that the number of norovirus outbreaks is underestimated (Ahmed et al., 2014). Note that waterborne and foodborne routes account for one-fifth of all-cause norovirus infections. A majority of norovirus infections spread through person-to-person transmission, especially within semiclosed settings such as hospitals, cruise ships, and schools (Table 2.3).

The number of recent studies reported in PubMed shows the trend and close relationship of norovirus and foodborne diseases and outbreaks (Fig. 2.3).

2.2 CHARACTERISTICS RELATED TO FOOD SAFETY

Noroviruses are highly transmissible; dosages as little as 100 particles can establish infection and cause disease, and the probability of a single norovirus particle causing an infection is approximately 0.5 (Teunis et al., 2008). The symptoms usually include vomiting and diarrhea. Although generally mild in otherwise healthy individuals, norovirus infections in at-risk patients such as young children and the elderly may require hospitalization and may be fatal. Outbreaks usually start with food contaminated by infected food workers, spread through person-to-person or

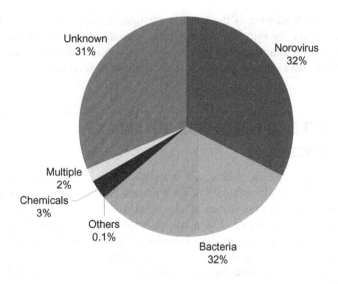

FIGURE 2.2

Number of foodborne disease outbreaks reported to the CDC, 2009–10. Total cases: 1521.

From: Centers for Disease Control and Prevention (CDC), 2013. Surveillance for foodborne disease outbreaks—United States, 2009–2010. Morb. Mort. Wkly. Rep. 62 (3), 41. Available from: <http://dx.doi.org/10.1016/j.annemergmed.2009.11.004>.

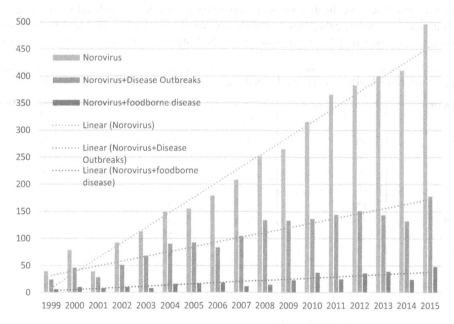

FIGURE 2.3

PubMed articles on norovirus, with "disease outbreak" and "foodborne diseases" as keywords, 1999–15.

From: PubMed. Retrieved December 20, 2015.

surface-to-person modes. Sanitation is the key to containing virus transmission. However, because the viruses are excreted during symptomatic and asymptomatic phases of illness, and survive well in environments outside the human body, it is nearly impossible to eliminate them without closing the food facilities. Next, we review noroviruses in the context of food safety.

2.3 FOODS RELATED TO NOROVIRUS OUTBREAKS

2.3.1 TYPES OF FOODS

Norovirus is the leading cause of illness and outbreaks from contaminated food in the United States. Approximately 50% of all outbreaks of food-related illness are caused by noroviruses. Food can become contaminated with noroviruses at any point during food production when it is being grown, shipped, handled, or prepared. Extensive outbreak analyses showed that water and food handlers are the primary sources of norovirus infections. Foods washed with water or prepared by food handlers and consumed raw without cooking constitute the main source of norovirus food-borne outbreaks. These foods include oysters, shellfish, fruits, vegetables, and salads and sandwiches prepared with these ingredients.

The CDC compiles searchable lists of norovirus outbreaks that can be retrieved from the Foodborne Outbreak Online Database (FOOD Tool; http://www.cdc.gov/foodborneoutbreaks). Our analysis of the norovirus outbreak data from the FOOD Tool for 5 years from 2010 to 2014 showed that food vehicles that have been commonly involved in norovirus outbreaks are salads, sandwiches, fruit, lettuce, oyster, cake, fish, shellfish, coleslaw, and chicken (Table 2.1). This analysis confirmed that any food that is served raw or handled after cooking can become contaminated.

Table 2.1 Norovirus Outbreaks in the United States From 2010 to 2014, by Food Vehicle

Food Vehicle	No. of Outbreaks	No. of Cases	No. of Hospitalizations	No. of Deaths
Salad	131	3,296	26	1
Sandwiches	40	709	14	0
Fruit	30	910	4	1
Lettuce[a]	19	443	8	0
Oyster	15	187	1	0
Cake	15	426	5	0
Fish/shellfish[b]	10	161	3	0
Coleslaw	8	342	7	0
Chicken[c]	7	322	0	1
Others	144	3,047	25	0
Vehicle not known	947	17,930	175	3
Total	1366	27,773	268	6

[a]Not including those involved in salad and sandwiches.
[b]Shellfish other than oyster.
[c]Not including those involved in salad and sandwiches.
CDC Foodborne Outbreak Online Database. Available from http://www.cdc.gov/foodsafety/outbreaks.

However, it is not uncommon for an implicated food vehicle not to be identified in an outbreak. For example, of 33 outbreaks during which more than 100 people became sick, implicated food vehicles were identified in only 13; in the remaining 20, food vehicles could not be determined. Table 2.1 provides that in most outbreaks (69%), the food vehicle could not be determined (947 out of 1366 total cases). The norovirus outbreak that affected most people during the study period, 294 in total, occurred in 2014 in Michigan and was caused by unspecified sauces. The common foods implicated in outbreaks of noroviruses include different kinds of salads, sandwiches, fruits, and shellfish including oysters. The ingredients most implicated in salads and sandwiches are lettuce and other vegetables. These foods pose significant risk because they can be contaminated by water with noroviruses, are usually handled by food service workers, and are usually eaten raw.

A search of PubMed studies with various food items as keywords gave similar results (Table 2.2).

Table 2.2 Number of Norovirus Reports Retrieved From PubMed by Food Items as Keywords (1981–2015)

Food Vehicle	No. of PubMed Reports in Past 5 Years/All Years[a]
Shellfish	79/210
Oyster	67/214
Fruits	43/77
Berries	36/65
Vegetables	50/82
Lettuce	56/87

[a]All years, 1981–2015; past 5 years, 2011–15.
PubMed. Retrieved December 20, 2015.

Table 2.3 Norovirus Outbreaks in the United States From 2010 to 2014, by Nature of Outbreak Setting

Outbreak Setting	No. of Outbreaks	No. of Cases	No. of Hospitalizations	No. of Deaths
Restaurant	836	13,307	150	2
Caterer	133	4,011	25	1
Banquet	113	3,607	24	0
Private home	83	1,511	21	0
Long-term/nursing home	23	746	22	2
School/college/university	14	744	2	0
Others	164	3,847	24	1
Total	1366	27,773	268	6

Data calculated from CDC Foodborne Outbreak Online Database. Available from http://www.cdc.gov/foodsafety/outbreaks.

These statistics may be representative for other developed countries such as those in the European Union, Australia, and New Zealand. However, the common food vehicles of norovirus outbreaks may be different in developing countries.

2.3.2 SOURCES AND CHARACTERISTICS OF FOOD CONTAMINATION

2.3.2.1 Water

Norovirus has been reported to cause waterborne gastroenteritis outbreaks. There are many water sources of outbreaks, including potable water, groundwater, municipal water systems, commercial ice, and recreation waters (Cho et al., 2014; Di Bartolo et al., 2015). Outbreaks have also been caused by foods contaminated with norovirus-containing water used in food preparation. Foods consumed raw are particularly susceptible to contamination through water. These foods include shellfish, especially raw oysters; fresh vegetables; and fruits. Raw oysters can be contaminated in their growth environment. Fresh vegetables and fruits can be contaminated by irrigation water or by washing water. It has been very difficult to test for the presence of noroviruses in the highly diverse sources of water (Sokolova et al., 2012). One of the most important norovirus sources is wastewater treatment plant effluents, and the use of such wastewater for irrigation of vegetables will seed contamination. There are different methods to remove and reduce noroviruses in wastewater systems, including the use of waste stabilization ponds, the application of activated sludge, or the use of submerged-membrane bioreactor treatments (da Silva et al., 2008; Victoria et al., 2010; Miura et al., 2015; Butler et al., 2015). Using a probabilistic quantitative microbial risk assessment model, norovirus removal in wastewater treatment systems has been reviewed (Verbyla and Mihelcic, 2015; Pouillot et al., 2015).

2.3.2.2 Fresh vegetables

Currently, it is trendy to eat healthy due to healthy lifestyle recommendations. One item included in healthy eating is fresh vegetables. They are consumed as a major component in salads and sandwiches, mostly in raw, uncooked forms. This trend is consistent with increasing rates of norovirus outbreaks in the United States and the European Union (Callejón et al., 2015). Using multiple correspondence analysis, norovirus was shown to be linked mainly with consumption of salad, followed by leafy vegetables and tomatoes, in the United States; in the European Union, leafy vegetables were the major vehicle, followed by salad (Callejón et al., 2015). Most norovirus outbreaks linked to fresh produce are reported in food service establishments (60% in the United States and 45% in the European Union). Modeling on fresh produce supply chains, Bouwknegt et al. (2015) showed that the risk of consumer exposure to noroviruses is mainly from food handlers' hands contaminating the produce. The risks were estimated to be less than 1 in 1000 for each norovirus exposure (Bouwknegt et al., 2015). Using murine norovirus (MNV-1) as a surrogate to examine cross-contamination of fresh produce by food handlers in a food service setting, Grove and others (2015) showed that MNV-1 bound differently to surfaces of various materials. MNV-1 attached to human hands and chopped lettuce more tightly than to utensils with hard surfaces, including chopping boards, knifes, and spigots. The washing of hands does not seem to be effective in eliminating MNV-1 but instead transfers MNV-1 from the contaminated hand to the clean hand (Grove et al., 2015).

2.3.2.3 Tropical fruits

Due to the globalization of food distribution, tropical fruits are now consumed throughout the world. The fruits are provided in a variety of forms—whole, fresh cut, dried, juice, blends, frozen, pulp, and nectars. Noroviruses are the leading pathogen in outbreaks associated with tropical fruits (Kim et al., 2008; Strawn et al., 2011). The major routes from tropical fruits to diseases are unclear (Strawn et al., 2011). Recent examples involve consumption of berries, avocados, bananas, and pineapples. Berries are the major fruits involved in norovirus outbreaks. A detailed discussion of berries as a source of norovirus outbreak is presented later in this book.

2.3.2.4 Seafood

Seafood is another major agent associated with norovirus outbreaks. Apart from oysters as a leading cause, mussels have been considered to be an important seafood item implicated in norovirus outbreaks in many countries (Henigman et al., 2015). Henigman et al. (2015) analyzed noroviruses in the harvesting areas of mussels implicated in Slovenia. Hundreds of mussel samples were collected in 2006—08 and 2010—12. The prevalence of noroviruses in the two time periods was similar, approximately 10—25% for norovirus GI and GII. They are phylogenetically similar to those from other countries, suggesting the spread of noroviruses among countries. Depuration—removal of contaminated viruses, bacteria, and other impurities—is legislated or required as a preventive measure for safe consumption of shellfish in many countries (Regulation, E.C., 2004).

2.4 LOCATION OF FOOD PREPARATION AND OUTBREAKS

Matthews et al. (2012) systematically reviewed norovirus outbreaks that occurred from 1993 to 2011. They found that foodborne transmission was the most common reported cause (362/666; 54%), and food service was the most common setting (294/830; 35%).

Although norovirus gastroenteritis outbreaks on cruise ships are as common as in other settings, outbreaks on ships make more news headlines (Freeland et al., 2016). WHO (2012) noted that when a norovirus outbreak occurs on a cruise ship, more than 80% of passengers can be affected due to the closed setting.

2.5 NOROVIRUS OCCURRENCE IN CHINA

The current information on norovirus has been collected mainly from developed countries, especially the United States and those of the Europe Union. Similar information from developing countries is rare. The People's Republic of China, at least in some regions, can serve as an example of the developing countries. A prospective investigation carried out among pediatric outpatients and inpatients with acute diarrhea between August 2008 and July 2009 showed that approximately 26% of fecal samples tested positive for noroviruses (Zeng et al., 2012). A survey in Beijing that tested patients with sporadic or outbreaks of acute nonbacterial gastroenteritis from July 2007 to June 2008 found that 26.6% were positive for noroviruses. The proportion of norovirus was much higher than that of other enteric viruses (Liu et al., 2010).

The Chinese Center for Disease Control and Prevention published "Guidelines on Outbreak Investigation, Prevention and Control of Norovirus Infection" (Chinese CDC, 2015), in which it stated that 60–96% of Chinese "other infectious diarrheal outbreaks" were caused by noroviruses. This guideline also reported that according to the Chinese public health emergency management system, in 2015 there were at least 88 reports of norovirus outbreaks. There has not been any estimation of the burden of norovirus disease in China as a whole (Chinese CDC, 2015). Lu et al. (2015) studied norovirus outbreaks in Guangdong province and reported a total of 52 norovirus outbreaks with 4618 cases from January 2013 to January 2015. In a survey on the prevalence of norovirus infection associated with sporadic gastroenteritis cases in Guangzhou, stool specimens were tested during two consecutive cold seasons in 2013–15. Noroviruses were detected in 12% of the samples (Xue et al., 2016). A search of the keyword "诺如病毒" ("norovirus" in Chinese) in the "Greater China Food Safety Information Database" (Chen et al., 2016; http://kwanlab.bio.cuhk.edu.hk/FS) returned 256 news articles and reports with an increasing trend up to 2015.

2.6 PREVENTION AND CONTROL OF OUTBREAKS

Preventive and control measures proposed by various organizations in many countries are similar. For example, the Chinese CDC (2015) recommended prevention and control strategies to include case management, hand hygiene, environmental disinfection, food and water safety, risk assessment, and health education. The US CDC recommended hand hygiene, exclusion and isolation, and environmental disinfection (CDC, 2011). These measures apply to both foodborne outbreak prevention and control and subsequent person-to-person spread of the virus. Indeed, the prevention and control of noroviruses are very difficult because of the low infectious dose of noroviruses, difficulty in disinfecting the vomit of patients, and the persistence of noroviruses in the environment. Nonetheless, because most norovirus outbreaks start with contaminated water and food, prevention measures to ensure food and water safety and personal hygiene are most important.

2.7 CONCLUSIONS AND PERSPECTIVES

Foodborne norovirus infection follows a very simple path of transmission. Water is the primary source of infection. Foods prepared using norovirus-contaminated water and that are eaten raw without further cooking are the major sources of human infections. Secondary contamination by carriers can occur in all kinds of foods. Control for noroviruses initiation can be straightforward by simply cooking the foods before consumption. However, people's preference to eat some of foods raw makes such control unrealistic. People like fresh green vegetables in their salads, sandwiches, or just by themselves. Many people enjoy raw oysters as a delicatessen. Tropical fruits are also preferably consumed fresh. As long as these foods are eaten raw, noroviruses cannot be easily controlled at the source to prevent them from infecting humans. The high transmissibility of noroviruses makes them even more difficult to control. When a norovirus foodborne outbreak starts, it is very difficult to terminate without drastic interruption such as closure of facilities. Norovirus appears to be a perfect foodborne pathogen that demands our greatest effort to develop innovative ways to control.

REFERENCES

Ahmed, S.M., Hall, A.J., Robinson, A.E., Verhoef, L., Premkumar, P., Parashar, U.D., et al., 2014. Global prevalence of norovirus in cases of gastroenteritis: a systematic review and meta-analysis. Lancet Infect. Dis. 14 (8), 725−730. Available from: <http://dx.doi.org/10.1016/S1473-3099(14)70767-4>.

Bouwknegt, M., Verhaelen, K., Rzezutka, A., Kozyra, I., Maunula, L., von Bonsdorff, C.H., et al., 2015. Quantitative farm-to-fork risk assessment model for norovirus and hepatitis A virus in European leafy green vegetable and berry fruit supply chains. Int. J. Food Microbiol. 198, 50−58. Available from: <http://dx.doi.org/10.1016/j.ijfoodmicro.2014.12.013>.

Butler, E., Hung, Y.-T., Suleiman Al Ahmad, M., Yeh, R.Y.-L., Liu, R.L.-H., Fu, Y.-P., 2015. Oxidation pond for municipal wastewater treatment. Appl. Water Sci. Available from: <http://dx.doi.org/10.1007/s13201-015-0285-z>.

Callejón, R.M., Rodríguez-Naranjo, M.I., Ubeda, C., Hornedo-Ortega, R., Garcia-Parrilla, M.C., Troncoso, A.M., 2015. Reported foodborne outbreaks due to fresh produce in the United States and European Union: trends and causes. Foodborne Pathog. Dis. 12 (1), 32−38. Available from: <http://dx.doi.org/10.1089/fpd.2014.1821>.

Centers for Disease Control and Prevention (CDC), 2011. Updated norovirus outbreak management and disease prevention guidelines. Morb. Mort. Wkly. Rep. Recomm. Rep. 60 (3), 1−18.

Centers for Disease Control and Prevention (CDC), 2013. Surveillance for foodborne disease outbreaks—United States, 2009−2010. Morb. Mort. Wkly. Rep. 62 (3), 41. Available from: <http://dx.doi.org/10.1016/j.annemergmed.2009.11.004>.

Chen, S., Huang, D., Nong, W., Kwan, H.S., 2016. Development of a food safety information database for greater China. Food Contr. 65, 54−62. Available from: <http://dx.doi.org/10.1016/j.foodcont.2016.01.002>.

Chinese Center for Disease Control and Prevention, 2015. Guidelines on outbreak investigation, prevention and control of norovirus infection.. Infect. Dis. Rep. 3 (37), 1−44.

Cho, H.G., Lee, S.G., Kim, W.H., Lee, J.S., Park, P.H., Cheon, D.S., et al., 2014. Acute gastroenteritis outbreaks associated with ground-waterborne norovirus in South Korea during 2008−2012. Epidemiol. Infect. 142 (12), 2604−2609. Available from: <http://dx.doi.org/10.1017/S0950268814000247>.

da Silva, A.K., Le Guyader, F.S., Le Saux, J.-C., Pommepuy, M., Montgomery, M.A., Elimelech, M., 2008. Norovirus removal and particle association in a waste stabilization pond. Environ. Sci. Technol. 42 (24), 9151−9157. Available from: <http://dx.doi.org/10.1021/es802787v>.

Di Bartolo, I., Pavoni, E., Tofani, S., Consoli, M., Galuppini, E., Losio, M.N., et al., 2015. Waterborne norovirus outbreak during a summer excursion in Northern Italy. New Microbiol. 38 (1), 109−112. Retrieved from: <http://www.ncbi.nlm.nih.gov/pubmed/25742154>.

Freeland, A.L., Vaughan, G.H., Banerjee, S.N., 2016. Acute gastroenteritis on cruise ships—United States, 2008−2014. Morb. Mort. Wkly. Rep. 65 (1), 1−5.

Grove, S.F., Suriyanarayanan, A., Puli, B., Zhao, H., Li, M., Li, D., et al., 2015. Norovirus cross-contamination during preparation of fresh produce. Int. J. Food Microbiol. 198, 43−49. Available from: <http://dx.doi.org/10.1016/j.ijfoodmicro.2014.12.023>.

Hall, A.J., Eisenbart, V.G., Etingüe, A.L., Gould, L.H., Lopman, B.A., Parashar, U.D., 2012. Epidemiology of foodborne norovirus outbreaks, United States, 2001−2008. Emer. Infect. Dis. 18 (10), 1566−1573. Available from: <http://dx.doi.org/10.3201/eid1810.120833>.

Henigman, U., Biasizzo, M., Vadnjal, S., Toplak, I., Gombac, M., Steyer, A., et al., 2015. Molecular characterisation of noroviruses detected in mussels (Mytilus galloprovincialis) from harvesting areas in Slovenia. The new microbiologica 38, 225−233.

Kim, H.-Y., Kwak, I.-S., Hwang, I.-G., Ko, G., 2008. Optimization of methods for detecting norovirus on various fruit. J. Virol. Meth. 153 (2), 104−110. Available from: <http://dx.doi.org/10.1016/j.jviromet.2008.07.022>.

Liu, L.-J., Liu, W., Liu, Y.-X., Xiao, H.-J., Jia, N., Liu, G., et al., 2010. Identification of norovirus as the top enteric viruses detected in adult cases with acute gastroenteritis. Am. J. Trop. Med. Hyg. 82 (4), 717−722. Available from: <http://dx.doi.org/10.4269/ajtmh.2010.09-0491>.

Lu, J., Sun, L., Fang, L., Yang, F., Mo, Y., Lao, J., et al., 2015. Gastroenteritis outbreaks caused by norovirus GII.17, Guangdong Province, China, 2014−2015. Emerg. Infect. Dis. 21 (7), 1240−1242. Available from: <http://dx.doi.org/10.3201/eid2107.150226>.

Matthews, J.E., Dickey, B.W., Miller, R.D., Felzer, J.R., Dawson, B.P., Lee, A.S., et al., 2012. The epidemiology of published norovirus outbreaks: a review of risk factors associated with attack rate and genogroup. Epidemiol. Infect. 140 (7), 1161−1172. Available from: <http://dx.doi.org/10.1017/S0950268812000234>.

Miura, T., Okabe, S., Nakahara, Y., Sano, D., 2015. Removal properties of human enteric viruses in a pilot-scale membrane bioreactor (MBR) process. Water Res. 75, 282−291. Available from: <http://dx.doi.org/10.1016/j.watres.2015.02.046>.

Patel, M.M., Widdowson, M.A., Glass, R.I., Akazawa, K., Vinjé, J., Parashar, U.D., 2008. Systematic literature review of role of noroviruses in sporadic gastroenteritis. Emerg. Infect. Dis. 14 (8), 1224−1231. Available from: <http://dx.doi.org/10.3201/eid1408.071114>.

Pouillot, R., van Doren, J.M., Woods, J., Plante, D., Smith, M., Goblick, G., et al., 2015. Meta-analysis of the reduction of norovirus and male-specific coliphage concentrations in wastewater treatment plants. Appl. Environ. Microbiol. 81 (14), 4669−4681. Available from: <http://dx.doi.org/10.1128/AEM.00509-15>.

Regulation, E.C., 2004. No 853/2004 of the European Parliament and of the Council of 29 April 2004 laying down specific rules for food of animal origin. Off. J. EU L 226, 93−127.

Sokolova, E., Aström, J., Pettersson, T.J.R., Bergstedt, O., Hermansson, M., 2012. Estimation of pathogen concentrations in a drinking water source using hydrodynamic modelling and microbial source tracking. J. Water Heal. 10 (3), 358−370. Available from: <http://dx.doi.org/10.2166/wh.2012.183>.

Strawn, L.K., Schneider, K.R., Danyluk, M.D., 2011. Microbial safety of tropical fruits. Crit. Rev. Food Sci. Nutr. 51 (2), 132−145. Available from: <http://dx.doi.org/10.1080/10408390903502864>.

Teunis, P.F.M., Moe, C.L., Liu, P., Miller, S.E., Lindesmith, L., Baric, R.S., et al., 2008. Norwalk virus: how infectious is it? J. Med. Virol. 80 (8), 1468−1476. Available from: <http://dx.doi.org/10.1002/jmv.21237>.

Verbyla, M.E., Mihelcic, J.R., 2015. A review of virus removal in wastewater treatment pond systems. Water Res. 71, 107−124. Available from: <http://dx.doi.org/10.1016/j.watres.2014.12.031>.

Victoria, M., Guimarães, F.R., Fumian, T.M., Ferreira, F.F.M., Vieira, C.B., Shubo, T., et al., 2010. One year monitoring of norovirus in a sewage treatment plant in Rio de Janeiro, Brazil. J. Water Heal. 8 (1), 158−165. Available from: <http://dx.doi.org/10.2166/wh.2009.012>.

World Health Organization (WHO), 2012. International travel and health: communicable diseases. Available from: <http://www.who.int/ith/mode_of_travel/communicable_diseases/en/>.

World Health Organization (WHO), 2015a. WHO estimates of the global burden of foodborne diseases. Foodborne disease burden epidemiology reference group 2007−2015. Available from: <http://apps.who.int/iris/bitstream/10665/199350/1/9789241565165_eng.pdf>.

World Health Organization (WHO), 2015b. WHO estimates of the global burden of foodborne diseases. Available from: <https://extranet.who.int/sree/Reports?op = vs&path = /WHO_HQ_Reports/G36/PROD/EXT/FoodborneDiseaseBurden>.

Xue, L., Dong, R., Wu, Q., Li, Y., Cai, W., Kou, X., et al., 2016. Molecular epidemiology of noroviruses associated with sporadic gastroenteritis in Guangzhou, China, 2013−2015. Arch. Virol. 2013−2015. Available from: <http://dx.doi.org/10.1007/s00705-016-2784-0>.

Zeng, M., Xu, X., Zhu, C., Chen, J., Zhu, Q., Lin, S., et al., 2012. Clinical and molecular epidemiology of norovirus infection in childhood diarrhea in China. J. Med. Virol. 84 (1), 145−151. Available from: <http://dx.doi.org/10.1002/jmv.22248>.

SHELLFISH AND BERRIES: THE READY-TO-EAT FOOD MOST INVOLVED IN HUMAN NOROVIRUS OUTBREAKS

Calogero Terregino and Giuseppe Arcangeli

Istituto Zooprofilattico Sperimentale delle Venezie, V.le Università, Legnaro, Padova, Italy

3.1 BACKGROUND

Noroviruses (NoVs) are very contagious enteric viruses that can easily spread from person to person via the fecal—oral route. Both the feces and the vomit of an infected person can contain many virus particles, up to $10^5 - 10^{11}$ viral copies per gram (cpg) of feces, even among asymptomatic infections. This suggests that up to 5 billion infectious doses may be shed by an infected individual in each gram of feces (Teunis et al., 2008; Aoki et al., 2010; Hall, 2012) (Figs. 3.1 and 3.2).

People infected with NoVs are contagious from the moment they show the first symptoms of the infection to 2 or 3 days after recovery, and sometimes for as long as 2 weeks. In addition, high resistance of the virus in the environment, survival at temperatures as high as 140°F, and an extremely low infectious dose (≥ 18 viral particles) may explain why NoVs represent a severe risk to human health in case rivers or seawater polluted by discharges from densely populated and industrial areas contaminate the food chain (Johl et al., 1991; Van Olphen et al., 1991; Payment et al., 1991).

Ineffective sewage treatment systems, as well as the risk of dirty wastewater draining into watersheds, may pose a serious threat to shellfish contamination. Likewise, when raw sewage is used in berry cultivation, the risk of infection in consumers is high (Sorber, 1983; Formiga-Cruz et al., 2002) because these foods are usually marketed ready to eat.

Shellfish, particularly bivalve mollusks such as oysters and mussels, can potentially accumulate NoVs in their tissues because they are filter-feeding animals, as in the case of the mature Atlantic oyster (*Crassostrea virginica*), which filters 5 L of water per hour (NOAA, Chesapeake Bay Office, 2015). Other viruses, such as hepatitis E virus, astrovirus, rotavirus, sapovirus, adenovirus, and vaccine strains poliovirus and Aichi virus, have been associated with outbreaks of shellfish-associated illness, although their impact on shellfish farming is not as great (Cacopardo et al., 1997; Piña et al., 1998; Potasman et al., 2002; Le Guyader et al., 2008; Nakagawa-Okamoto et al., 2009).

Berries grow close to the surface of cultivated areas and are subjected to remarkable manipulation during harvesting, which makes them more exposed to NoVs compared to other fruits. Particular climatic conditions (e.g., heavy rainfall) can increase the transfer of NoVs from

The Norovirus. DOI: http://dx.doi.org/10.1016/B978-0-12-804177-2.00003-8

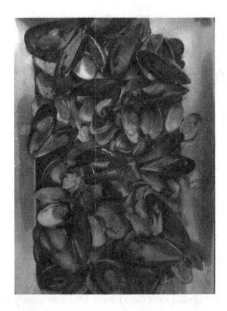

FIGURE 3.1

The complete opening of the shells after cooking is a guarantee for the NoV hazard.

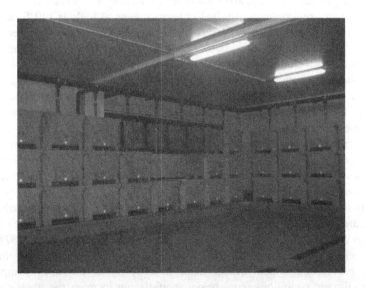

FIGURE 3.2

A modern purification system for bivalves: NoV load is not completely reduced by this treatment.

sewage to irrigation water sources or directly to berry cultures (Maunula et al., 2013; Verhaelen et al., 2013a,b).

The existing literature, which covers mainly North America and Europe, confirms that water is the main route of spread of NoVs. This means that among the categories most at risk of infection are bivalve mollusks and berries.

Large seafood-associated outbreaks have strongly affected oysters and clams harvested from sewage-contaminated waters (Sugieda et al., 1996; Simmons et al., 2007; Iwamoto et al., 2010; Wall et al., 2011). In 2002, an oyster-associated outbreak in Italy and France resulted in 327 confirmed cases (Le Guyader et al., 2006). In the same year, the consumption of raw fish contaminated with NoV was linked to an outbreak of gastroenteritis in Bari (southeast Italy) (Prato et al., 2004). NoV-contaminated oysters were responsible for another outbreak in British Columbia, Canada, which included 53 cases during a 3-month period (David et al., 2007). This chapter discusses cooked and chilled mollusks and proper cooking procedures, which should be sufficient to kill any norovirus present in the raw material. Webby et al. (2007) described multiple outbreaks of norovirus in Australia caused by frozen oyster meat. Later, other important events occurred in the United States and Europe (Westrell et al., 2010; Iwamoto et al., 2010; Smith et al., 2012), and it has been estimated that the annual cost of illness ascribable to seafood contaminated with NoV in the United States is approximately $184 million (Batz et al., 2011). It must also be considered that NoV illness resulting from shellfish consumption is probably underreported because in most cases the symptoms are mild and remain undiagnosed (Sugieda et al., 1996; Tam et al., 2003).

Numerous papers in the literature describe European NoV outbreaks in berries, with the first reported case dating back to 1988 (Pönkä et al., 1999a,b; Le Guyader et al., 2004; Cotterelle et al., 2005; Hjertqvist et al., 2006; Stals et al., 2011; Baert et al., 2011; Sarvikivi et al., 2012; Maunula et al., 2013; Mäde et al., 2013). In the United States, the first outbreaks caused by berry consumption date back to 2005 (CDC, 2013). Surely the largest recorded foodborne illness caused by berries occurred in Germany in 2012: 390 establishments, mainly schools and childcare facilities in five federal states, reported nearly 11,000 cases of gastroenteritis. All institutions had been supplied with food products almost exclusively by one large catering company. The analytical epidemiological studies consistently identified the dishes containing strawberries as the most likely vehicle of infection (Bernard et al., 2014).

3.2 SYSTEMS TO PREVENT NoV CONTAMINATION IN SHELLFISH AND BERRIES

3.2.1 PREVENTION SYSTEMS IN SHELLFISH—PREHARVESTING PHASE

Shellfish are filter-feeding animals and they can accumulate large concentrations of solutes that are present in water. This process is influenced by many environmental parameters, such as water temperature, salinity, the presence of phytoplankton, and turbidity (Riisgard et al., 2011).

The mechanism of accumulation consists of a first phase in which suspended particles are captured by gills that sweep the selected material toward the labial palps and mouth and into the stomach and digestive diverticula. The entry of viruses into bivalve hosts is perhaps mostly associated with normal feeding activities, but it is unclear how small virus particles such as NoVs (<50 nm) are captured by bivalve hosts because the ciliated structures of gills can be spaced to a maximum of 500—600 nm. It may be the case that viral particles can become electrostatically bound to sulfates on the mucopolysaccharides of the shellfish mucus and so they are entrapped in feeding structures when associated with marine aggregates large enough to be captured by the gill (Horin et al., 2015). Studies that have investigated the persistence of enteric viruses infecting humans that contaminate bivalve tissues suggest that certain acid-tolerant viruses (i.e., NoVs) can survive and remain infectious within bivalve hemocytes for extended periods, whereas other viruses disappear more rapidly (Ueki et al., 2007; McLeod et al., 2009). Studies on NoVs suggest that circulating hemocytes are the primary site of virus entry and persistence (Provost et al., 2011).

NoV is able to bind to different histo-blood group antigens, which are complex glycans present on many types of human cells (Tan and Jiang, 2011). Such ligands are also present in shellfish and account for NoV bioaccumulation in oysters and probably in other shellfish species (Tian et al., 2007; Zakhour et al., 2010; Maalouf et al., 2011).

The previously described accumulation behavior demonstrates the difficulty of eliminating NoV from bivalve mollusks once these have been bred in contaminated areas; therefore, it is important to minimize the presence of NoV in production areas. Semiclosed environments, such as lagoons, are probably the most affected areas; here, the enteric viruses can be transported through the supply of fresh water from rivers where they can remain for several weeks (Fong and Lipp, 2005). Although all water potentially contaminated by NoV and of urban derivation must be subjected to a purification treatment, this step is not always sufficient to guarantee the total removal of NoV.

Sewage water undergoes three main stages of purification: The first stage is intended to remove large objects, the second is a nitrification phase in a tank, and the third phase is an ultraviolet (UV) treatment, which is the only phase capable of eliminating NoVs. Unfortunately, not all purification plants meet this requirement (FSA, 2013). It must also be kept in mind that during heavy rainfall events, the capacity of purification plants is often compromised (La Rosa et al., 2010).

NoV may be detected in wastewater even when only a few cases of infection are reported. Thus, NoV and other enteric viruses can be used as an early warning of outbreaks. A large amount of NoV was detected in sewage waters in Sweden during an outbreak, and 2 or 3 weeks passed before most patients were diagnosed with this infection (Hellmér et al., 2014).

Once in brackish lagoons or in the sea, NoV undergoes a dilution effect. Therefore, shellfish farms located far from the coastline are at a lower risk of contamination (Croci et al., 2007).

Different tidal excursions must also be considered. Lagoons located farther away from the Equator are exposed to a greater tidal range and, consequently, to a greater change of water than those located farther south.

There is no significant difference between buried shellfish (i.e., clams) and suspended shellfish (i.e., mussels) with regard to the amount of NoV that they accumulate. Some studies show that there is a positive correlation between the presence of NoV in seawater and rainfall events (Miossec et al., 2000; Suffredini et al., 2008; Bruggink and Marshall, 2010).

For the previously discussed reasons, it is clear that it is important to prevent any form of contact between NoV and shellfish, particularly in the case of mollusks that are traditionally consumed raw, such as oysters. As such, it is important to identify potential sources of pollution in upstream production sites in order to evaluate whether a location may be suitable for farming purposes. Biomolecular quantitative analysis allows us to detect the viral load in production areas and, as a consequence, to identify those with a lower charge to be allocated to shellfish farming. Considering the possibility of developing the disease when NoV concentrations exceed 2000 genome cpg that outbreaks have also been associated with values greater than 1000 cpg, the current advice derived from a study referring to Ireland in particular is that 200 cpg can be taken as the reasonable limit of safety (Lowther et al., 2010; Hartnell et al., 2011; Food Safety Authority of Ireland, 2013; Suffredini et al., 2014).

3.2.2 PREVENTION SYSTEMS IN BERRIES—PREHARVESTING AND HARVESTING PHASES

Berries to be used for commercial purposes are grown in open fields, or they can also be picked from the wild (woods, highlands, grasslands, and wetlands). Protected cultures, particularly for raspberry, soil-less, or hydroponic cultivations, are also used, especially to reduce the contamination caused by animals and bad weather (EFSA, 2014a,b).

Each production site presents specific characteristics that can influence the presence and persistence of pathogens in the fields where berries are grown. Many berry fruits grow close to the ground and are more susceptible to contamination with irrigation water and soil; in addition, they cannot be harvested mechanically, which implies more direct contact with food handlers.

Although it is not clear how long NoVs persist on berries, evidence from outbreaks indicates that these viruses can persist for a prolonged period of time in frozen berries. The ability of viral particles to adhere to a surface depends on several factors, such as intrinsic surface properties, conformation of the surfaces, physicochemical characteristics of the surfaces, and environmental parameters (Deboosere et al., 2012).

The possibility for NoV to internalize in strawberry fruits via plant roots has been demonstrated (Di Caprio et al., 2015). Because of the high acidity of the internal tissues (pH 2.7−4.5), berries are unlikely to support the survival of bacteria. However, considering that NoVs tolerate low pH environments, they could persist in both fresh and frozen berries over extended periods. Internalized viruses would be protected from surface decontamination practices, thus posing a significant risk to public health.

Environmental factors, particularly climatic conditions (e.g., abundant precipitation), increase the transfer of NoVs from sewage to fields of leafy greens. Heavy rainfalls increase the risk of exposure of berries to pathogens, meaning that the contaminated soil may litter the fruit surfaces, or they could cause contamination through flooding whenever floodwater comes into direct contact with berries (EFSA, 2014a,b).

The use of sewage-contaminated irrigation water is another important risk factor that must be considered. Preharvest contamination of berry fruit with NoVs, if the fruit is spray-irrigated with fecally contaminated water or treated with contaminated liquid pesticides (Verhaelen et al., 2013b), is also a risk.

Poor hygiene practices by agricultural workers (including leaked fluid from transportable toilets and defecation in the field, as well as deliberate contamination with fecal material) were also identified as significant sources of contamination of fresh products (Suslow et al., 2003), which significantly increased the risk of contaminating berries as well. A recently developed risk assessment model confirmed that hand contact is the most dominant NoV contamination source for berries (Bouwknegt et al., 2015).

In order to prevent contamination, production areas should be carefully evaluated to identify hazards that may compromise hygiene and food safety, with particular attention to potential sources of fecal contamination. If the levels of contamination in a specific area are considered to compromise the safety of crops, adequate strategies to limit cultivators from using these terrains for berry production should be applied. Implementation of food safety management systems, such as good agricultural practices (GAP), good hygiene practices (GHP), and good manufacturing practices (GMP), as well as the selection of appropriate irrigation sources and the ban of use of uncontrolled water sources, should be the primary goals of operators producing berries.

Water treatment and functioning drainage systems may be used to prevent possible dissemination of contaminated water. If possible, only potable water should be used. The quality of the water used in manufacturing establishments should be adequately controlled and monitored using tests for detecting organisms and/or foodborne and waterborne pathogens. Clean equipment and cleaning preventive measures should be adopted to avoid contamination associated with growing and harvesting for berry production. Compliance with hygiene requirements, particularly hand hygiene, is an absolute necessity for berry handlers to reduce the risks of contamination; furthermore, all those involved in berry production and harvest should receive appropriate hygiene training and periodic evaluation (EFSA, 2014a,b).

3.3 SYSTEMS TO ELIMINATE NoV ACCUMULATED IN SHELLFISH AND BERRIES

3.3.1 ELIMINATION SYSTEMS IN SHELLFISH—POSTHARVESTING PHASE

3.3.1.1 Purification system

The purification (or depuration) system is a treatment that consists of the relay of shellfish in clean environmental waters or in tanks with recirculating treated water; this allows purification of the shellfish flesh from sewage contaminants.

Purification may be achieved if normal filter-feeding activity takes place. To avoid mortality, it is important to create the correct physiological conditions for the shellfish to be purified. For this reason, the following parameters need to be controlled: dissolved oxygen level, shellfish loading, water flow, salinity, temperature, and turbidity. Four systems are usually used to maintain clean water: chlorination, UV light, ozonation, and iodophors (WHO, 2010). In the United Kingdom, a minimum purification time of 42 hours is currently required; in other countries, such as Italy, due to higher environmental temperature, generally a purification time of 18−24 hours is sufficient.

The practice of shellfish purification began more than a century ago and has significantly lowered the incidence of shellfish-borne illnesses (Herdman and Scott, 1896). This process was developed to reduce the load of fecal bacteria accumulated in shellfish, and it is less effective for other organisms, such as enteric viruses. Numerous laboratory studies support the resistance of human enteric viruses in shellfish during the depuration process (Grohmann et al., 1981; Richards, 1988; Power and Collins, 1989, 1990; Sobsey and Jaykus, 1991; Jaykus et al., 1994; Doré and Lees, 1995; Ang, 1998; Le Guyader et al., 2008). Research on NoV has led to the same conclusions (Schwab et al., 1998). Ueki et al. (2007) detected NoV in oysters 10 days after the depuration process, and other studies show the permanence of NoV in oysters after depuration periods of 23 hours at 20°C (McLeod et al., 2009) and 10 days at 10°C (Nappier et al., 2008).

The inefficiency of the purification treatment requires the production of oysters in especially clean water, with extremely low levels of fecal pollution. In the case of other mollusks that are traditionally eaten cooked, such restrictions are not binding (EFSA, 2011).

3.3.1.2 Relaying system

The term "relay" refers to the transfer of shellfish from a contaminated area to clean water, where they are placed on the seafloor or into containers laid on the seafloor, or suspended in racks, generally for a period of at least 2 months. This practice is not commonly used in the European Union and the United States because it is much more expensive than use of the inland purification system.

In 2010, Dorè et al. applied a relaying period to oysters naturally contaminated by NoV. In this case, NoV level decreased from 2900 viral genome copies to 492 during a 17-day period. This system, combined with a final purification process, allowed the achievement of a NoV load less than 200 viral genome cpg.

3.3.1.3 Cooking

A rigorous cooking treatment eliminates enteric viruses, including NoVs. According to the Codex Alimentarius (note CAC/GL 79–2012), cooking at 85–90°C for 90 seconds is enough to inactivate enteric viruses. The application of this treatment in the United Kingdom has proven that NoV inactivation is effective, as evidenced by a decrease in human illness resulting from the consumption of bivalve mollusks (Lees, 2000) (Table 3.1).

Specific tests have recently been performed to evaluate the thermal resistance of NoV with the following outcome: The digestive glands of mussels contaminated with feline calicivirus (FCV) were still infectious after exposure at 80°C for 15 minutes (Croci et al., 2012). An inactivation equal to 5 $\log_{10}$ was obtained using murine norovirus (MNV) after treatment in PBS at 72°C for 3 minutes (Wolf et al., 2009). Evidence from home cooking in a pan of manila clams contaminated with NoV shows that 10 minutes is enough to guarantee the inactivation of the virus (Toffan et al., 2014a,b).

The product can be considered safe as long as the suggested temperatures reach the core of the product, keeping in mind that the shell has a certain resistance to heat penetration. Cases of infection by NoV due to the consumption of undercooked shellfish are described in the literature (Alfano-Sobsey et al., 2012).

Strict regulations (in force in the United States and the European Union) detail the precautions that need to be taken to monitor the presence of fecal bacteria (*Escherichia coli*) in live bivalve mollusks; however, enteric viruses (i.e., NoV) are not included in the list of dangerous pathogens. Nevertheless, several manufacturers independently choose to print on the labels of their products "to be cooked before consumption" as a precaution against the possible presence of NoV and other heat-sensitive pathogens.

3.3.1.4 Other systems

High-pressure processing (HPP) is a method usually applied to facilitate the shucking of oysters and extend the shelf-life of the products. High hydrostatic pressure (HHP) is also called the "cold-pasteurization" method because it is able to inactivate the vegetative cells of the normal bacterial

Table 3.1 Parameters for NoV Inactivation in Shellfish

Virus	Inactivation Method Applied	Matrix	Log Reduction	Reference
FCV	Boiling water, 30 s	Cockle	1.7	Slomka and Appleton (1998)
FCV	Heating, 65°C/30 s	Mussel homogenate	7.5	Cekmer (2014)
FCV	Fermentation, 15 days (5% NaCl)	Oyster	3.01	Seo et al. (2014)
MNV-1	400 MPa, 5°C, 5 min	Oyster	4	Kingsley et al. (2007)
MNV-1	Heating, 90°C, 90 s	Soft-shell clam	3.3	Sow et al. (2011)
MNV-1	500 MPa, 10°C, 1 min	Manila clam	4	Arcangeli et al. (2012)
MNV-1	Fermentation, 15 days (5% NaCl)	Oyster	1.6	Seo et al. (2014)
MNV-1	Heating, 100°C, 2 min	Manila clam	4	Toffan et al. (2014a, b)
MNV-1	Heating, 72°C, 20 s	Mussel homogenate	6.7	Cekmer (2014)
MNV-1	Heating, 85°C, 6 min	Mussel dried	3.2	Park et al. (2014)
Human NV[a]	450 MPa, 1°C, 5 min	Oyster and clam homogenates	4	Ye et al. (2014)

[a]*NV vitality estimated by indirect method: binding to porcine gastric mucin-conjugated magnetic beads (PGM-MBs).*

flora, including pathogens such as salmonella and vibrios. Specific experiments involving NoV and the related FCV indicate a $4 \log_{10}$ decrease in virus infectivity after pressure treatment of oysters for 5 minutes at 400 MPa (Kingsley et al., 2007). Ye et al. (2014) demonstrated that a treatment at 450 MPa at 1°C for 5 minutes achieved a greater than $4 \log_{10}$ reduction of NoV in both oyster and clam homogenates.

UV irradiation at 120 J/m^2 reduced the infectivity of FCV by $3 \log_{10}$y (de Roda Husman et al., 2004). In PBS, MNV-1 was readily inactivated by UV (the amount of UV was not specified) (Wolf et al., 2009). In another study, the inactivation of MNV-1 in oysters by electron beam (E-beam) irradiation was investigated. The reduction of potential infection risks was quantified for E-beam irradiation technology employed on raw oysters at various virus contamination levels. The E-beam dose required to reduce the MNV by 90% (D_{10} value) in whole oysters was 4.05 kGy (Praveen et al., 2013). Note that consumers have expressed a certain degree of doubt about the safety of irradiated foods.

Other techniques, such as cooling, freezing, marinating, and pasteurization, do not appear to be particularly effective for NoV inactivation (Mormann et al., 2010).

3.3.2 ELIMINATION SYSTEMS IN BERRIES—POSTHARVESTING PHASE

After harvest, the risk factors for berries are the persistence of live viruses acquired during cultivation and harvest, as well as contamination during processing from the environment (e.g., water sources), from equipment, or from NoV-infected workers who do not meet adequate sanitation measures and personal hygiene.

Cross-contamination with foodborne pathogens can be associated with harvesting methods, and these can be transferred via dirt (soil, debris, dust, etc.) on the berries during and after harvesting (EFSA, 2014a,b).

Differences in the viral persistence among different berries have been observed. Possible factors that may influence the infectivity of virus particles are temperature, relative humidity, and the fruit matrix. The fruit matrix may influence virus infectivity for the presence of antiviral compounds, proteolytic enzymes, or by physiological parameters such as respiration rate. For example, raspberries are characterized by a higher respiration rate compared to strawberries when kept at a temperature of 20°C, which produces a higher humidity level in the microclimate of raspberries (Verhaelen et al., 2012). Therefore, viruses may be protected from dryness on raspberries but not on strawberries (Cannon et al., 2006). The surface structure may be another important factor affecting viral persistence on berry fruits. The presence of hydrophobic pockets can affect the efficacy of washing treatments in removing virus particles on fresh produce (Adams et al., 1989).

The presence of dirt in the processing plant and cross-contamination between processed products and wastes or contaminated materials are also important risk factors. Water can be a vehicle of contamination when berries are washed. Other uses of water (refreshing, fungicide application, and ice) may also account for other ways of contamination.

The risk from workers is similar for leafy greens as well as for any other sector processing ready-to-eat foods (EFSA, 2014a,b). Berries, particularly frozen fruits, undergo considerable handling before processing; they must often be graded and trimmed by hand. Work surfaces can be contaminated by workers handling contaminated products or by infected workers; therefore, NoV can be transferred to uncontaminated berries through fruit contact materials (Stals et al., 2013).

NoV cannot grow on food; therefore, the contamination level cannot increase during processing or storage. However, the possibility of inducing illness should be considered even with low viral loads due to high infectivity (Carter, 2005; Koopmans and Duizer, 2004) and resistance of NoVs, especially in particular environmental conditions. The following treatments can be used to sanify berries:

Freezing: Freezing has no significant effect on the infectivity of NoV due to the fact that the structural integrity and the genome remain stable after freezing or after several freeze–thaw cycles (Richards et al., 2012). The presence of NoV in frozen raspberries and strawberries has often been linked to outbreaks of gastroenteritis (Sarvikivi et al., 2012; Mäde et al., 2013); it is therefore likely that lowering the temperature of berry fruits will not reduce the potential for NoV to remain infectious.

Washing: Removal of viruses by washing abundantly depends both on the produce type and the viral load. In general, not more than 1 or 2 logs of microorganisms can be removed by washing fruits or vegetables with water (Beuchat, 1998). The application of chlorine in treating strawberries at levels not affecting their sensory aspect did not result in an additional reduction of NoV (Gulati et al., 2001). Even prolongation of treatment with chlorine is not useful for significantly increasing the effectiveness of chlorination (Duizer et al., 2004; Gulati et al., 2001). Use to peroxyacetic acid to treat strawberries resulting in a maximum 2 log reduction of NoV compared to washing with water (Gulati et al., 2001). Electrolyzed oxidizing water (EOW) is a new effective disinfection method that is easy to use, relatively economic, and environmentally friendly (Huang, 2008). In the future, EOW may represent a valid method of inactivation of viruses in food products.

High hydrostatic pressure (HHP): HHP is used to stabilize nonthermally treated fruit juices (Nguyen-The, 2012). After treatment of artificially contaminated blueberries with HHP at 600 MPa for 2 minutes at 21°C, a receptor-binding reduction in NoV higher than 3 log on water-immersed blueberries but less than 1 log in those on dried blueberries was observed (Li et al., 2013).

Heating: The use of surrogates demonstrated that NoV infectivity could be reduced by heating at pasteurization temperatures (Baert, 2013). In studies conducted using substrates other than berries, different inactivation rates of FCV and canine calicivirus (CaCV) at temperatures ranging from 37°C to 100°C were observed (Duizer et al., 2004). Thermal inactivation levels were also observed for FCV and murine NoV (M-NV1) at 63°C and 72°C (Cannon et al., 2006). To reduce the risk of foodborne viral infections caused by the consumption of frozen berries, sanitary authorities of some European countries have recommended that berries must be cooked at boiling temperature (100°C) before consumption for at least 2 minutes.

UV: UV light treatment can be used as a sanitation method for berries. A 3 log reduction was obtained for FCV and CaCV in cell culture medium after exposure to UV at a dose of 12 and 20 mW s/cm^2, respectively (De Roda Husman et al., 2004). When used at a dose of 200 Gy, gamma irradiation reduced CaCV and FCV, respectively by 2.4 and 1.6 log (De Roda Husman et al., 2004). Water-assisted UV treatment can be used as an alternative to chlorine washing for blueberries, and it has proven to have higher efficacy than dry UV treatment (Liu et al., 2015).

Ozone: Promising results have been obtained by treating berries with ozone. Predmore et al. (2015) studied the effectiveness of gaseous ozone for the sanitization of two human norovirus surrogates (MNoV-1 and Tulane virus) from both liquid media and strawberries. Gaseous ozone significantly reduced the two human NoV surrogate viral titers in both liquid virus stock and food matrix through the disruption of the virion structure and the degradation of proteins on the surface of the virus, while leaving genomic RNA intact.

Given that many of the treatments used so far to sanitize berries have shown limited efficacy, prevention of contamination is a critical issue. As mentioned previously, NoV-infected food handlers are the main risk factor for contamination during the postharvesting production stages. As such, only workers who have been trained in hygienic handling procedures should be assigned to process berries. All workers involved in the handling of berries should receive training appropriate to their tasks and undergo periodic assessment to ensure that they are working in accordance with GHP (EFSA, 2014a,b).

3.4 CONCLUSIONS AND PERSPECTIVES

Waterborne outbreaks of gastroenteritis associated with NoVs are reported worldwide. Shellfish, especially bivalve mollusks such as oysters and mussels, can potentially accumulate NoVs in their tissues because they are filter-feeding animals. Berries grow close to the surface of cultivated areas and undergo a remarkable manipulation process during harvesting, which makes them more exposed to NoVs than other fruits. Once contaminated, it is difficult to eliminate NoVs from the food and only drastic treatments such as cooking are effective for eliminating the virus. The most effective way to control this hazard is to prevent viral contamination. Therefore, the methods of production and harvesting, if they effectively control contamination sources and apply good hygienic processing practices, protect the health of consumers.

REFERENCES

Adams, M.R., Hartley, A.D., Cox, L.J., 1989. Factors affecting the efficacy of washing procedures used in the production of prepared salads. Food Microbiol. 6, 6977.

Alfano-Sobsey, E., Sweat, D., Hall, A., Breedlove, F., Rodriguez, R., Greene, S., et al., 2012. Norovirus outbreak associated with undercooked oysters and secondary household transmission. Epidemiol. Infect. 140 (2), 276–282.

Ang, L.H., 1998. An outbreak of viral gastroenteritis associated with eating raw oysters. Commun. Dis. Public Health 1, 38–40.

Aoki, Y., Suto, A., Mizuta, K., Ahiko, T., Osaka, K., Matsuzaki, Y., 2010. Duration of norovirus excretion and the longitudinal course of viral load in norovirus-infected elderly patients. J. Hospital Infect. 75, 42–46.

Arcangeli, G., Terregino, C., De Benedictis, P., Zecchin, B., Manfrin, A., et al., 2012. Effect of high hydrostatic pressure on murine norovirus in manila clams. Lett. Appl. Microbiol. 54, 325–329.

Baert, L., 2013. Foodborne virus inactivation by thermal and non-thermal processes. In: Cook, N. (Ed.), Viruses in Food and Water. Woodhead Publishing, pp. 237–260.

Baert, L., Mattison, K., Loisy-Hamon, F., Harlow, J., Martyres, A., Lebeau, B., et al., 2011. Review: norovirus prevalence in Belgian, Canadian and French fresh produce: a threat to human health? Int. J. Food Microbiol. 151, 261–269.

Batz, M.B., Hoffmann, S., Morris, J.G., 2011. Ranking the risks: the 10 pathogen–food combinations with the greatest burden on public health. Emerging Pathogens Institute, University of Florida, Gainesville, FL.

Bernard, H., Faber, M., Wilking, H., Haller, S., Höhle, M., Schielke, A., et al. (2014) Large multistate outbreak of norovirus gastroenteritis associated with frozen strawberries, Germany, 2012. Euro Surv.19 (8), pii = 20719. Available from: <http://www.eurosurveillance.org/ViewArticle.aspx?ArticleId=20719> (accessed 16.09.15.).

Beuchat, L.R. 1998. Surface decontamination of fruits and vegetables eaten raw: a review. Food Safety Unit, World Health Organization, WHO/FSF/FOS/98.2.

Bouwknegt, M., Verhaelen, K., Rzeżutka, A., Kozyra, I., Maunula, L., Von, et al., 2015. Quantitative farm-to-fork risk assessment model for norovirus and hepatitis A virus in European leafy green vegetable and berry fruit supply chains. Int. J. Food Microbiol. 198, 50–58.

Bruggink, L.D., Marshall, J.A., 2010. The incidence of norovirus-associated gastroenteritis outbreaks in Victoria, Australia (2002–2007) and their relationship with rainfall. Int. J. Environ. Res. Public Health 7, 2822–2827.

Cacopardo, B., Russo, R., Preiser, W., Benanti, F., Brancati, F., Nunnari, A., 1997. Acute hepatitis E in Catania (eastern Sicily) 1980–1994. Role Hepatitis E Virus. Infec. 25, 313–316.

Cannon, J.L., Papafragkou, E., Park, G.W., Osborne, J., Jaykus, L.A., Vinje, J., 2006. Surrogates for the study of norovirus stability and inactivation in the environment: a comparison of murine norovirus and feline calicivirus. J. Food Protect. 69, 2761–2765.

Carter, M.J., 2005. Enterically infecting viruses: pathogenicity, transmission and significance for food and waterborne infection. J. Appl. Microbiol. 98, 1354–1380.

Cekmer, H.B., 2014. Thermal inactivation of human norovirus surrogates and hepatitis A virus in foods, Doctoral Dissertations, University of Tennessee—Knoxville. Available from: <http://trace.tennessee.edu/> (accessed 11.15).

Centers for Disease Control and Prevention (CDC)., 2013. Foodborne outbreak online database. Available from: <http://wwwn.cdc.gov/foodborneoutbreaks/Default.aspx> (accessed 3.10.15).

Cotterelle, B., Drougard, C., Rolland, J., Becamel, M., Boudon, M., Pinede, S., et al., 2005. Outbreak of norovirus infection associated with the consumption of frozen raspberries, France. Euro Surv. 10 (17), pii = 2690. Available from: <http://www.eurosurveillance.org/ViewArticle.aspx?ArticleId=2690> (accessed 8.11.15).

Croci, L., Losio, M.N., Suffredini, E., Pavoni, E., Di Pasquale, S., Fallacara, F., et al., 2007. Assessment of human enteric viruses in shellfish from the Northern Adriatic sea. Int. J. Food Microbiol. 114, 252–257.

Croci, L., Suffredini, E., Di Pasquale, S., Cozzi, L., 2012. Detection of norovirus and feline calicivirus in spiked molluscs subjected to heat treatments. Food Contr. 25, 17–22.

David, S.T., Mcintyre, L., Macdougal, L., Kelly, D., Liem, S., Schallie, K., et al., 2007. An outbreak of norovirus caused by consumption of oysters from geographically dispersed harvest sites, British Columbia, Canada, 2004. Foodborne Path. Dis. 4, 349–358.

Deboosere, N., Pinon, A., Caudrelier, Y., Delobel, A., Merle, G., Perelle, S., et al., 2012. Adhesion of human pathogenic enteric viruses and surrogate viruses to inert and vegetal food surfaces. Food Microbiol. 32, 48–56.

De Roda Husman, A.M., Bijkerk, P., Lodder, W., Van Den Berg, H., Pribil, W., Cabaj, et al., 2004. Calicivirus inactivation by nonionizing (253.7-nanometerwavelength [UV]) and ionizing (gamma) radiation. Appl. Environ. Microbiol. 70, 5089–5093.

Di Caprio, E., Culbertson, D., Li, J., 2015. Evidence of the internalization of animal caliciviruses via the roots of growing strawberry plants and dissemination to the fruit. Appl. Environ. Microbiol. 81 (8), 2727–2734.

Doré, B., Keaveney, S., Flannery, J., Rajko-Nenow, P., 2010. Management of health risks associated with oysters harvested from a norovirus contaminated area, Ireland. Euro Surv. 15 (19), pii = 19567. Available from: <http://www.eurosurveillance.org/ViewArticle.aspx?ArticleId=19567> (accessed 9.11.15).

Doré, W.J., Lees, D.N., 1995. Behaviour of *Escherichia coli* and male-specific bacteriophage in environmentally contaminated bivalve molluscs before and after depuration. Appl. Environ. Microbiol. 61, 2830–2834.

Duizer, E., Bijkerk, P., Rockx, B., De Groot, A., Twisk, F., et al., 2004. Inactivation of caliciviruses. Appl. Environ. Microbiol. 70, 4538–4543.

EFSA Panel on Biological Hazards (Biohaz), 2011. Scientific opinion on an update on the present knowledge on the occurrence and control of foodborne viruses. EFSA J. 9 (7), 2190. Available from: <http://doi:10.2903/j.efsa.2011.2190> (accessed 12.11.15)

EFSA (European Food Safety Authority), 2014a. Scientific opinion on the risk posed by pathogens in food of non-animal origin. Part 2 (salmonella and norovirus in berries). EFSA J. 12 (6), 3706.

EFSA (European Food Safety Authority), 2014b. Scientific opinion on the risk posed by pathogens in food of non-animal origin. Part 2: Salmonella and norovirus in berries. EFSA J. 12 (6), 3706. Available from: <http://www.efsa.europa.eu/sites/default/files/scientific_output/files/main_documents/3706.pdf> (accessed 12.11.15)

Fong, T.T., Lipp, E.R.I.N. K., 2005. Enteric viruses of humans and animals in aquatic environments: health risks, detection, and potential water quality assessment tools. Microbiol. Mol. Biol. Rev. 69 (2), 357–371.

Food Safety Authority of Ireland 2013. Risk management of norovirus in oysters, opinion by the Food Safety Authority of Ireland Scientific Committee. Available from: <https://www.fsai.ie/publications_norovirus_opinion/> (accessed 02.11.15.).

Formiga-Cruz, M., Tofin-o-Quesada, G., Bofill-Mas, S., Lees, D.N., Henshilwood, K., Allard, A.K., et al., 2002. Distribution of human virus contamination in shellfish from different growing areas in Greece, Spain, Sweden, and the United Kingdom. Appl. Environ. Microbiol. 68 (12), 5990–5998.

FSA, 2013. Proceedings of the Food Standards Agency's Foodborne Viruses Research Conference. January 2013, Holiday Inn London, Bloomsbury, London.

Grohmann, G.S., Murphy, A.M., Christopher, P.J., Auty, G., Greenberg, H.B., 1981. Norwalk virus gastroenteritis in volunteers consuming depurated oysters. Austr. J. Exp. Biol. Med. Sci. 59, 219–228.

Gulati, B.R., Allwood, P.B., Hedberg, C.W., Goyal, S.M., 2001. Efficacy of commonly used disinfectants for the inactivation of calicivirus on strawberry, lettuce, and a food-contact surface. J. Food Prot. 64, 1430–1434.

Hall, A.J., 2012. Noroviruses: the perfect human pathogens? J. Infect. Dis. 205 (11), 1622−1624. Available from: <http://dx.doi.org/10.1093/infdis/jis251>. (accessed 17.09.15).

Hartnell, R., Avant, J., Lowther, J., Stockley, L., Lees, D.N., Russe, J.E., 2011. Comparative testing and reference materials in molluscan shellfish microbiology. VIII International Conference on Molluscan Shellfish Safety (ICMSS). Abstract Proceedings. June 12−17, Charlottetown, Canada.

Hellmér, M., Paxéus, N., Magnius, L., Enache, L., Arnholm, B., Johansson, A., et al., 2014. Detection of pathogenic viruses in sewage provided early warnings of hepatitis A virus and norovirus outbreaks. Appl. Environ. Microbiol. 80 (21), 6771−6781.

Herdman, W.A., Scott, A., 1896. Report on the investigations carried out in 1895 in connection with the Lancashire Sea—Fisheries Laboratory at the University College, Liverpool. Proc. Trans. Liverpool Biol. Soc. 10, 103−117.

Hjertqvist, M., Johansson, A., Svensson, N., Abom, P.E., Magnusson, C., Olsson, M., et al., 2006. Four outbreaks of norovirus gastroenteritis after consuming raspberries, Sweden. Euro Surv. 11 (36), pii = 3038. Available from: <http://www.eurosurveillance.org/ViewArticle.aspx?ArticleId = 3038>. (accessed 17.11.15).

Horin, T.B., Bidegain, G., Huey, L., Narvaez, D.A., Bushek, D., 2015. Parasite transmission through suspension feeding. J. Invert. Pathol. Available from: <http://dx.doi.org/10.1016/j.jip.2015.07.006> (accessed 12.11.15).

Huang, Y.R., 2008. Application of electrolyzed water in the food industry. Food Contr. 19, 329−345.

Iwamoto, M., Ayers, T., Mahon, B.E., Swerdlow, D.L., 2010. Epidemiology of seafood—associated infections in the United States. Clin. Microbiol. Rev. 23, 399−411.

Jaykus, L.A., Hemard, M.T., Sobsey, M.D., 1994. Human enteric pathogenic viruses. In: Hackney, C.R., Pierson, M.D. (Eds.), Environmental Indicators and Shellfish Safety. Chapman and Hall, London, UK, pp. 92−153.

Johl, M., Kerkmann, M.L., Kramer, U., Walter, R., 1991. Virological investigation of the river Elbe. Water Sci. Technol. 24, 205−208.

Kingsley, D.H., Holliman, D.R., Calci, K.R., Chen, H., Flick, G.J., 2007. Inactivation of a norovirus by high-pressure processing. Appl. Environ. Microbiol. 73, 581−585.

Koopmans, M., Duizer, E., 2004. Foodborne viruses: an emerging problem. Int. J. Food Microbiol. 90, 23−41.

La Rosa, G., Iaconelli, M., Pourshaban, M., Fratini, M., Muscillo, M., 2010. Molecular detection and genetic diversity of norovirus genogroup IV: a yearlong monitoring of sewage throughout Italy. Arch. Virol. 155 (4), 589−593.

Lees, D., 2000. Viruses and bivalve shellfish. Int. J. Food Microbiol. 59, 81−116.

Le Guyader, F.S., Mittelholzer, C., Haugarreau, L., Hedlund, K.O., Alsterlund, R., Pommepuy, et al., 2004. Detection of noroviruses in raspberries associated with a gastroenteritis outbreak. Int. J. Food Microbiol. 97, 179−186.

Le Guyader, F.S., Bon, F., Demedici, D., Parnaudeau, S., Bertone, A., Crudeli, et al., 2006. Detection of multiple noroviruses associated with an international gastroenteritis outbreak linked to oyster consumption. J. Clin. Microbiol. 44, 3878−3882.

Le Guyader, F.S., Le Saux, J.C., Ambert-Balay, K., Krol, J., Serais, O., Parnaudeau, S., et al., 2008. Aichi virus, notovirus, astrovirus, enterovirus, and rotavirus involved in clinical cases from a French oyster-related gastroenteritis outbreak. J. Clin. Microbiol. 46, 4011−4017.

Li, X., Chen, H., Kingsley, D.H., 2013. The influence of temperature, pH, and water immersion on the high hydrostatic pressure inactivation of GI.1 and GII.4 human noroviruses. Int. J. Food Microbiol. 167, 138−143.

Liu, C., Li, X., Chen, H., 2015. Application of water-assisted ultraviolet light processing on the inactivation of murine norovirus on blueberries. Int. J. Food Microbiol. 214, 18−23.

Lowther, J.A., Gustar, N.E., Hartnell, E., Lees, D.N., 2010. Comparison of norovirus RNA levels in outbreak-related oysters with background environmental levels. J. Food Prot. 75, 389–393.

Maalouf, H., Schaeffer, J., Parnaudeau, S., Le Pendu, J., Atmar, R.L., et al., 2011. Strain-dependent norovirus bioaccumulation in oysters. Appl. Environ. Microbiol. 77, 3189–3196.

Mäde, D., Trübner, K., Neubert, E., Höhne, M., Johne, R., 2013. Detection and typing of norovirus from frozen strawberries involved in a large-scale gastroenteritis outbreak in Germany. Food Environ. Virol. 5, 162–168.

Maunula, L., Kaupke, A., Vasickova, P., Soderberg, K., Kozyra, I., Lazic, S., et al., 2013. Tracing enteric viruses in the European berry fruit supply chain. Int. J. Food Microbiol. 167, 177–185.

Mcleod, C., Hay, B., Grant, C., Greening, G., Day, D., 2009. Inactivation and elimination of human enteric viruses by Pacific oysters. J. Appl. Microbiol. 107, 1809–1818.

Miossec, L., Le Guyader, F., Haugarreau, L., Pommepuy, M., 2000. Importance de la pluviométrie sur la contamination virale du milieu littoral lors de phénomènes épidémiques dans la population. Revue d'Epidémiologie et de Santé Publique 48, 62–71.

Mormann, S., Dabisch, M., Becker, B., 2010. Effects of technological processes on the tenacity and inactivation of norovirus genogroup II in experimentally contaminated foods. Appl. Environ. Microbiol. 76 (2), 536–545.

Nakagawa-Okamoto, R., Arita-Nishida, T., Todo, S., Kato, H., Iwata, H., Akiyama, M., et al., 2009. Detection of multiple sapovirus genotypes and genogroups in oyster-associated outbreaks. Jpn. J. Infect. Dis. 62, 63–66.

Nappier, S.P., Graczyk, T.K., Schwab, K.J., 2008. Bioaccumulation, retention, and depuration of enteric viruses by *Crassostrea virginica* and *Crassostrea ariakensis* oysters. Appl. Environ. Microbiol. 74, 6825–6831.

Nguyen-The, C., 2012. Biological hazards in processed fruits and vegetables. Risk factors and impact of processing techniques. Food Sci. Technol. 49, 172–177.

NOAA (National Oceanic And Atmospheric Administration), 2015. Chesapeake bay office. Oysters. Available from: <http://chesapeakebay.noaa.gov/fish-facts/oysters> (accessed 10.10.15).

Park, S.Y., Kim, S.H., Ju, J.S., Cho, J.I., Ha, S.D., 2014. Thermal inactivation of murine norovirus-1 in suspension and in dried mussels (Mytilus edulis). J. Food Saf. 34, 193–198.

Payment, P., Richardson, L., Siemiatycki, J., Dewar, R., Edwardes, M., Franco, E., 1991. A randomized trial to evaluate the risk of gastrointestinal disease due to consumption of drinking water meeting current microbiological standards. Am. J. Public Health. 81, 703–707.

Piña, S., Puig, M., Lucena, F., Jofre, J., Girones, R., 1998. Viral pollution in the environment and in shellfish: human adenovirus detection by PCR as an index of human viruses. Appl. Environ. Microbiol. 64 (9), 3376–3382.

Pönkä, A., Maunula, L., Von Bonsdorff, C.H., Lyytikäinen, O., 1999a. Outbreak of calicivirus gastroenteritis associated with eating frozen raspberries. Euro Surv. 4 (6), pii = 56. Available from: <http://www.eurosurveillance.org/ViewArticle.aspx?ArticleId=56> (accessed 12.10.15.).

Pönkä, A., Maunula, L., Von Bonsdorff, C.H., Lyytikäinen, O., 1999b. An outbreak of calicivirus associated with consumption of frozen raspberries. Epidemiol. Infect. 123 (3), 469–474.

Potasman, I., Paz, A., Odeh, M., 2002. Infectious outbreaks associated with bivalve shellfish consumption: a worldwide perspective Israel. Clin. Infect. Dis. 35, 921–928.

Power, U.F., Collins, J.K., 1989. Differential depuration of poliovirus *Escherichia coli* and a coliphage by the common mussel mytilus-edulis. Appl. Environ. Microbiol. 55, 1386–1390.

Power, U.F., Collins, J.K., 1990. Elimination of coliphages and *Escherichia-coli* from mussels during depuration under varying conditions of temperature salinity and food availability. J. Food Protect. 53, 208–226.

Prato, R., Lopalco, P.L., Chironna, M., Barbuti, G., Germinario, C., Quarto, M., 2004. Norovirus gastroenteritis general outbreak associated with raw shellfish consumption in South Italy. BMC (Bio Medical Center) Infect. Dis. 4, 37−42.

Praveen, C., Dancho, B.A., Kingsley, D.H., Calci, K.R., Meade, G.K., Mena, K.D., et al., 2013. Susceptibility of murine norovirus and hepatitis A virus to electron beam irradiation in oysters and quantifying the reduction in potential infection risks. Appl. Environ. Microbiol. 79 (12), 3796−3801.

Predmore, A., Sanglay, G., Li, J., Lee, K., 2015. Control of human norovirus surrogates in fresh foods by gaseous ozone and a proposed mechanism of inactivation. Food Microbiol. 50, 118−125.

Provost, K., Ozbay, G., Anderson, R., Richards, G.P., Kingsley, D.H., 2011. Hemocytes are sites of persistence for virus-contaminated oysters. Appl. Environ. Microbiol. 77, 8360−8369.

Richards, G.P., 1988. Microbial purification of shellfish a review of depuration and relaying. J. Food Protect. 51, 218−251.

Richards, G.P., Watson, M.A., Meade, G.K., Hovan, G.L., Kingsley, D.H., 2012. Resilience of norovirus GII.4 to freezing and thawing: implications for virus infectivity. Food Environ. Virol. 4, 192−197.

Riisgard, H.U., Egede, P.P., Saavedra, I.B., 2011. Feeding behaviour of the Mussel, Mytilus edulis: new observations, with a minireview of current knowledge. J. Marine Biol. 312459, 13. Available from: <http://dx.doi.org/10.1155/2011/312459>. (accessed 13.10.15).

Sarvikivi, E., Roivainen, M., Maunula, L., Niskanen, T., Korhonen, T., Lappalainen, M., et al., 2012. Multiple norovirus outbreaks linked to imported frozen raspberries. Epidemiol. Infect. 140, 260−267.

Schwab, K.J., Neill, F.H., Estes, M.K., Metcalf, T.G., Atmar, R.L., 1998. Distribution of Norwalk virus within shellfish following bioaccumulation and subsequent depuration by detection using RT-PCR. J. Food Protect. 61, 1674−1680.

Seo, D.J., Lee, M.H., Seo, J., Do Ha, S., Choi, C., 2014. Inactivation of murine norovirus and feline calicivirus during oyster fermentation. Food Microbiol. 44, 81−86.

Simmons, G., Garbutt, C., Hewitt, J., Greening, G., 2007. A New Zealand outbreak of norovirus gastroenteritis linked to the consumption of imported raw Korean oysters. NZ Med. J. 120, U2773.

Slomka, M.J., Appleton, H., 1998. Feline calicivirus as a model system for heat inactivation studies of small round structured viruses in shellfish. Epidemiol. Infect. 121, 401−407.

Smith, A.J., Mccarthy, N., Saldana, L., Ihekweazu, C., Mcphedran, K., Adak, G.K., et al., 2012. A large food-borne outbreak of norovirus in diners at a restaurant in England between January and February 2009. Epidemiol. Infect. 140, 1695−1701.

Sobsey, M.D., Jaykus, L.A., 1991. Human enteric viruses and depuration of bivalve mollusks. In: Otwell, W.S., Rodrick, G.E., Martin, R.E. (Eds.), Molluscan Shellfish Depuration. CRC Press, Boca Raton, FL, pp. 71−114.

Sorber, C.A., 1983. Removal of viruses from wastewater and effluent by treatment processes. In: Berg, G. (Ed.), Viral Pollution of the Environment. CRC Press, Boca Raton, FL, pp. 39−52.

Sow, H., Desbiens, M., Morales-Royas, R., Ngazoa, S.E., Jean, J., 2011. Heat inactivation of hepatitis A virus and a norovirus surrogate in soft-shell clams (Mya arenaria). Foodborne Path. Dis. 8, 387−393.

Stals, A., Baert, L., Jasson, V., Van Coillie, E., Uyttendaele, M., 2011. Screening of fruit products for norovirus and the difficulty of interpreting positive PCR results. J. Food Protect. 74, 425−431.

Stals, A., Uyttendaele, M., Baert, L., Van Coillie, E., 2013. Norovirus transfer between foods and food contact materials. J. Food Protect. 76, 1202−1209.

Suffredini, E., Corrain, C., Arcangeli, G., Fasolato, L., Manfrin, A., Rossetti, E., et al., 2008. Occurrence of enteric viruses in shellfish and relation to climatic-environmental factors. Lett. Appl. Microbiol. 20, 462−468.

Suffredini, E., Lanni, L., Arcangeli, G., Pepe, T., Mazzette, R., Ciccaglioni, G., et al., 2014. Qualitative and quantitative assessment of viral contamination in bivalve molluscs harvested in Italy. Int. J. Food Microbiol. 184, 21−26.

Sugieda, M., Nakajima, K., Nakajima, S., 1996. Outbreaks of Norwalk-like virus-associated gastroenteritis traced to shellfish: coexistence of two genotypes in one specimen. Epidemiol. Infect. 116, 339—346.

Suslow, T.V., Oria, M.P., Beuchat, L.R., Garrett, E.H., Parish, M.E., Harris, L.J., et al., 2003. Production practices as risk factors in microbial food safety of fresh and fresh-cut produce. Comprehensive Rev. Food Sci. Food Saf. 2 (S1), 38—77.

Tam, C.C., Rodrigues, L., O'brien, S.J., 2003. The study of infectious intestinal disease in England: what risk factors for presentation to general practice tell us about potential for selection bias in case—control studies of reported cases of diarrhoea. Int. J. Epidemiol. 32, 99—105.

Tan, M., Jiang, X., 2011. Norovirus—host interaction: multi-selections by human histoblood group antigens. Trends Microbiol. 19, 382—388.

Teunis, P.F., Moe, C.L., Liu, P., Miller, S.E., Lindesmith, L., Baric, R.S., et al., 2008. Norwalk virus: how infectious is it?. J. Med. Virol. 80 (8), 1468—1476. Available from: <http://dx.doi.org/10.1002/jmv.21237> (accessed 13.11.15).

Tian, P., Engelbrektson, A.L., Jiang, X., Zhong, W., Mandrell, R.E., 2007. Norovirus recognizes histo-blood group antigens on gastrointestinal cells of clams, mussels, and oysters: a possible mechanism of bioaccumulation. J. Food Protect. 70, 2140—2147.

Toffan, A., Brutti, A., De Pasquale, A., Cappellozza, E., Pascoli, F., Cigarini, M., et al., 2014a. The effectiveness of domestic cook on inactivation of murine norovirus in experimentally infected Manila clams (*Ruditapes philippinarum*). J. Appl. Microbiol. 116 (1), 191—198.

Toffan, A., Brutti, A., De Pasquale, A., Cappellozza, E., Pascoli, F., et al., 2014b. The effectiveness of domestic cook on inactivation of murine norovirus in experimentally infected Manila clams (*Ruditapes philippinarum*). J. Appl. Microbiol. 116 (1), 191—198.

Ueki, Y., Shoji, M., Suto, A., Tanabe, T., Okimura, Y., Kikuchi, Y., et al., 2007. Persistence of caliciviruses in artificially contaminated oysters during depuration. Appl. Environ. Microbiol. 73, 5698—5701.

Van Olphen, M., De Bruin, H.A.M., Havelaar, A.H., Schijven, J.F., 1991. The virological quality of recreational waters in the Netherlands. Water Sci. Technol. 24 (2), 209—211.

Verhaelen, K., Bouwknegt, M., Lodder-Verschoor, F., Rutjes, S.A., De Roda Husman, A.M., 2012. Persistence of human norovirus GII.4 and GI.4, murine norovirus, and human adenovirus on soft berries as compared with PBS at commonly applied storage conditions. Int. J. Food Microbiol. 160, 137—144.

Verhaelen, K., Bouwknegt, M., Carratala, A., Lodder-Verschoor, F., Diez-Valcarce, M., Rodriguez-Lazaro, D., et al., 2013a. Virus transfer proportions between gloved fingertips, soft berries, and lettuce, and associated health risks. Int. J. Food Microbiol. 166, 419—425.

Verhaelen, K., Bouwknegt, M., Rutjes, S.A., De Roda Husman, A.M., 2013b. Persistence of human norovirus in reconstituted pesticides—pesticide application as a possible source of viruses in fresh produce chains. Int. J. Food Microbiol. 160, 323—328.

Wall, R., Dymond, N., Bell, A., Thornley, C., Buik, H., Cumming, D., et al., 2011. Two New Zealand outbreaks of norovirus gastroenteritis linked to commercially farmed oysters. NZ Med. J. 124, 63—71.

Webby, R.J., Carville, K.S., Kirk, M.D., Greening, G., Ratcliff, R.M., Crerar, S.K., et al., 2007. Internationally distributed frozen oyster meat causing multiple outbreaks of norovirus infection in Australia. Clin. Infect. Dis. 44, 1026—1031. Available from: <http://dx.doi.org/10.1086/512807> (accessed 14.11.15).

Westrell, T., Dusch, V., Ethelberg, S., Harris, J., Hjertqvist, M., Jourdan-Da Silva, N., et al. 2010. Norovirus outbreaks linked to oyster consumption in the United Kingdom, Norway, France, Sweden and Denmark. Euro Surv. 15. pii = 19524. Available from: <http://www.eurosurveillance.org/ViewArticle.aspx?ArticleId19524> (accessed 30.10.15).

WHO (World Health Organization), 2010. Safe Management of Shellfish and Harvest Waters. IWA Publishing, Alliance House, UK, pp. 145—181.

Wolf, S., Rivera-Aban, M., Greening, G.E., 2009. Long-range reverse transcription as a useful tool to assess the genomic integrity of norovirus. Food Environ. Virol. 1, 129−136.

Ye, M., Li, X., Kingsley, D.H., Jiang, X., Chen, H., 2014. Inactivation of human norovirus in contaminated oysters and clams by high hydrostatic pressure. Appl. Environ. Microbiol. 80 (7), 2248−2253.

Zakhour, M., Maalouf, H., Di Bartolo, I., Haugarreau, L., Le Guyader, F.S., et al., 2010. Bovine norovirus ligand, environmental contamination and potential cross-species transmission via oyster. Appl. Environ. Microbiol. 76, 6404−6411.

PATHOGEN

STRUCTURE AND GENOTYPES OF NOROVIRUSES

4

Martin C.W. Chan, Hoi Shan Kwan and Paul K.S. Chan
The Chinese University of Hong Kong, Hong Kong, China

4.1 INTRODUCTION

Infection with human noroviruses is a leading cause of acute gastroenteritis affecting all age groups worldwide. According to a 2015 World Health Organization report on the estimates of global burden of foodborne diseases from 2007 to 2015, noroviruses and *Campylobacter* spp. are the top two causes (among biological and nonbiological agents) of foodborne illnesses. This highlights the public health importance of noroviruses with regard to the worldwide human population. Understanding the structure of noroviruses may provide important insights into why this group of enteric viruses is highly stable under hostile external environment and is very successful in person-to-person transmission. Noroviruses are genetically very diverse, and how this diversity influences public health and shapes the epidemiology are of clinical and research interest. Finally, as with most, if not all, viruses, noroviruses are continuously evolving, and it is not surprising that new variants of norovirus with better survival fitness occasionally emerge. What do we expect to see when a new norovirus variant emerges? Will a new variant reshape the current epidemiological landscape of norovirus gastroenteritis? In this chapter, we discuss the structure and genotypes of noroviruses as well as the latest research developments with an aim to provide more clues for those who are interested in pursuing the ultimate answers to these questions.

4.2 STRUCTURE

4.2.1 GENOME ORGANIZATION

Human noroviruses belong to the family *Caliciviridae* and the genus *Norovirus*. They have a relatively small, single-stranded, positive-sense, linear RNA genome approximately 7500 nucleotides in length. The first complete genome of Norwalk virus, the prototype (GI.1) of noroviruses, was deciphered in 1990 (Xi et al., 1990) (Fig. 4.1). The genome is organized into three overlapping open reading frames (ORF1−ORF3). ORF1, with a size of approximately 5100 bases, encodes for a polyprotein including structural protein VPg and nonstructural proteins such as 3C-like protease and 3D-like RNA-dependent RNA polymerase. ORF2, with a size of approximately 1600 bases, encodes for the major capsid protein called viral protein 1 (VP1), which is further subdivided into

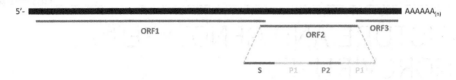

FIGURE 4.1

Genome organization of human noroviruses into three overlapping open reading frames (ORF1−ORF3). ORF1, -2, and -3 encode for polyprotein, major capsid protein VP1, and minor capsid protein viral protein 2, respectively. The diagram is not drawn in scale. P1, protruding domain 1; P2, protruding domain 2; S, shell.

the shell (S), protruding 1 (P1), and P2 subdomains (Fig. 4.1) (Prasad et al., 1999). ORF3, with a size of approximately 720 bases, encodes for the minor capsid protein called VP2, which may function to stabilize the capsid virion (Bertolotti-Ciarlet et al., 2003; Vongpunsawad et al., 2013). The 5′ end of the genome is covalently linked to VPg (Daughenbaugh et al., 2006), and the 3′ end contains a polyadenylated tail. Transfection of complete norovirus RNA genome can produce intact virus particles, suggesting that the genome itself is infectious (Guix et al., 2007).

4.2.2 VIRION STRUCTURE AND ENVIRONMENTAL STABILITY

Norovirus virion is nonenveloped and approximately 27 nm in diameter. Each virion is composed of 90 dimers of VP1 arranged on a T = 3 icosahedral symmetry with a cup-shaped morphology under electron microscopy (Chen et al., 2004; Dolin et al., 1982; Prasad et al., 1999). The P2 domain of VP1 is the most surface-exposed part of the virion and contains histo-blood group antigen binding interface (putative host attachment factor for noroviruses) and antigenic epitopes linked to immune escape (Cao et al., 2007; Chen et al., 2006; Choi et al., 2008; de Rougemont et al., 2011; Donaldson et al., 2008; Lindesmith et al., 2012; Prasad et al., 1999). Human noroviruses are highly resistant to harsh external environments. Repeated freeze−thaw process up to 14 cycles and long storage in frozen form up to 120 days did not have any notable effect on norovirus capsid integrity, as reflected by the measurement of the quantity of encapsulated virus RNA (Richards et al., 2012). In a volunteer challenge study, Norwalk virus inoculum treated with up to 10 mg/L of chlorine retained infectiousness as reflected by inducing typical symptoms of acute gastroenteritis (Keswick et al., 1985). Using in vitro-expressed virus-like particles, norovirus capsid was found to be highly stable in a wide range of pH from 3 to 7 and at elevated temperature up to nearly 60°C (Ausar et al., 2006). It was speculated that temperature, pH, and ionic strength affect the stability of the secondary and tertiary structure of the virus capsid protein, which in turn mediates virus infectivity and binding capability to inanimate surfaces (Samandoulgou et al., 2015).

4.3 GENOTYPES
4.3.1 OVERVIEW

Human noroviruses are still regarded as noncultivable despite a recent breakthrough that demonstrated limited human norovirus replication in B cells cocultured with bacteria expressing

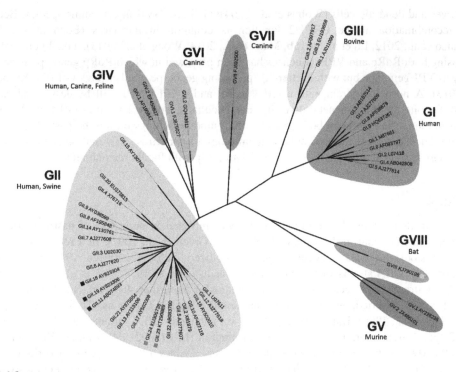

FIGURE 4.2

Classification of norovirus into eight genogroups (GI−GVIII) and 44 genotypes using neighbor-joining phylogenetic inference on complete amino acid sequences of VP1. One tentative new genogroup (GVIII from bats) and two tentative new genotypes (GII.23 and GII.24) not described in Vinje (2015) are indicated by blue (light gray in print versions) and magenta (dark gray in print versions) squares, respectively. Each sequence is denoted as genogroup.genotype or as only genogroup if there is just one genotype within the genogroup, followed by GenBank accession number. The animal host of each genogroup is shown in gray text underneath genogroup designation. All genotypes within GII infect humans except GII.11, GII.18, and GII.19, which infect pigs (black squares). For clarity, bootstrap values at nodes and branch lengths are omitted.

histo-blood group antigens (Jones et al., 2014, 2015). Because an efficient cell culture system is not available, serotyping of human noroviruses by neutralization assay is not yet possible; thus, "serotype" is not applicable to noroviruses. Currently, classification of norovirus is largely based on complete amino acid sequences of VP1 (Vinje, 2015; Zheng et al., 2006). Norovirus is genetically very diverse and can be classified into at least seven genogroups (GI−GVII) and 41 genotypes (e.g., GI.1) according to the latest scheme proposed by Dr. Jan Vinje of the National Calicivirus Laboratory of the US Centers for Disease Control and Prevention (CDC) (Vinje, 2015) (Fig. 4.2). Recently, an additional genogroup (GVIII) has been described (Wu et al., 2015). GI and GII infect humans only; GII.11, GII.18, and GII.19 infect porcine species. GIII infects bovine species. GIV infects canine and feline species. Human infections of GIV are very rare (Ao et al., 2014; Eden et al., 2012). GV infects murine species and is the only norovirus genogroup that can be cultivated in vitro efficiently in macrophages and dendritic cells (Wobus et al., 2004). GVI and GVII infect canine species. Because genetic recombination at the ORF1/2 junction is common in norovirus (Eden et al., 2013; Giammanco et al., 2012; Lu et al., 2015b; Mans et al., 2014; Wong et al., 2013), a dual nomenclature system using both RdRp and VP1 sequences has been proposed in which RdRp genotype is denoted similarly as VP1 genotype but with a letter "P" preceding genotype number (e.g., GII.P3) (Kroneman et al., 2013). A norovirus strain with a GII.3 RdRp and a GII.6 VP1 will be designated as GII.P3_GII.6. Despite the broad genetic diversity, one peculiar genotype known as GII.4 has been predominant in human infections in both sporadic and outbreak settings during the past 20 years. The following section describes the molecular epidemiology of norovirus GII.4 and other important and emerging norovirus genotypes, as well as their relationship with foodborne outbreaks.

4.3.2 **GII.4**

The first strain that belonged to norovirus GII.4 was reported in outbreaks of gastroenteritis in a nursing home in Maryland in the winter of 1987–88 (Green et al., 2002). In a retrospective study on archived stool materials collected from hospitalized children between 1974 and 1991 in Washington, DC, GII.4 strains were found in samples as early as 1974 (Bok et al., 2009), suggesting that GII.4 strains have been circulating in humans for more than 40 years. Since then, sporadic detection has been reported, and the first pandemic GII.4 variant, known as 95/96-US, was reported in 1999 (Noel et al., 1999). Dating back to 1996, six pandemic GII.4 variants have been identified: 95/96-US (years of circulation, 1995–2002), Farmington Hills (2002–04), Hunter (2004–06), Den Haag (2006–09), New Orleans (2009 to present), and Sydney (2012 to present) (Pringle et al., 2015) (Fig. 4.3). A new GII.4 variant has emerged every 2–4 years, replacing the previously circulating GII.4 variant (Bull and White, 2011; Eden et al., 2013). Interestingly, the emergence of some new GII.4 variants has been associated with a surge in norovirus outbreaks in the community. For example, an international surveillance network of 10 European countries reported an unusual surge in norovirus gastroenteritis outbreaks in the summer of 2002 that temporally coincided with the emergence of the then novel GII.4 Farmington Hill variant (Lopman et al., 2004). Similar

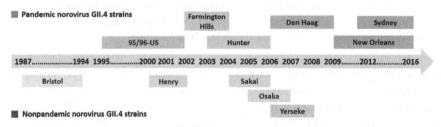

FIGURE 4.3

Schematic diagram showing the years of circulation of 11 key norovirus GII.4 variants detected since the 1980s. The long arrow in the middle denotes the timeline. Pandemic and nonpandemic GII.4 variants are shown above and below the timeline, respectively. Truncated years are indicated by serial dots. Some GII.4 variants have multiple names: Bristol (also known as Lordsdale, Camberwell, and MD145-12), 95/96-US (Grimsby), Farmington Hills (2002 variant), Hunter (2004 variant), Sakai (Chiba and Asia_2003), Yerseke (2006a and Laurens), and Den Haag (2006b and Minerva).

observations have been reported in other countries such as Australia (Bull et al., 2006). In 2006, atypical norovirus activities observed in Europe and Asia were associated with the emergence of the then novel GII.4 Den Haag variant (Ho et al., 2007; Kroneman et al., 2006). However, not all newly emerged GII.4 variants lead to increased norovirus activities in the community. In a study during the winter of 2009−10 in the United States, there was no increase in norovirus outbreaks amid of the emergence of the then novel GII.4 New Orleans variant (Yen et al., 2011). The current circulating GII.4 Sydney variant was also not found to associate with higher norovirus activity in the winter of 2012−13 in the United States (Leshem et al., 2013).

Norovirus GII.4 variants pose substantial disease burden of clinical significance in all age groups, especially young children and the elderly. In a 2-year cohort study of hospitalized norovirus gastroenteritis conducted between 2012 and 2014 in Hong Kong, 80% of cases were attributed to GII.4 variants (Chan et al., 2015b). A U-shaped age distribution in hospitalization incidence was observed, with the highest rate in young children aged 5 years or younger, followed by elderly aged older than 84 years. In a meta-analysis of more than 200 published articles on norovirus outbreaks of different virus genogroups and genotypes, GII.4 was found to be associated with more severe clinical manifestations in terms of hospitalization and death rates (Desai et al., 2012). Elderly aged older than 84 years are at risk of fatal norovirus infections (van Asten et al., 2012). Norovirus GII.4 also exhibits a higher concentration of fecal virus shedding compared to other genotypes (Costantini et al., 2016). The clinical relevance of fecal viral concentration remains largely elusive and contradictory. In an observational study of 40 inpatients hospitalized with norovirus GII.4 infections, longer duration of diarrhea was observed in cases with higher fecal viral concentration (Lee et al., 2007). However, in a retrospective study of nosocomial outbreaks, no correlation between symptom duration and fecal viral concentration was observed (Partridge et al., 2012).

4.3.3 GII.17

Norovirus GII.17 has been the focus of the field recently. The story started from a report that found that GII.17 accounted for more than 80% of outbreaks of gastroenteritis in different settings (kindergartens, colleges, and factories) among 10 cities in Guangdong province of China in the winter of 2014−15 (Lu et al., 2015a). This is in sharp contrast to the previous winter of 2013−14, during which GII.4 Sydney 2012 was predominant. Phylogenetic analysis suggested that the emergent GII.17 was a new variant, and it was named Kawasaki 2014 (also known as Kawasaki308-like) by the NoroNet (de Graaf et al., 2015). A similar surge in activity of the emerging norovirus GII.17 in the same period was reported in other cities in China, including Beijing, Hong Kong, Huzhou, Jiangsu, and Shanghai (Chan et al., 2015a; Chen et al., 2015; Fu et al., 2015; Gao et al., 2015; Han et al., 2015). This new variant was also associated with a waterborne outbreak in Hebei, China (Qin et al., 2016). Displacement of the contemporary GII.4 Sydney 2012 by the GII.17 Kawasaki 2014 outside China, however, was reported only in Japan (Matsushima et al., 2015). Although there were reports of sporadic detection of GII.17 Kawasaki 2014 in North America and Europe, large-scale outbreaks or evidence of GII.4 displacement have been lacking (Dinu et al., 2016; Medici et al., 2015; Parra and Green, 2015). The current geographical restriction of GII.17 Kawasaki 2014 to a portion of Asia is intriguing. It will be very interesting to determine whether or not this new GII.17 variant will persist in the 2016−17 winter season in China and whether it will spread globally in a way resembling the pandemic GII.4 strains.

Our current understanding of this previously rare norovirus GII.17 genotype is very limited. Prior to the sudden emergence and predominance in China, norovirus GII.17 genotype had been only sporadically reported in clinical cases (de Graaf et al., 2015). One study reported frequent detection of norovirus GII.17 in environmental water samples (Kiulia et al., 2014). Currently, several pieces of evidence suggest that the emergent GII.17 Kawasaki 2014 is of public health concern. First, older children and adults aged 5−65 years comprise a high proportion (up to 50%) of observed hospitalized cases of gastroenteritis infected with the new GII.17 variant (Chan et al., 2015a; Chen et al., 2015). This shift in age distribution suggests that GII.17 may be associated with a higher susceptibility or more severe clinical presentation in older children and adults. GII.17 Kawasaki 2014 may be able to escape immunity acquired from previous GII.4 infections. This speculation is supported by recent elucidation of the crystal structure of this new GII.17 variant (Singh et al., 2016). Frequent hospitalization of immunocompetent older children and adults may also reflect higher virulence of this new GII.17 variant. Second, saliva binding analysis reveals that the new GII.17 Kawasaki 2014 is capable of recognizing a wide spectrum of histo-blood group antigens present on the host cell surface that can serve as an attachment factor for noroviruses, suggesting an expanded susceptible human population for GII.17 (Chan et al., 2015a; Zhang et al., 2015). Third, using molecular clock analysis on complete VP1 sequences, norovirus GII.17 was found to evolve at a rate one order of magnitude faster than that of GII.4 during the past decade (Chan et al., 2015a). Although the mechanism remains elusive, the fast-mutating nature of GII.17 will fuel norovirus GII.17 with a high potential to further acquire virulence and transmissibility in the future. International collaborative effort to monitor the global spread of this emerging GII.17 variant is urgently needed.

4.3.4 NEW GENOGROUPS AND GENOTYPES

The first systematic classification of noroviruses into five genogroups (GI−GV) was reported in 2006 (Zheng et al., 2006). Since then, three tentatively new genogroups, GVI−GVIII, have been identified (Fig. 4.1). Using the traditional Sanger sequencing approach, two canine norovirus-like sequences were identified from fecal matter of diarrheal dogs and were tentatively designated GVI and GVII (Martella et al., 2008; Tse et al., 2012). Recently, with advancements in the increasingly affordable high-throughput next-generation sequencing (NGS) technology, human and animal viromes are being rapidly explored and sequenced (Berg et al., 2015; Hoffmann et al., 2015; Sasaki et al., 2014; Woo et al., 2014). In a study of bat virome using anal and pharyngeal swab samples collected from more than 4000 bats representing 40 bat species in China, six bat calicivirus-like sequences were identified, including two that were most closely related to noroviruses (Wu et al., 2015). Phylogenetic analysis suggests that the bat sequences may represent a novel norovirus genogroup, tentatively designated GVIII. It may seem that the search for novel noroviruses has been more fruitful in nonhuman animal species. This is not true. In a community-based cohort of Ecuadorian children, a norovirus belonging to a novel GII genotype, tentatively called GII.23, was reported (Lopman et al., 2015). In 2016, a complete norovirus genome (GenBank accession number KU306738), belonging to another novel GII genotype, tentatively called GII.24, was released in GenBank by the National Calicivirus Laboratory of the CDC. Currently, there is very little information about this GII.24 genome except that it was collected from a stool sample in Nicaragua and was sequenced using NGS. It is anticipated that the wide utilization of state-of-the-art molecular sequencing technology in both research and clinical laboratories will reveal more norovirus strains and expand our understanding of the species distribution of noroviruses in the future.

4.3.5 NOROVIRUS GENOTYPE AND FOODBORNE OUTBREAKS

One characteristic feature of norovirus-associated foodborne outbreaks is the presence of multiple norovirus genotypes. In a meta-analysis of data submitted to FBVE/NoroNet of the Netherlands, CaliciNet of the CDC, and ESR-Epi-Surv of New Zealand from 1999 to 2012, 10% of foodborne outbreaks were attributed to genotype GII.4 and 27% to other single non-GII.4 genotypes, whereas 37% were caused by mixed GII.4 and non-GII.4 genotypes (Verhoef et al., 2015). It also appears that non-GII.4 genotypes are more likely to associate with foodborne outbreaks. In an analysis of 3960 norovirus outbreaks reported to CaliciNet of the CDC between 2009 and 2013, several non-GII.4 genotypes in genogroup I (GI.3, GI.6, and GI.7) and genogroup II (GII.3, GII.6, and GII.12) were found to associate with foodborne outbreaks (Vega et al., 2014). Oyster- and other shellfish-associated foodborne outbreaks are notoriously known to involve multiple norovirus genotypes, including GI.1, GI.2, GI.4, GI.5, GI.6, GI.7, GII.3, GII.4, GII.6, GII.7, GII.11, GII.12, GII.13, GII.14, and GII.17 (Cho et al., 2016; Ma et al., 2013; Rajko-Nenow et al., 2013, 2014; Wang et al., 2015). This is because norovirus can bind to histo-blood group antigens present on the intestinal cells of oysters and other bivalves, including clams and mussels (Tian et al., 2006, 2007, 2008). The filter-feeding nature of oysters also leads to bioaccumulation of noroviruses from the living water environment contaminated with human sewage. In contrast, foodborne outbreaks associated with other food types such as fruits are more likely to involve a single norovirus non-GII.4 genotype (Hoffmann et al., 2013; Muller et al., 2015; Ruan et al., 2013), probably via contamination from asymptomatic, norovirus-shedding food handlers (Barrabeig et al., 2010; Franck et al., 2015).

4.4 CONCLUSIONS AND PERSPECTIVES

Human noroviruses are ubiquitous and highly infectious. Structural determinants of their super environmental stability remain poorly understood, partly due to the lack of a robust and efficient in vitro culture system to assess virus infectivity. Research priority should be given to optimize existing norovirus culture models. The mechanism of norovirus adsorption onto food surfaces is a largely unexplored research area. Given that some norovirus genotypes are more likely to be found in foodborne outbreaks, one may assume that different norovirus genotypes have different preferences for attachment factors on food surfaces. What are these factors? Are they proteins or carbohydrates or both? Noroviruses are found in a diverse array of mammalian species, including bats, which are long-recognized super-carriers of many ancient viruses such as coronaviruses. This suggests that noroviruses may have an ancient origin. Some animal noroviruses (e.g., porcine GII.11, GII.18, and GII.19) are closely related to human noroviruses. Although there are no reports of human infections of animal noroviruses, zoonotic potential of norovirus transmission from other mammals, especially those farmed for human consumption, to humans via the food chain cannot be neglected. The prevalence of noroviruses in animal species needs to be systematically monitored.

REFERENCES

Ao, Y.Y., Yu, J.M., Li, L.L., Jin, M., Duan, Z.J., 2014. Detection of human norovirus GIV.1 in China: a case report. J. Clin. Virol. 61 (2), 298−301. Available from: http://dx.doi.org/10.1016/j.jcv.2014.08.002.

Ausar, S.F., Foubert, T.R., Hudson, M.H., Vedvick, T.S., Middaugh, C.R., 2006. Conformational stability and disassembly of Norwalk virus-like particles. Effect of pH and temperature. J. Biol. Chem. 281 (28), 19478−19488. Available from: http://dx.doi.org/10.1074/jbc.M603313200.

Barrabeig, I., Rovira, A., Buesa, J., Bartolome, R., Pinto, R., Prellezo, H., et al., 2010. Foodborne norovirus outbreak: the role of an asymptomatic food handler. BMC Infect. Dis. 10, 269. Available from: http://dx. doi.org/10.1186/1471-2334-10-269.

Berg, M.G., Lee, D., Coller, K., Frankel, M., Aronsohn, A., Cheng, K., et al., 2015. Discovery of a novel human pegivirus in blood associated with hepatitis C virus co-infection. PLoS Pathog. 11 (12), e1005325. Available from: http://dx.doi.org/10.1371/journal.ppat.1005325.

Bertolotti-Ciarlet, A., Crawford, S.E., Hutson, A.M., Estes, M.K., 2003. The 3′ end of Norwalk virus mRNA contains determinants that regulate the expression and stability of the viral capsid protein VP1: a novel function for the VP2 protein. J. Virol. 77 (21), 11603−11615.

Bok, K., Abente, E.J., Realpe-Quintero, M., Mitra, T., Sosnovtsev, S.V., Kapikian, A.Z., et al., 2009. Evolutionary dynamics of GII.4 noroviruses over a 34-year period. J. Virol. 83 (22), 11890−11901. Available from: http://dx.doi.org/10.1128/JVI.00864-09.

Bull, R.A., White, P.A., 2011. Mechanisms of GII.4 norovirus evolution. Trend. Microbiol. 19 (5), 233−240. Available from: http://dx.doi.org/10.1016/j.tim.2011.01.002.

Bull, R.A., Tu, E.T., McIver, C.J., Rawlinson, W.D., White, P.A., 2006. Emergence of a new norovirus genotype II.4 variant associated with global outbreaks of gastroenteritis. J. Clin. Microbiol. 44 (2), 327−333. Available from: http://dx.doi.org/10.1128/JCM.44.2.327-333.2006.

Cao, S., Lou, Z., Tan, M., Chen, Y., Liu, Y., Zhang, Z., et al., 2007. Structural basis for the recognition of blood group trisaccharides by norovirus. J. Virol. 81 (11), 5949−5957. Available from: http://dx.doi.org/ 10.1128/JVI.00219-07.

Chan, M.C., Lee, N., Hung, T.N., Kwok, K., Cheung, K., Tin, E.K., et al., 2015a. Rapid emergence and predominance of a broadly recognizing and fast-evolving norovirus GII.17 variant in late 2014. Nature Commun. 6, 10061. Available from: http://dx.doi.org/10.1038/ncomms10061.

Chan, M.C., Leung, T.F., Chung, T.W., Kwok, A.K., Nelson, E.A., Lee, N., et al., 2015b. Virus genotype distribution and virus burden in children and adults hospitalized for norovirus gastroenteritis, 2012−2014, Hong Kong. Sci. Rep. 5, 11507. Available from: http://dx.doi.org/10.1038/srep11507.

Chen, R., Neill, J.D., Noel, J.S., Hutson, A.M., Glass, R.I., Estes, M.K., et al., 2004. Inter- and intragenus structural variations in caliciviruses and their functional implications. J. Virol. 78 (12), 6469−6479. Available from: http://dx.doi.org/10.1128/JVI.78.12.6469-6479.2004.

Chen, R., Neill, J.D., Estes, M.K., Prasad, B.V., 2006. X-ray structure of a native calicivirus: structural insights into antigenic diversity and host specificity. Proc. Natl. Acad. Sci. USA 103 (21), 8048−8053. Available from: http://dx.doi.org/10.1073/pnas.0600421103.

Chen, H., Qian, F., Xu, J., Chan, M., Shen, Z., Zai, S., et al., 2015. A novel norovirus GII.17 lineage contributed to adult gastroenteritis in Shanghai, China, during the winter of 2014−2015. Emerg. Microb. Infect. 4 (11), e67.

Cho, H.G., Lee, S.G., Lee, M.Y., Hur, E.S., Lee, J.S., Park, P.H., et al., 2016. An outbreak of norovirus infection associated with fermented oyster consumption in South Korea, 2013. Epidemiol. Infect. 1−6. Available from: http://dx.doi.org/10.1017/S0950268816000170.

Choi, J.M., Hutson, A.M., Estes, M.K., Prasad, B.V., 2008. Atomic resolution structural characterization of recognition of histo-blood group antigens by Norwalk virus. Proc. Natl. Acad. Sci. USA 105 (27), 9175−9180. Available from: http://dx.doi.org/10.1073/pnas.0803275105.

Costantini, V.P., Cooper, E.M., Hardaker, H.L., Lee, L.E., Bierhoff, M., Biggs, C., et al., 2016. Epidemiologic, virologic, and host genetic factors of norovirus outbreaks in long-term care facilities. Clin. Infect. Dis. 62 (1), 1−10. Available from: http://dx.doi.org/10.1093/cid/civ747.

Daughenbaugh, K.F., Wobus, C.E., Hardy, M.E., 2006. VPg of murine norovirus binds translation initiation factors in infected cells. J. Virol. 3, 33. Available from: http://dx.doi.org/10.1186/1743-422X-3-33.

de Graaf, M., van Beek, J., Vennema, H., Podkolzin, A.T., Hewitt, J., Bucardo, F., et al., 2015. Emergence of a novel GII.17 norovirus—end of the GII.4 era? Eurosurveillance 20 (26), pii = 21178.

de Rougemont, A., Ruvoen-Clouet, N., Simon, B., Estienney, M., Elie-Caille, C., Aho, S., et al., 2011. Qualitative and quantitative analysis of the binding of GII.4 norovirus variants onto human blood group antigens. J. Virol. 85 (9), 4057−4070. Available from: http://dx.doi.org/10.1128/JVI.02077-10.

Desai, R., Hembree, C.D., Handel, A., Matthews, J.E., Dickey, B.W., McDonald, S., et al., 2012. Severe outcomes are associated with genogroup 2 genotype 4 norovirus outbreaks: a systematic literature review. Clin. Infect. Dis. 55 (2), 189−193. Available from: http://dx.doi.org/10.1093/cid/cis372.

Dinu, S., Nagy, M., Negru, D.G., Popovici, E.D., Zota, L., Oprisan, G., 2016. Molecular identification of emergent GII.P17-GII.17 norovirus genotype, Romania, 2015. Eurosurveillance 21 (7). Available from: http://dx.doi.org/10.2807/1560-7917.ES.2016.21.7.30141.

Dolin, R., Reichman, R.C., Roessner, K.D., Tralka, T.S., Schooley, R.T., Gary, W., et al., 1982. Detection by immune electron microscopy of the Snow Mountain agent of acute viral gastroenteritis. J. Infect. Dis. 146 (2), 184−189.

Donaldson, E.F., Lindesmith, L.C., Lobue, A.D., Baric, R.S., 2008. Norovirus pathogenesis: mechanisms of persistence and immune evasion in human populations. Immun. Rev. 225, 190−211. Available from: http://dx.doi.org/10.1111/j.1600-065X.2008.00680.x.

Eden, J.S., Lim, K.L., White, P.A., 2012. Complete genome of the human norovirus GIV.1 strain Lake Macquarie virus. J. Virol. 86 (18), 10251−10252. Available from: http://dx.doi.org/10.1128/JVI.01604-12.

Eden, J.S., Tanaka, M.M., Boni, M.F., Rawlinson, W.D., White, P.A., 2013. Recombination within the pandemic norovirus GII.4 lineage. J. Virol. 87 (11), 6270−6282. Available from: http://dx.doi.org/10.1128/JVI.03464-12.

Franck, K.T., Lisby, M., Fonager, J., Schultz, A.C., Bottiger, B., Villif, A., et al., 2015. Sources of calicivirus contamination in foodborne outbreaks in Denmark, 2005−2011—the role of the asymptomatic food handler. J. Infect. Dis. 211 (4), 563−570. Available from: http://dx.doi.org/10.1093/infdis/jiu479.

Fu, J., Ai, J., Jin, M., Jiang, C., Zhang, J., Shi, C., et al., 2015. Emergence of a new GII.17 norovirus variant in patients with acute gastroenteritis in Jiangsu, China, September 2014 to March 2015. Eurosurveillance 20 (24), pii = 21157.

Gao, Z., Liu, B., Huo, D., Yan, H., Jia, L., Du, Y., et al., 2015. Increased norovirus activity was associated with a novel norovirus GII.17 variant in Beijing, China during winter 2014−2015. BMC Infect. Dis. 15 (1), 574. Available from: http://dx.doi.org/10.1186/s12879-015-1315-z.

Giammanco, G.M., Rotolo, V., Medici, M.C., Tummolo, F., Bonura, F., Chezzi, C., et al., 2012. Recombinant norovirus GII.g/GII.12 gastroenteritis in children. Infect. Genet. Evol. 12 (1), 169−174. Available from: http://dx.doi.org/10.1016/j.meegid.2011.10.021.

Green, K.Y., Belliot, G., Taylor, J.L., Valdesuso, J., Lew, J.F., Kapikian, A.Z., et al., 2002. A predominant role for Norwalk-like viruses as agents of epidemic gastroenteritis in Maryland nursing homes for the elderly. J. Infect. Dis. 185 (2), 133−146. Available from: http://dx.doi.org/10.1086/338365.

Guix, S., Asanaka, M., Katayama, K., Crawford, S.E., Neill, F.H., Atmar, R.L., et al., 2007. Norwalk virus RNA is infectious in mammalian cells. J. Virol. 81 (22), 12238−12248. Available from: http://dx.doi.org/10.1128/JVI.01489-07.

Han, J., Ji, L., Shen, Y., Wu, X., Xu, D., Chen, L., 2015. Emergence and predominance of norovirus GII.17 in Huzhou, China, 2014−2015. J. Virol. 12 (1), 139. Available from: http://dx.doi.org/10.1186/s12985-015-0370-9.

Ho, E.C., Cheng, P.K., Lau, A.W., Wong, A.H., Lim, W.W., 2007. Atypical norovirus epidemic in Hong Kong during summer of 2006 caused by a new genogroup II/4 variant. J. Clin. Microbiol. 45 (7), 2205−2211. Available from: http://dx.doi.org/10.1128/JCM.02489-06.

Hoffmann, D., Mauroy, A., Seebach, J., Simon, V., Wantia, N., Protzer, U., 2013. New norovirus classified as a recombinant GII.g/GII.1 causes an extended foodborne outbreak at a university hospital in Munich. J. Clin. Virol. 58 (1), 24−30. Available from: http://dx.doi.org/10.1016/j.jcv.2013.06.018.

Hoffmann, B., Tappe, D., Hoper, D., Herden, C., Boldt, A., Mawrin, C., et al., 2015. A variegated squirrel bornavirus associated with fatal human encephalitis. New Engl. J. Med. 373 (2), 154−162. Available from: http://dx.doi.org/10.1056/NEJMoa1415627.

Jones, M.K., Watanabe, M., Zhu, S., Graves, C.L., Keyes, L.R., Grau, K.R., et al., 2014. Enteric bacteria promote human and mouse norovirus infection of B cells. Science 346 (6210), 755−759. Available from: http://dx.doi.org/10.1126/science.1257147.

Jones, M.K., Grau, K.R., Costantini, V., Kolawole, A.O., de Graaf, M., Freiden, P., et al., 2015. Human norovirus culture in B cells. Nat. Prot. 10 (12), 1939−1947. Available from: http://dx.doi.org/10.1038/nprot.2015.121.

Keswick, B.H., Satterwhite, T.K., Johnson, P.C., DuPont, H.L., Secor, S.L., Bitsura, J.A., et al., 1985. Inactivation of Norwalk virus in drinking water by chlorine. Appl. Environ. Microbiol. 50 (2), 261−264.

Kiulia, N.M., Mans, J., Mwenda, J.M., Taylor, M.B., 2014. Norovirus GII.17 predominates in selected surface water sources in Kenya. Food Environ. Virol. 6, 221−231. Available from: http://dx.doi.org/10.1007/s12560-014-9160-6.

Kroneman, A., Vennema, H., Harris, J., Reuter, G., von Bonsdorff, C.H., Hedlund, K.O., et al., 2006. Increase in norovirus activity reported in Europe. Eurosurveillance 11 (12), E061214-061211.

Kroneman, A., Vega, E., Vennema, H., Vinje, J., White, P.A., Hansman, G., et al., 2013. Proposal for a unified norovirus nomenclature and genotyping. Arch. Virol. 158 (10), 2059−2068. Available from: http://dx.doi.org/10.1007/s00705-013-1708-5.

Lee, N., Chan, M.C., Wong, B., Choi, K.W., Sin, W., Lui, G., et al., 2007. Fecal viral concentration and diarrhea in norovirus gastroenteritis. Emerg. Infect. Dis. 13 (9), 1399−1401. Available from: http://dx.doi.org/10.3201/eid1309.061535.

Leshem, E., Wikswo, M., Barclay, L., Brandt, E., Storm, W., Salehi, E., et al., 2013. Effects and clinical significance of GII.4 Sydney norovirus, United States, 2012−2013. Emerg. Infect. Dis. 19 (8), 1231−1238. Available from: http://dx.doi.org/10.3201/eid1908.130458.

Lindesmith, L.C., Beltramello, M., Donaldson, E.F., Corti, D., Swanstrom, J., Debbink, K., et al., 2012. Immunogenetic mechanisms driving norovirus GII.4 antigenic variation. PLoS Pathog. 8 (5), e1002705. Available from: http://dx.doi.org/10.1371/journal.ppat.1002705.

Lopman, B., Vennema, H., Kohli, E., Pothier, P., Sanchez, A., Negredo, A., et al., 2004. Increase in viral gastroenteritis outbreaks in Europe and epidemic spread of new norovirus variant. Lancet 363 (9410), 682−688, doi: 10.1016/S0140-6736(04)15641-9.

Lopman, B.A., Trivedi, T., Vicuna, Y., Costantini, V., Collins, N., Gregoricus, N., et al., 2015. Norovirus infection and disease in an Ecuadorian birth cohort: association of certain norovirus genotypes with host FUT2 secretor status. J. Infect. Dis. 211 (11), 1813−1821. Available from: http://dx.doi.org/10.1093/infdis/jiu672.

Lu, J., Sun, L., Fang, L., Yang, F., Mo, Y., Lao, J., et al., 2015a. Gastroenteritis outbreaks caused by norovirus GII.17, Guangdong Province, China, 2014−2015. Emerg. Infect. Dis. 21 (7), 1240−1242. Available from: http://dx.doi.org/10.3201/eid2107.150226.

Lu, Q.B., Huang, D.D., Zhao, J., Wang, H.Y., Zhang, X.A., Xu, H.M., et al., 2015b. An increasing prevalence of recombinant GII norovirus in pediatric patients with diarrhea during 2010−2013 in China. Infect. Genet. Evol. 31, 48−52. Available from: http://dx.doi.org/10.1016/j.meegid.2015.01.008.

Ma, L.P., Zhao, F., Yao, L., Li, X.G., Zhou, D.Q., Zhang, R.L., 2013. The presence of genogroup II norovirus in retail shellfish from seven coastal cities in China. Food Environ. Virol. 5 (2), 81–86. Available from: http://dx.doi.org/10.1007/s12560-013-9102-8.

Mans, J., Murray, T.Y., Taylor, M.B., 2014. Novel norovirus recombinants detected in South Africa. Virol. J. 11 (1), 168. Available from: http://dx.doi.org/10.1186/1743-422X-11-168.

Martella, V., Lorusso, E., Decaro, N., Elia, G., Radogna, A., D'Abramo, M., et al., 2008. Detection and molecular characterization of a canine norovirus. Emerg. Infect. Dis. 14 (8), 1306–1308. Available from: http://dx.doi.org/10.3201/eid1408.080062.

Matsushima, Y., Ishikawa, M., Shimizu, T., Komane, A., Kasuo, S., Shinohara, M., et al., 2015. Genetic analyses of GII.17 norovirus strains in diarrheal disease outbreaks from December 2014 to March 2015 in Japan reveal a novel polymerase sequence and amino acid substitutions in the capsid region. Eurosurveillance 20 (26), pii = 21173.

Medici, M.C., Tummolo, F., Calderaro, A., Chironna, M., Giammanco, G.M., De Grazia, S., et al., 2015. Identification of the novel Kawasaki 2014 GII.17 human norovirus strain in Italy, 2015. Eurosurveillance 20 (35), pii = 30010. Available from: http://dx.doi.org/10.2807/1560-7917.ES.2015.20.35.30010.

Muller, L., Schultz, A.C., Fonager, J., Jensen, T., Lisby, M., Hindsdal, K., et al., 2015. Separate norovirus outbreaks linked to one source of imported frozen raspberries by molecular analysis, Denmark, 2010–2011. Epidemiol. Infect. 143 (11), 2299–2307. Available from: http://dx.doi.org/10.1017/S0950268814003409.

Noel, J.S., Fankhauser, R.L., Ando, T., Monroe, S.S., Glass, R.I., 1999. Identification of a distinct common strain of "Norwalk-like viruses" having a global distribution. J. Infect. Dis. 179 (6), 1334–1344. Available from: http://dx.doi.org/10.1086/314783.

Parra, G.I., Green, K.Y., 2015. Genome of emerging norovirus GII.17, United States, 2014. Emerg. Infect. Dis. 21 (8), 1477–1479.

Partridge, D.G., Evans, C.M., Raza, M., Kudesia, G., Parsons, H.K., 2012. Lessons from a large norovirus outbreak: impact of viral load, patient age and ward design on duration of symptoms and shedding and likelihood of transmission. J. Hosp. Infect. 81 (1), 25–30. Available from: http://dx.doi.org/10.1016/j.jhin.2012.02.002.

Prasad, B.V., Hardy, M.E., Dokland, T., Bella, J., Rossmann, M.G., Estes, M.K., 1999. X-ray crystallographic structure of the Norwalk virus capsid. Science 286 (5438), 287–290.

Pringle, K., Lopman, B., Vega, E., Vinje, J., Parashar, U.D., Hall, A.J., 2015. Noroviruses: epidemiology, immunity and prospects for prevention. Future Microbiol. 10 (1), 53–67. Available from: http://dx.doi.org/10.2217/fmb.14.102.

Qin, M., Dong, X.G., Jing, Y.Y., Wei, X.X., Wang, Z.E., Feng, H.R., et al., 2016. A waterborne gastroenteritis outbreak caused by norovirus GII.17 in a hotel, Hebei, China, December 2014. Food Environ. Virol. Available from: http://dx.doi.org/10.1007/s12560-016-9237-5.

Rajko-Nenow, P., Waters, A., Keaveney, S., Flannery, J., Tuite, G., Coughlan, S., et al., 2013. Norovirus genotypes present in oysters and in effluent from a wastewater treatment plant during the seasonal peak of infections in Ireland in 2010. Appl. Environ. Microbiol. 79 (8), 2578–2587. Available from: http://dx.doi.org/10.1128/AEM.03557-12.

Rajko-Nenow, P., Keaveney, S., Flannery, J., Mc, I.A., Dore, W., 2014. Norovirus genotypes implicated in two oyster-related illness outbreaks in Ireland. Epidemiol. Infect. 142 (10), 2096–2104. Available from: http://dx.doi.org/10.1017/S0950268813003014.

Richards, G.P., Watson, M.A., Meade, G.K., Hovan, G.L., Kingsley, D.H., 2012. Resilience of norovirus GII.4 to freezing and thawing: implications for virus infectivity. Food Environ. Virol. 4 (4), 192–197. Available from: http://dx.doi.org/10.1007/s12560-012-9089-6.

Ruan, F., Tan, A.J., Man, T.F., Li, H., Mo, Y.L., Lin, Y.X., et al., 2013. Gastroenteritis outbreaks caused by norovirus genotype II.7 in a college in China (Zhuhai, Guangdong) in 2011. Foodborne Pathog. Dis. 10 (10), 856–860. Available from: http://dx.doi.org/10.1089/fpd.2013.1519.

Samandoulgou, I., Hammami, R., Morales Rayas, R., Fliss, I., Jean, J., 2015. Stability of secondary and tertiary structures of virus-like particles representing noroviruses: effects of pH, ionic strength, and temperature and implications for adhesion to surfaces. Appl. Environ. Microbiol. 81 (22), 7680–7686. Available from: http://dx.doi.org/10.1128/AEM.01278-15.

Sasaki, M., Orba, Y., Ueno, K., Ishii, A., Moonga, L., Hang'ombe, B.M., et al., 2014. Metagenomic analysis of shrew enteric virome reveals novel viruses related to human stool-associated viruses. J. Gen. Virol. Available from: http://dx.doi.org/10.1099/vir.0.071209-0.

Singh, B.K., Koromyslova, A.D., Hefele, L., Gurth, C., Hansman, G., 2016. Structural evolution of the emerging 2014–2015 GII.17 noroviruses. J. Virol. 90 (5), 2710–2715.

Tian, P., Bates, A.H., Jensen, H.M., Mandrell, R.E., 2006. Norovirus binds to blood group A-like antigens in oyster gastrointestinal cells. Lett. Appl. Microbiol. 43 (6), 645–651. Available from: http://dx.doi.org/10.1111/j.1472-765X.2006.02010.x.

Tian, P., Engelbrektson, A.L., Jiang, X., Zhong, W., Mandrell, R.E., 2007. Norovirus recognizes histo-blood group antigens on gastrointestinal cells of clams, mussels, and oysters: a possible mechanism of bioaccumulation. J. Food Prot. 70 (9), 2140–2147.

Tian, P., Engelbrektson, A.L., Mandrell, R.E., 2008. Seasonal tracking of histo-blood group antigen expression and norovirus binding in oyster gastrointestinal cells. J. Food Prot. 71 (8), 1696–1700.

Tse, H., Lau, S.K., Chan, W.M., Choi, G.K., Woo, P.C., Yuen, K.Y., 2012. Complete genome sequences of novel canine noroviruses in Hong Kong. J. Virol. 86 (17), 9531–9532. Available from: http://dx.doi.org/10.1128/JVI.01312-12.

van Asten, L., van den Wijngaard, C., van Pelt, W., van de Kassteele, J., Meijer, A., van der Hoek, W., et al., 2012. Mortality attributable to 9 common infections: significant effect of influenza A, respiratory syncytial virus, influenza B, norovirus, and parainfluenza in elderly persons. J. Infect. Dis. 206 (5), 628–639. Available from: http://dx.doi.org/10.1093/infdis/jis415.

Vega, E., Barclay, L., Gregoricus, N., Shirley, S.H., Lee, D., Vinje, J., 2014. Genotypic and epidemiologic trends of norovirus outbreaks in the United States, 2009 to 2013. J. Clin. Microbiol. 52 (1), 147–155. Available from: http://dx.doi.org/10.1128/JCM.02680-13.

Verhoef, L., Hewitt, J., Barclay, L., Ahmed, S.M., Lake, R., Hall, A.J., et al., 2015. Norovirus genotype profiles associated with foodborne transmission, 1999–2012. Emerg. Infect. Dis. 21 (4), 592–599. Available from: http://dx.doi.org/10.3201/eid2104.141073.

Vinje, J., 2015. Advances in laboratory methods for detection and typing of norovirus. J. Clin. Microbiol. 53 (2), 373–381. Available from: http://dx.doi.org/10.1128/JCM.01535-14.

Vongpunsawad, S., Venkataram Prasad, B.V., Estes, M.K., 2013. Norwalk virus minor capsid protein VP2 associates within the VP1 shell domain. J. Virol. 87 (9), 4818–4825. Available from: http://dx.doi.org/10.1128/JVI.03508-12.

Wang, Y., Zhang, J., Shen, Z., 2015. The impact of calicivirus mixed infection in an oyster-associated outbreak during a food festival. J. Clin. Virol. 73, 55–63. Available from: http://dx.doi.org/10.1016/j.jcv.2015.10.004.

Wobus, C.E., Karst, S.M., Thackray, L.B., Chang, K.O., Sosnovtsev, S.V., Belliot, G., et al., 2004. Replication of norovirus in cell culture reveals a tropism for dendritic cells and macrophages. PLoS Biol. 2 (12), e432. Available from: http://dx.doi.org/10.1371/journal.pbio.0020432.

Wong, T.H., Dearlove, B.L., Hedge, J., Giess, A.P., Piazza, P., Trebes, A., et al., 2013. Whole genome sequencing and de novo assembly identifies Sydney-like variant noroviruses and recombinants during the winter 2012/2013 outbreak in England. J. Virol. 10, 335. Available from: http://dx.doi.org/10.1186/1743-422X-10-335.

Woo, P.C., Lau, S.K., Teng, J.L., Tsang, A.K., Joseph, M., Wong, E.Y., et al., 2014. Metagenomic analysis of viromes of dromedary camel fecal samples reveals large number and high diversity of circoviruses and pico-birnaviruses. Virology 471−473, 117−125. Available from: http://dx.doi.org/10.1016/j.virol.2014.09.020.

Wu, Z., Yang, L., Ren, X., He, G., Zhang, J., Yang, J., et al., 2015. Deciphering the bat virome catalog to better understand the ecological diversity of bat viruses and the bat origin of emerging infectious diseases. ISME J. Available from: http://dx.doi.org/10.1038/ismej.2015.138.

Xi, J.N., Graham, D.Y., Wang, K.N., Estes, M.K., 1990. Norwalk virus genome cloning and characterization. Science 250 (4987), 1580−1583.

Yen, C., Wikswo, M.E., Lopman, B.A., Vinje, J., Parashar, U.D., Hall, A.J., 2011. Impact of an emergent norovirus variant in 2009 on norovirus outbreak activity in the United States. Clin. Infect. Dis. 53 (6), 568−571. Available from: http://dx.doi.org/10.1093/cid/cir478.

Zhang, X.F., Huang, Q., Long, Y., Jiang, X., Zhang, T., Tan, M., et al., 2015. An outbreak caused by GII.17 norovirus with a wide spectrum of HBGA-associated susceptibility. Sci. Rep. 5, 17687. Available from: http://dx.doi.org/10.1038/srep17687.

Zheng, D.P., Ando, T., Fankhauser, R.L., Beard, R.S., Glass, R.I., Monroe, S.S., 2006. Norovirus classification and proposed strain nomenclature. Virology 346 (2), 312−323. Available from: http://dx.doi.org/10.1016/j.virol.2005.11.015.

WHOLE GENOME SEQUENCING APPROACH TO GENOTYPING AND EPIDEMIOLOGY

5

Julianne R. Brown[1] and Judith Breuer[2]

[1]Great Ormond Street Hospital for Children NHS Foundation Trust, London, United Kingdom
[2]University College London, London, United Kingdom

5.1 BACKGROUND

Norovirus is a global cause of acute gastroenteritis capable of causing large outbreaks in enclosed settings such as schools, cruise ships, and health care and military facilities. Outbreaks can be person-borne or foodborne, with foodborne outbreaks sometimes affecting several towns, states, or countries. To establish transmission events, classic epidemiological investigations rely primarily on linking cases in time and space. However, in the case of multiregion foodborne outbreaks, cases caused by the same contaminated foodstuff may not be recognized as part of a wider outbreak using classical epidemiology alone. Conversely, because the number of cases of norovirus characteristically peaks during winter, it can be difficult to distinguish a true outbreak occurring in an institution from a collection of unlinked cases that just happen to have caught norovirus in the community at the same time. Molecular epidemiology uses genetic information of a pathogen to investigate the cause and course of transmission and allows us to compare viral genome sequences between cases, thus excluding cases from an outbreak or linking previously unrecognized transmission events. The application of molecular epidemiology to elucidate transmission was elegantly demonstrated in a Dutch hospital, in which the comparison of sequences from patients infected with norovirus revealed that outpatients, who visit the hospital for short appointments and therefore were assumed to have infections from the community, were shown in fact to be linked to outbreaks within the hospital. This consequently allowed targeting of infection control practices in outpatient departments, which were previously not recognized as a risk for nosocomial transmission (Sukhrie et al., 2011).

The use of whole genome sequencing for molecular epidemiology increases our understanding of the transmission dynamics of norovirus. This can be applied to develop evidence-based interventions and target infection control practices, thus, minimizing transmission and reducing the burden of norovirus disease. This chapter describes the utility of norovirus genotyping and whole genome sequencing in molecular epidemiology and also the methods for achieving each of these.

The Norovirus. DOI: http://dx.doi.org/10.1016/B978-0-12-804177-2.00005-1

5.2 UTILITY OF GENOTYPING

The 7.5-kb norovirus genome is composed of three open reading frames (ORFs). ORF1 codes for a nonstructural polyprotein including the RNA-dependent RNA polymerase, ORF2 for a major capsid protein VP1, and ORF3 for a minor capsid protein VP2.

Noroviruses are classified into seven genogroups (GI–GVII), of which GI and GII, and rarely GIV, cause infections in humans (Vinje, 2015). GI and GII are further categorized into 9 and 22 genotypes, respectively (GI.1–GI.9 and GII.1–GII.22). Due to recombination between genotypes at the ORF1/ORF2 junction, noroviruses have a dual-typing system based on the polymerase (ORF1) and major capsid (ORF2) sequences. Thus, a norovirus with a GII.4 polymerase and capsid type will be designated GII.P4_GII.4, whereas a recombinant sequence with a GII.3 RdRp and a GII.4 capsid type will be designated GII.P3_GII.4. Orphan polymerase sequences, which are novel polymerase types that have only been seen in combination with established ORF2 genotypes, are designated a letter, such as GII.Pc, GII.Pe, and GII.Pg (e.g., GII.Pc_GII.3). Despite the occurrence of recombination and the recommendation of a dual-typing system involving both polymerase and capsid sequences (Kroneman et al., 2013), norovirus genotyping is often still based on capsid typing alone.

5.2.1 GENOTYPING AND GLOBAL EPIDEMIOLOGY

Genotyping is a good indicator of the global epidemiology of norovirus. Since the mid-1990s, GII.4 has been the dominant circulating genotype (Vinje, 2015), often implicated in more than 90% of outbreaks (Chen and Chiu, 2012). The genotypes causing the non-GII.4 proportion of outbreaks vary between season, with GII.2, GII.3, GII.6, and GII.7 detected most frequently (Gallimore et al., 2007; Franck et al., 2015); GII.3 is reported more frequently in children.

The norovirus major capsid consists of the N-terminal shell (S) domain and the protruding (P) domain. The P domain has two subdomains, P1 and P2. P2 contains the receptor-binding region and is the most exposed antigenic site; consequently, it has the greatest sequence variation and can be used to differentiate GII.4 variant types. GII.4 is the only genotype further categorized into variants; every 2 or 3 years, a novel GII.4 variant emerges, replacing the previously predominant variant as listed in Table 5.1. This results in global epidemics, a season of heightened norovirus

Table 5.1 Norovirus GII.4 Epidemic Variants	
Variant Name	**Year First Emerged**
US95_96	1995
Farmington_Hills_2002	2002
Asia_2003	2003
Hunter_2004	2004
Yerseke_2006a	2006
Den Haag_2006b	2006
New Orleans_2009	2009
Sydney_2012	2012

activity, or an increase in cases outside the usual winter peak, and it correlates with residue changes in immunogenic epitopes of the P2 domain (Debbink et al., 2012; Lindesmith et al., 2012).

For the first time in almost 20 years, in China and Japan, GII.4 has been outcompeted by an emerging genotype, GII.17 Kawasaki 2014 (de Graaf et al., 2015). In Hong Kong during the winter of 2014−2015, GII.17 caused 66% of hospitalized norovirus cases compared to 19% caused by GII.4. GII.17 reportedly causes more infections in elderly people, causing infection in only 16% of children younger than age 5 years but 37% of people older than age 65 years, in contrast to 70% and 11%, respectively, caused by GII.4. GII.17 is reported to be an immune-escape variant with a high evolutionary rate (4.4×10^{-2} nucleotide substitutions per site per year; 10-fold higher than GII.4), which could account for its rapid emergence in Asia (Chan et al., 2015). It remains to be determined whether GII.17 will replace GII.4 globally; nevertheless, early detection of GII.17, facilitated by genotyping, allows public health bodies to prepare for potential heightened norovirus activity in coming seasons.

5.2.2 GENOTYPING CAN INDICATE THE SOURCE OF AN OUTBREAK

GII.4 dominates outbreaks of norovirus globally and is likely to represent person-to-person trans-mission (Verhoef et al., 2010); conversely, its association with person-borne transmission means that only 10% of foodborne outbreaks are associated with GII.4 (Verhoef et al., 2015). GIs, on the other hand, are rarely detected in hospital settings; they were associated with only 2% of hospital infections in Denmark between 2002 and 2010 (Franck et al., 2015). Instead, GIs are more frequently detected in, and therefore more likely to indicate, foodborne outbreaks (Verhoef et al., 2010). In the United States, GI.3, GI.6, GI.7, GII.3, GII.6, and GII.12 are two to seven times more likely to be detected in foodborne rather than person-to-person transmission (Vega et al., 2014).

Whereas only 14% of all norovirus outbreaks globally are foodborne, 37% of outbreaks involving mixed genotypes are considered foodborne (Verhoef et al., 2015); a diversity of geno-types is likely to indicate contamination at source with sewage (Gallimore et al., 2005; Wang et al., 2015; Hohne et al., 2015). The detection of mixed genotypes in sewage suggests that there is a far greater diversity of norovirus genotypes circulating in the community than in hospital settings. Community-acquired infections (CAIs) that are detected in hospitalized patients show a broader range of genotypes compared to infections that are hospital-acquired, with 17% compared to 6% non-GII.4 infections, respectively (Franck et al., 2015). However, CAIs that are detected in hospital are not a true reflection of the norovirus genotypes circulating in the community because they signify a presentation bias; they do not represent acute sporadic infections in patients without comorbidities. A comprehensive community cohort study was undertaken in the United Kingdom in which a community cohort was followed up weekly for 1 year. This study revealed that there are 147 community cases of infectious intestinal disease, of which norovirus is the most common, for every case reported to national surveillance (Tam et al., 2012). Norovirus genotyping was not reported in this study; therefore, the true distribution of norovirus genotypes in the community is not known.

In instances in which foodborne outbreaks are dominated by a single, rare, genotype, genotyp-ing can be used to link cases across geographical regions. For instance, a peak in norovirus cases in Denmark during a 3-month period in 2010 and 2011 was initially attributed to six independent outbreaks. However, genotyping using partial polymerase and capsid sequences across these outbreaks revealed a shared genotype, GI.Pb_GI.6, which was also detected in a batch of imported frozen raspberries, thus linking the outbreaks and implicating the raspberries as the common source (Muller et al., 2015).

5.2.3 SEQUENCING HYPERVARIABLE SITES IDENTIFY TRANSMISSION CLUSTERS IN SINGLE-GENOTYPE OUTBREAKS

Outbreaks in health care settings are often dominated by a single genotype, most commonly GII.4. Therefore, genotyping allows patients with a different genotype to be excluded from the outbreak. However, because of the lack of diversity in the polymerase and capsid shell domains used for genotyping, these regions provide insufficient information for tracking outbreaks within a single genotype (Lopman et al., 2006).

In lieu of full genomes, due to its high level of diversity, the P2 region of the major capsid is the most informative region in norovirus outbreak investigation (Verhoef et al., 2012). In immunocompetent people, the P2 region is expected to be 100% identical between patients in whom a transmission event has occurred (Xerry et al., 2008), with a 10% probability of one or two nucleotide changes in samples collected 3 weeks postinfection (Sukhrie et al., 2013). Therefore, in acute norovirus outbreaks among immunocompetent persons, P2 sequencing can identify independent clusters of transmission among patients infected with the same genotype and, conversely, identify transmission events that were missed based on traditional epidemiological data alone (Sukhrie et al., 2013; Holzknecht et al., 2015; Xerry et al., 2008; Sukhrie et al., 2011).

In immunocompromised patients, however, transmission may occur after in vivo evolution; therefore, single nucleotide polymorphisms (SNPs) are observed between linked patients (Holzknecht et al., 2015), which makes interpretation of phylogenies based on P2 sequences alone challenging and less reliable.

5.3 CAPSID AND POLYMERASE GENOTYPING METHODS

Conventional genotyping is based on polymerase chain reaction (PCR) amplification and sequencing of 330- to 650-nt fragments of the norovirus polymerase or major capsid genes, as illustrated in Fig. 5.1. Capsid genotyping is achieved by PCR amplification of the shell domain using genogroup-specific primers. The broad-range nature of these primers, necessary due to sequence variation between genotypes, results in limited sensitivity; therefore, a nested PCR approach is often required. Following capillary sequencing of the capsid shell domain amplicon, the genotype is determined by reconstructing a phylogeny of the unknown sequence with reference sequences of known genotypes. The genotype is assigned based on clustering with a known reference with bootstrap support greater than 70 (Kroneman et al., 2013). The same PCR and phylogeny approach is used for polymerase typing. Both analyses can be done using the Norovirus Genotyping Tool (http://www.rivm.nl/mpf/norovirus/typingtool) (Kroneman et al., 2011), a publicly available online repository of norovirus sequences to which one submits the polymerase and/or capsid sequence of an unknown sample, and the tool automatically reconstructs a phylogeny for each and reports the genotype.

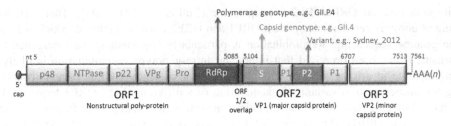

FIGURE 5.1

Schematic of norovirus genome, with genotyping regions highlighted. Nucleotide numbering is based on a GII.4 genome. p48, unknown function; NTP, nucleoside triphosphatase 2C-like protein; p22, 3A-like protein; VPG, viral genome-linked protein (5′ cap); 3C, protease; RdRp, RNA-dependent RNA polymerase; S, shell domain; P1, protruding domain 1; P2, protruding domain 2.

Once the genotype is determined, genotype-specific primers are used to amplify the variable P2 region. Universal GI and GII primers to amplify P2 have been reported, negating the need for different primer sets to amplify each of the 31 known norovirus GI and GII genotypes. These broad-range primers can successfully amplify the P2 region of several genotypes but with only a 71% success rate. Once sequenced, the P2 region can be compared to the P2 region from other samples of interest using in-house bioinformatics pipelines for phylogenetic reconstruction and pairwise sequence identity. Similar to the polymerase and shell domain sequences, the P2 sequence from a GII.4 norovirus can be compared to known reference sequences in a phylogeny to determine the GII.4 variant type—for example, Sydney_2012 or NewOrleans_2009—via the Norovirus Genotyping Tool.

5.4 UTILITY OF WHOLE GENOME SEQUENCING

Traditional polymerase and major capsid genotyping by PCR and additional sequencing of the P2 region for outbreak investigations is a labor-intensive process requiring several rounds of PCR and sequencing, each requiring genogroup- or genotype-specific primers, and yields only partial genome sequences at the end. Moreover, whereas the P2 domain can identify linked outbreak events with 64−73% specificity (assuming bootstrap support >70 or <70, respectively), the full capsid sequence can identify linked outbreak events with 100% specificity (Verhoef et al., 2012) and thus is more informative.

Whole genome sequencing simplifies investigation of norovirus molecular epidemiology by generating all the regions of interest in one step, thus allowing identification of the genotype, variant type, and full capsid sequence, negating the need for sequential PCR and sequencing reactions.

5.4.1 FULL GENOMES REVEAL INTER- AND INTRA-GENOTYPE RECOMBINATION

Whole genome sequencing generates a full capsid sequence but, crucially, also the full ORF1 sequence. This is important because recombination between norovirus genomes occurs with a breakpoint in or near the ORF1/ORF2 overlap region (Bull et al., 2005, 2007). Therefore, to get a full picture of norovirus epidemiology, both ORF1 and ORF2 must be analyzed, which is facilitated by whole genome sequencing. Recombination is particularly important in the emergence of new GII.4 variants. It has been proposed that inter- and intra-genotype recombination is likely to be an important force in driving the evolution and emergence of novel GII.4 variants by affecting the antigenic properties of a variant (via acquisition of a different ORF2/ORF3 sequences) or by altering the balance of replication and mutation rates, thus increasing viral fitness (via acquisition of a different ORF1). All of the GII.4 variants since FarmingtonHills_2002 have been influenced by recombination, either as the parent of a new recombinant or as a recombinant itself; the current dominant variant, GII.4 Sydney_2012, is a recombinant of Osaka_2007 (ORF1) and Apeldoorn_2008 (ORF2/ORF3) (Eden et al., 2013).

The utility of whole genome sequencing for identifying recombinant strains was demonstrated by Wong et al. (2013), who sequenced 32 stool samples from patients infected with norovirus GII.4 in England during the 2012−13 winter season, achieving full genome sequences in 23 of the 32 samples. During the winter of 2012−13, GII.4 variant Sydney_2012 replaced the previously circulating variant NewOrleans_2009; Wong and colleagues used full genome sequences to identify two samples with Sydney_2012/NewOrleans_2009 recombinant sequences, suggesting that during cocirculation of the two variants, coinfection and recombination had occurred. Wong et al. identified the recombination breakpoint in the ORF1/ORF2 overlap region, which confirms the breakpoint previously identified using partial genome sequences by Bull et al. Full genome sequences have also been used to identify a GII.12/GII.13 recombinant sequence in a stool sample from South Korea (Won et al., 2013), although the prevalence of this recombinant strain has not been investigated.

Detection of recombination is important for local epidemiology, as well as global epidemiology. An outbreak investigation that utilizes capsid sequences alone will not identify recombinant sequences; patients infected with recombinant virus will be misidentified as belonging to one transmission cluster when in fact they are linked to more than one, as illustrated in Fig. 5.2.

5.4.2 INTRA-HOST MINORITY VARIANTS INDICATE DIRECTION OF TRANSMISSION

One additional utility of generating full genome sequences using deep sequencing methods is that it allows analysis of minority variants.

RNA viruses lack proofreading polymerases, resulting in a high mutation frequency of 10^{-3} to 10^{-5} substitution per nucleotide per replication cycle (Steinhauer et al., 1992; Domingo et al., 1996). Intra-host viral populations consequently exist as a heterogeneous population with a consensus sequence and minority variant sequences, known as quasispecies. During a norovirus transmission event between an infected donor and an uninfected recipient, only some of those variants will establish a new infection in the recipient (Bull et al., 2012). By comparing the consensus sequence and minority variants between two linked patients, it is possible to infer the direction of transmission (i.e., which is the donor and which is the recipient) by demonstrating that minority variant sequences in one patient (the donor) are seen as the consensus sequence in the other patient (the recipient), as illustrated in Fig. 5.3. Full genomes are required for this kind of analysis because the minority variant sites can be spread across the genome (Kundu et al., 2013).

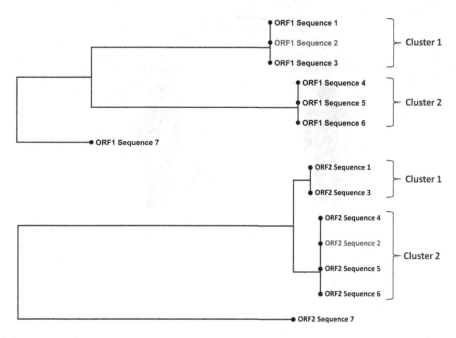

FIGURE 5.2

Phylogenetic reconstruction (neighbor joining tree) of norovirus ORF1 and ORF2 sequences, derived from full genome sequences. Each sequence (sequences 1−7) is taken from a different patient. The tree topology suggests sequences 1 and 3 form one transmission cluster (cluster 1) and sequences 4 and 5 a separate transmission cluster (cluster 2). Sequence 7 is not linked to any other sequences and therefore is not part of the outbreak. ORF1 and ORF2 of sequence 2 cluster with different sequences in each tree, suggesting that this is a recombinant genome, with ORF1 derived from cluster 1 and ORF2 from cluster 2.

5.4.3 EVOLUTIONARY RATES DIFFER BETWEEN GENOMIC REGIONS

The largest number of norovirus whole genome sequences generated to date in a single study has allowed estimations of norovirus evolutionary rates (Cotten et al., 2014). More than 100 whole genome sequences ($n = 112$) from stool samples collected in Vietnam between 2009 and 2011 suggest that the evolutionary rate across the whole genome is $5.34-6.15 \times 10^{-3}$ substitutions per site per year, which supports previous estimates generated using partial genome sequences. Analysis of full genomes showed that ORF1, encoding a nonstructural polyprotein including polymerase, exhibited a lower evolutionary rate than the major capsid protein encoding ORF2. Moreover, for the first time, the evolutionary rate was calculated for ORF3, which is a minor capsid protein with poorly understood function. It was demonstrated that ORF3 was the region with the highest evolutionary rate across the genome ($7.4-9.0 \times 10^{-3}$ substitutions per site per year). The authors proposed that ORF3 could therefore be a possible site of virus−host interaction under selective pressure. Without full genome sequences, this would remain unrecognized. In addition, whole genome sequencing of several genotypes in this study suggests similar evolutionary rates in GII.3 and GII.4 sequences. Infections with GII.4 are far more prevalent than those with GII.3; it has

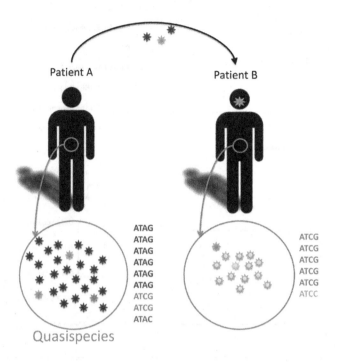

FIGURE 5.3

Illustration of norovirus minority variant analysis and transmission dynamics. A minority variant from Patient A is transmitted to Patient B, in whom an infection is established. Deep sequencing of the quasispecies in each patient shows that the nucleotide sequence corresponding to the minority variant in Patient A is seen as the majority (consensus) sequence in Patient B.

previously been suggested that this could be due to a higher evolutionary rate in GII.4 viruses (Bull et al., 2010). A similar evolutionary rate in the two genotypes suggests that the difference in prevalence could instead be a sampling bias caused by infections with GII.4 genotypes presenting more frequently to health care facilities, although there are no genotyping data available from community cohorts to corroborate this.

5.5 WHOLE GENOME SEQUENCING METHODS

Unlike bacteria, which can be isolated in pure culture, norovirus is as yet unculturable. Recent success in culturing human norovirus in a B lymphocyte cell line in the presence of H antigen (Jones et al., 2014) is promising; however, it has yet to be replicated (Jones et al., 2015) and would not be a pure isolate because it would include DNA from the cell line. Due to this lack of in vitro culture system, norovirus whole genome sequencing must be achieved directly from clinical specimens. This presents a challenge because stool specimens are heavily contaminated with DNA and RNA from other sources, such as enteric bacteria and host cells.

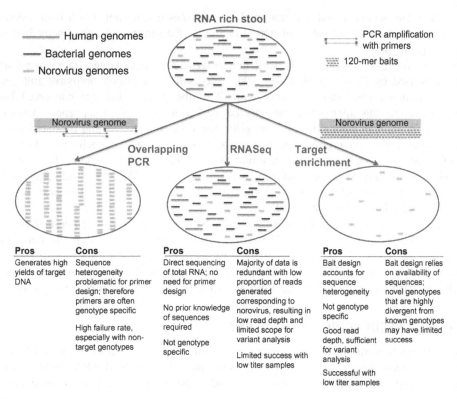

RNA rich stool

———— Human genomes
——— Bacterial genomes
- - - Norovirus genomes

PCR amplification
with primers
120-mer baits

Norovirus genome

Norovirus genome

Overlapping
PCR

RNASeq

Target
enrichment

Pros	Cons	Pros	Cons	Pros	Cons
Generates high yields of target DNA	Sequence heterogeneity problematic for primer design; therefore primers are often genotype specific	Direct sequencing of total RNA; no need for primer design	Majority of data is redundant with low proportion of reads generated corresponding to norovirus, resulting in low read depth and limited scope for variant analysis	Bait design accounts for sequence heterogeneity	Bait design relies on availability of sequences; novel genotypes that are highly divergent from known genotypes may have limited success
	High failure rate, especially with non-target genotypes	No prior knowledge of sequences required		Not genotype specific	
		Not genotype specific	Limited success with low titer samples	Good read depth, sufficient for variant analysis	
				Successful with low titer samples	

FIGURE 5.4

Schematic overview of the three principal methods used to generate norovirus full genome sequences with summary of advantages and disadvantages for each method.

Three principal methods have been applied to sequence norovirus full genomes from clinical specimens: sequencing of overlapping PCR fragments, direct sequencing of total RNA, and target enrichment. These are summarized in Fig. 5.4. The latter two methods have been achieved with the advent of next-generation deep sequencing.

5.5.1 OVERLAPPING PCR AMPLICON SEQUENCING

The advantage of PCR for sequencing from clinical specimens is that over the course of 30–40 amplification cycles, the target sequence, in this case norovirus, is amplified exponentially, generating a high yield of DNA for sequencing. The nontarget sequences become insignificant. The generated amplicons can then be sequenced either by capillary sequencing or with a next-generation sequencing (NGS) platform.

The norovirus genome is 7.5 kb. Because this is beyond the upper size limit of a PCR reaction, the genome must be amplified in several overlapping fragments, referred to as tiled PCR. PCR amplification works using specific primers that are designed to be complementary to a conserved region of the target sequence and will not amplify sequences that do not match both forward and reverse primers. This is problematic for norovirus due to the sequence heterogeneity both within and between genotypes.

Smaller fragments (<1 kb) amplify with greater efficiency than larger fragments; thus, this approach was used by Kundu et al. (2013), who successfully amplified norovirus full genomes using 22 overlapping fragments. However, not all of the primer sites are conserved between genotypes; therefore, this approach could only be used to amplify GII.4 sequences. Larger fragments (2−3 kb), although more difficult to amplify, require fewer primers and thus are more likely to be successful across genotypes. Nonetheless, due to sequence heterogeneity both between and within genotypes, this approach retains a limited success rate, as demonstrated by Cotten et al. (2014), who successfully amplified full genome sequences from 83%, 88%, 92%, and 100% of GII.13, GII.6, GII.4, and GII.9 samples, respectively, but only 20%, 40%, 50%, and 77% of GI, GII.2, GII.12, and GII.3, respectively, and 0% of GII.7 samples.

Norovirus whole genome sequencing from a single 7.5 kb amplicon has been described and used to generate 25 full genome sequences (Eden et al., 2013). Although the authors do not report the success rate using this approach, it is generally very difficult to amplify fragments of such a size. The long dwell times of the PCR cycling often result in nonspecific amplification, and the technique relies on purifying intact full-length RNA genomes; fragmented genomes are not amplified.

5.5.2 DIRECT SEQUENCING OF TOTAL RNA

The most straightforward method to sequence norovirus genomes direct from stool is whole transcriptome sequencing, or RNASeq. This involves purifying the total RNA content of a stool specimen and preparing a sequencing library with all of the RNA, which is then sequenced on an NGS platform.

The advantage of RNASeq is that there is no requirement for PCR primers; therefore, it is completely unbiased. Although all whole genomes by RNASeq reported to date are GII.4, it is theoretically possible to sequence all genotypes with equal success.

The major limitation of RNASeq is also its very reason for success. The unbiased nature of RNASeq means that all RNA present in the sample, which will include host and bacterial RNA transcripts as well as norovirus RNA, will be sequenced. The proportion of norovirus to other RNA can be very low; therefore, great sequencing capacity is required to capture the norovirus sequences in each sample. Because sequencing platforms generate an approximately fixed amount of data, which are shared among the number of samples sequenced on one run, to generate the read depth required to recover norovirus genomes, the number of samples sequenced per run is very limited. For instance, to generate norovirus full genomes, Illumina's bench-top sequencing platform MiSeq, which generates approximately 15 Gb of data and 25 million reads, can accommodate only six stool samples per run (Batty et al., 2013).

The data generated by RNASeq are sufficient to generate almost complete norovirus genome sequences; 40−99% of reported samples achieved greater than 90% genome coverage. However, due to the low proportion of reads that belong to norovirus, a median of 2−3% across all reported samples, the average read depth per sample sequenced on a MiSeq is only 9−259 (Nakamura et al., 2009; Wong et al., 2013; Batty et al., 2013). Although this read depth is, in most cases, sufficient for a reliable consensus sequence, it does not allow variant analysis. Sequencing on a higher-throughput platform, such as the Illumina HiSeq, which generates up to 750 Gb and 2.5 billion reads, allows up to 96 samples to be sequenced on a single run. Although the proportion of reads generated that corresponds to norovirus is still only 3%, the increased sequencing output allows greater read depth per sample, in some cases up to 1000-fold. Nevertheless, the median reported mean depth remains approximately 100-fold (Batty et al., 2013).

Unbiased sequencing of nontarget RNA results in low read depths but also has a financial implication. For instance, the reagents for a single MiSeq and single HiSeq sequencing run (not including library preparation) cost approximately $800 and $5300, respectively; when shared between few samples, this does not make whole genome sequencing cost-effective.

5.5.3 TARGET ENRICHMENT

The proportion of norovirus RNA in stool samples can be very low, which leads to limited read depth in direct sequencing of total RNA. The purpose of target enrichment is to purify the RNA of interest in the specimen, in this case norovirus, and discard the rest. Consequently, the specimen is enriched for the genomes of interest and sequencing is not wasted on nontarget genomes, such as host or bacteria. Target enrichment uses overlapping RNA or DNA oligonucleotide probes to pull out target DNA. This system was initially developed for human exome sequencing, the premise of which was to enrich specimens for all the protein-coding genes (the exome), thus discarding and preventing sequencing of noncoding regions. This has now been applied to DNA and RNA pathogens, including norovirus. Instead of enriching for regions of interest in the human genome, the objective is to enrich for whole genomes of a specific pathogen in a background of other, nontarget, genomes (Brown et al., 2015; Christiansen et al., 2014; Depledge et al., 2011).

In our hands, enrichment makes use of 120-mer RNA baits that are complimentary to the norovirus genome. The baits are designed using a database of all publicly available norovirus sequences, across all GI and GII genotypes. Baits are tiled across the genome so that every position in the genome has a complimentary bait. The major advantage of this technique is that unlike PCR, which uses a single primer at each site, multiple baits are designed to cover each position, thus accounting for sequence variation between norovirus genomes. This allows unbiased sequencing across genotypes in a single reaction, without prior knowledge of the genotype presents in the specimen. The limitation of this technique is that if a novel genotype is not included in the bait design, then enrichment for this genotype may be limited if it is highly divergent to existing genotypes. Because ORF1 is relatively conserved between genotypes, this region of the genome may still be enriched, but it is possible that the divergent capsid genes (ORF2 and ORF3) will not.

To enrich stool specimens for norovirus genomes, total RNA is incubated with biotinylated norovirus-specific RNA baits, which will hybridize to norovirus genomes present in the sample. Streptavidin-coated magnetic beads will in turn bind to the hybridized baits, which can then be separated from all nontarget cDNA using magnetic bead capture. The RNA baits are then digested, leaving an enriched library of norovirus cDNA that can be sequenced on an NGS platform.

Target enrichment eliminates the majority of non-norovirus genomes; therefore, the median proportion of generated sequencing reads that correspond to norovirus is 81%. Consequently, the average read depth is greatly improved compared to total RNA sequencing; the median read depth on an Illumina MiSeq is 8000. This generates robust consensus sequences and allows minority variant analysis.

Moreover, because target enrichment prevents sequencing of nontarget genomes, efficiency is increased by allowing up to 96 samples to be sequenced on a single MiSeq run compared to 6 using RNASeq; thus, it is more cost-effective. Using this method, we are able to recover full norovirus genomes with a minimum 100-fold read depth in greater than 90% of norovirus-positive stool samples with a diagnostic cycle threshold (Ct) value less than 35.

5.6 CONCLUSIONS AND PERSPECTIVES

A full understanding of transmission dynamics is critical for prevention and control of norovirus transmission in both foodborne and health care settings. Classical epidemiology, which links cases in time and space, is important in identifying outbreaks and, based on circumstantial evidence, may give an indication of the source of transmission. Nevertheless, circumstantial evidence may incorrectly link cases or, conversely, not identify transmission between cases that are not traditionally linked in time or space. The implication of these scenarios is potential misallocation of infection control resources in the former or unrecognized transmission, potentially leading to a wider outbreak, in the latter.

Knowledge of the viral genome in the context of transmission and outbreaks, termed molecular epidemiology, provides an evidence base for outbreak investigations and thus the implementation of interventions. Classical genotyping techniques provide useful information, particularly for identifying the genotypes causing infection. However, the techniques are time-consuming and provide only a snapshot of information; in particular, genotyping is of limited use when a predominant genotype is in circulation, as is the case with norovirus GII.4 globally. Full genome sequences, on the other hand, provide far greater resolution. In addition to the known regions of interest used in conventional genotyping, such as the RNA polymerase and capsid sequences, full genomes allow us to identify recombination events and to analyze minority variants in the intra-host viral population. The data generated from full genome sequencing can unequivocally include or exclude cases from an outbreak and, especially in foodborne point source outbreaks, confirm the source of infection.

The advancement of sequencing techniques, from PCR with capillary sequencing to target enrichment with deep sequencing, has facilitated the use of norovirus full genomes in clinical practice. In conjunction with increasing expertise, lower costs, and faster turnaround times, sequencing of full genomes can now be done cost-effectively and quickly, which makes full genome sequencing a reality not just in academic settings but also for informing public health practice in real time.

REFERENCES

Batty, E.M., Wong, T.H., Trebes, A., Argoud, K., Attar, M., Buck, D., et al., 2013. A modified RNA-Seq approach for whole genome sequencing of RNA viruses from faecal and blood samples. PLoS ONE 8, e66129.

Brown, A.C., Bryant, J.M., Einer-Jensen, K., Holdstock, J., Houniet, D.T., Chan, J.Z., et al., 2015. Rapid whole-genome sequencing of *Mycobacterium tuberculosis* isolates directly from clinical samples. J. Clin. Microbiol. 53, 2230–2237.

Bull, R.A., Hansman, G.S., Clancy, L.E., Tanaka, M.M., Rawlinson, W.D., White, P.A., 2005. Norovirus recombination in ORF1/ORF2 overlap. Emerg. Infect. Dis. 11, 1079−1085.

Bull, R.A., Tanaka, M.M., White, P.A., 2007. Norovirus recombination. J. Gen. Virol. 88, 3347−3359.

Bull, R.A., Eden, J.S., Rawlinson, W.D., White, P.A., 2010. Rapid evolution of pandemic noroviruses of the GII.4 lineage. PLoS Pathog. 6, e1000831.

Bull, R.A., Eden, J.S., Luciani, F., Mcelroy, K., Rawlinson, W.D., White, P.A., 2012. Contribution of intra- and interhost dynamics to norovirus evolution. J. Virol. 86, 3219−3229.

Chan, M.C., Lee, N., Hung, T.N., Kwok, K., Cheung, K., Tin, E.K., et al., 2015. Rapid emergence and predominance of a broadly recognizing and fast-evolving norovirus GII.17 variant in late 2014. Nat. Commun. 6, 10061.

Chen, S.Y., Chiu, C.H., 2012. Worldwide molecular epidemiology of norovirus infection. Paediatr. Int. Child Health. 32, 128−131.

Christiansen, M.T., Brown, A.C., Kundu, S., Tutill, H.J., Williams, R., Brown, J.R., et al., 2014. Whole-genome enrichment and sequencing of *Chlamydia trachomatis* directly from clinical samples. BMC Infect. Dis. 14, 591.

Cotten, M., Petrova, V., Phan, M.V., Rabaa, M.A., Watson, S.J., Ong, S.H., et al., 2014. Deep sequencing of norovirus genomes defines evolutionary patterns in an urban tropical setting. J. Virol. 88, 11056−11069.

De Graaf, M., Van Beek, J., Vennema, H., Podkolzin, A.T., Hewitt, J., Bucardo, F., et al., 2015. Emergence of a novel GII.17 norovirus—end of the GII.4 era? Euro. Surveill. 20.

Debbink, K., Donaldson, E.F., Lindesmith, L.C., Baric, R.S., 2012. Genetic mapping of a highly variable norovirus GII.4 blockade epitope: potential role in escape from human herd immunity. J. Virol. 86, 1214−1226.

Depledge, D.P., Palser, A.L., Watson, S.J., Lai, I.Y., Gray, E.R., Grant, P., et al., 2011. Specific capture and whole-genome sequencing of viruses from clinical samples. PLoS ONE 6, e27805.

Domingo, E., Escarmis, C., Sevilla, N., Moya, A., Elena, S.F., Quer, J., et al., 1996. Basic concepts in RNA virus evolution. FASEB J. 10, 859−864.

Eden, J.S., Tanaka, M.M., Boni, M.F., Rawlinson, W.D., White, P.A., 2013. Recombination within the pandemic norovirus GII.4 lineage. J. Virol. 87, 6270−6282.

Franck, K.T., Nielsen, R.T., Holzknecht, B.J., Ersboll, A.K., Fischer, T.K., Bottiger, B., 2015. Norovirus genotypes in hospital settings: differences between nosocomial and community-acquired infections. J. Infect. Dis. 212, 881−888.

Gallimore, C.I., Pipkin, C., Shrimpton, H., Green, A.D., Pickford, Y., Mccartney, C., et al., 2005. Detection of multiple enteric virus strains within a foodborne outbreak of gastroenteritis: an indication of the source of contamination. Epidemiol. Infect. 133, 41−47.

Gallimore, C.I., Iturriza-Gomara, M., Xerry, J., Adigwe, J., Gray, J.J., 2007. Inter-seasonal diversity of norovirus genotypes: emergence and selection of virus variants. Arch. Virol. 152, 1295−1303.

Hohne, M., Niendorf, S., Mas Marques, A., Bock, C.T., 2015. Use of sequence analysis of the P2 domain for characterization of norovirus strains causing a large multistate outbreak of norovirus gastroenteritis in Germany 2012. Int. J. Med. Microbiol. 305, 612−618.

Holzknecht, B.J., Franck, K.T., Nielsen, R.T., Bottiger, B., Fischer, T.K., Fonager, J., 2015. Sequence analysis of the capsid gene during a genotype II.4 dominated norovirus season in one university hospital: identification of possible transmission routes. PLoS ONE 10, e0115331.

Jones, M.K., Watanabe, M., Zhu, S., Graves, C.L., Keyes, L.R., Grau, K.R., et al., 2014. Enteric bacteria promote human and mouse norovirus infection of B cells. Science 346, 755−759.

Jones, M.K., Grau, K.R., Costantini, V., Kolawole, A.O., Graaf, M.D.E., Freiden, P., et al., 2015. Human norovirus culture in B cells. Nat. Protocol. 10, 1939−1947.

Kroneman, A., Vennema, H., Deforche, K., V D Avoort, H., Penaranda, S., et al., 2011. An automated genotyping tool for enteroviruses and noroviruses. J. Clin. Virol. 51, 121−125.

Kroneman, A., Vega, E., Vennema, H., Vinje, J., White, P.A., Hansman, G., et al., 2013. Proposal for a unified norovirus nomenclature and genotyping. Arch. Virol. 158, 2059–2068.

Kundu, S., Lockwood, J., Depledge, D.P., Chaudhry, Y., Aston, A., Rao, K., et al., 2013. Next-generation whole genome sequencing identifies the direction of norovirus transmission in linked patients. Clin. Infect. Dis. 57, 407–414.

Lindesmith, L.C., Beltramello, M., Donaldson, E.F., Corti, D., Swanstrom, J., Debbink, K., et al., 2012. Immunogenetic mechanisms driving norovirus GII.4 antigenic variation. PLoS Pathog. 8, e1002705.

Lopman, B.A., Gallimore, C., Gray, J.J., Vipond, I.B., Andrews, N., Sarangi, J., et al., 2006. Linking health-care associated norovirus outbreaks: a molecular epidemiologic method for investigating transmission. BMC Infect. Dis. 6, 108.

Muller, L., Schultz, A.C., Fonager, J., Jensen, T., Lisby, M., Hindsdal, K., et al., 2015. Separate norovirus outbreaks linked to one source of imported frozen raspberries by molecular analysis, Denmark, 2010–2011. Epidemiol. Infect. 143, 2299–2307.

Nakamura, S., Yang, C.S., Sakon, N., Ueda, M., Tougan, T., Yamashita, A., et al., 2009. Direct metagenomic detection of viral pathogens in nasal and fecal specimens using an unbiased high-throughput sequencing approach. PLoS ONE 4, e4219.

Steinhauer, D.A., Domingo, E., Holland, J.J., 1992. Lack of evidence for proofreading mechanisms associated with an RNA virus polymerase. Gene 122, 281–288.

Sukhrie, F.H., Beersma, M.F., Wong, A., Van Der Veer, B., Vennema, H., et al., 2011. Using molecular epidemiology to trace transmission of nosocomial norovirus infection. J. Clin. Microbiol. 49, 602–606.

Sukhrie, F.H., Teunis, P., Vennema, H., Bogerman, J., VAN Marm, S., et al., 2013. P2 domain profiles and shedding dynamics in prospectively monitored norovirus outbreaks. J. Clin. Virol. 56, 286–292.

Tam, C.C., Rodrigues, L.C., Viviani, L., Dodds, J.P., Evans, M.R., Hunter, P.R., et al., 2012. Longitudinal study of infectious intestinal disease in the UK (IID2 study): incidence in the community and presenting to general practice. Gut 61, 69–77.

Vega, E., Barclay, L., Gregoricus, N., Shirley, S.H., Lee, D., Vinje, J., 2014. Genotypic and epidemiologic trends of norovirus outbreaks in the United States, 2009 to 2013. J. Clin. Microbiol. 52, 147–155.

Verhoef, L., Vennema, H., Van Pelt, W., Lees, D., Boshuizen, H., et al., 2010. Use of norovirus genotype profiles to differentiate origins of foodborne outbreaks. Emerg. Infect. Dis. 16, 617–624.

Verhoef, L., Williams, K.P., Kroneman, A., Sobral, B., Van Pelt, W., Koopmans, M., 2012. Selection of a phylogenetically informative region of the norovirus genome for outbreak linkage. Virus Genes 44, 8–18.

Verhoef, L., Hewitt, J., Barclay, L., Ahmed, S.M., Lake, R., Hall, A.J., et al., 2015. Norovirus genotype profiles associated with foodborne transmission, 1999–2012. Emerg. Infect. Dis. 21, 592–599.

Vinje, J., 2015. Advances in laboratory methods for detection and typing of norovirus. J. Clin. Microbiol 53, 373–381.

Wang, X., Yong, W., Shi, L., Qiao, M., He, M., Zhang, H., et al., 2015. An outbreak of multiple norovirus strains on a cruise ship in China, 2014. J. Appl. Microbiol 120, 226–233.

Won, Y.J., Park, J.W., Han, S.H., Cho, H.G., Kang, L.H., Lee, S.G., et al., 2013. Full-genomic analysis of a human norovirus recombinant GII.12/13 novel strain isolated from South Korea. PLoS ONE 8, e85063.

Wong, T.H., Dearlove, B.L., Hedge, J., Giess, A.P., Piazza, P., Trebes, A., et al., 2013. Whole genome sequencing and de novo assembly identifies Sydney-like variant noroviruses and recombinants during the winter 2012/2013 outbreak in England. Virol. J. 10, 335.

Xerry, J., Gallimore, C.I., Iturriza-Gomara, M., Allen, D.J., Gray, J.J., 2008. Transmission events within outbreaks of gastroenteritis determined through analysis of nucleotide sequences of the P2 domain of genogroup II noroviruses. J. Clin. Microbiol. 46, 947–953.

PART

III

PATHOGEN AND THE HOST

CLINICAL MANIFESTATIONS

6

Way-Seah Lee[1] and Edmond A.S. Nelson[2]

[1]*University of Malaya, Kuala Lumpur, Malaysia* [2]*The Chinese University of Hong Kong, Hong Kong, China*

6.1 INTRODUCTION

Norovirus infection, also known as "winter vomiting disease," is characterized by a high incidence of vomiting and diarrhea, and it occurs predominantly during the winter season. Norovirus is emerging as the leading cause of viral gastroenteritis worldwide and affects people of all ages. In the following sections of rotavirus vaccination, it has become the most common cause of gastroenteritis in both children and adults.

Norovirus infection due to norovirus can lead to a spectrum of manifestations, including asymptomatic infection, mild illness with fever and watery stools, and more severe illness with fever, vomiting, headache, and constitutional symptoms (Chen, C.J. et al., 2015a; Tian et al., 2014). Key features of norovirus infection include the following:

- Short incubation period (12−72 hours).
- Short duration of illness (2−3 days).
- Vomiting followed by diarrhea are the principal symptoms.
- Dehydration is the main complication.
- Peripheral white blood cell count is generally normal or mildly elevated, and relative lymphopenia may be observed.
- Immunocompromised patients may develop persistent infection.
- Suspected rare extraintestinal involvement includes convulsion, hepatitis, and urticaria.

6.2 CLINICAL MANIFESTATIONS IN CHILDREN

Asymptomatic infection has been observed, probably as a result of exposure to low inoculum, lack of genetic susceptibility of the host, as well as variability in host immune response.

6.2.1 INCUBATION PERIOD

The incubation period is generally between 24 and 48 hours (range, 12−72 hours). The onset of symptoms is characteristically sudden (Table 6.1). Clinical disease typically lasts for 2 or 3 days,

The Norovirus. DOI: http://dx.doi.org/10.1016/B978-0-12-804177-2.00006-3

81

Table 6.1 Clinical Features of Acute Gastroenteritis in Taiwanese Children Caused by Norovirus and Other Viruses

Features	Norovirus ($n = 320$)	Rotavirus ($n = 498$)	Adenovirus ($n = 80$)
Cool season (November to April; %)	71.6	67.6	55.0
Upper respiratory tract symptoms (%)	56.3	65.5	63.8
Duration of fever (days; mean ± SD)	2.8 ± 2.8	3.2 ± 2.2	3.4 ± 3.0
Duration of vomiting (days; mean ± SD)	1.7 ± 1.9	1.7 ± 1.5	1.6 ± 2.0
Maximum episodes of vomiting/24 hours (mean ± SD)	4.5 ± 4.0	4.8 ± 3.3	2.9 ± 2.7
Duration of diarrhea (days; mean ± SD)	5.6 ± 2.6	5.1 ± 2.0	6.9 ± 3.4
Maximum episodes of diarrhea/24 hours (mean ± SD)	7.3 ± 4.4	7.7 ± 4.1	6.9 ± 3.4
Duration of hospital stay (days; mean ± SD)	4.7 ± 2.3	4.5 ± 2.1	5.0 ± 2.6
White cell counts ($\times 10^9$/L)	11.2 ± 5.5	10.9 ± 6.1	12.3 ± 5.0
C-reactive protein (mg/L)	18.2 ± 35.1	14.1 ± 30.6	23.5 ± 39.6

Adapted from Chen, C.J., et al., 2015a. Clinical and epidemiologic features of severe viral gastroenteritis in children: a 3-year surveillance, multicentered study in Taiwan with partial rotavirus immunization. Medicine 94 (33), e1372. Available from <http://www.ncbi.nlm.nih.gov/pmc/articles/PMC4616446>.

and the recovery is rapid. The duration of illness may persist longer in younger children and immunosuppressed patients.

6.2.2 CLINICAL FEATURES

Slightly more than half of children with norovirus may develop prodromal symptoms such as coryza and cough. These are followed by fever, vomiting, and diarrhea (Table 6.1). Vomiting usually stops within 2 days after the onset of illness, although diarrhea may last considerably longer (Table 6.1). There are considerable similarities in the clinical features of infection caused by norovirus and other viruses that cause acute gastroenteritis, such as rotavirus and adenovirus (Table 6.1).

The stools in children with norovirus are typically moderate in amount. Blood and mucus are usually absent because the gastroenteritis caused by norovirus is typically a noninvasive process. There may be other constitutional symptoms, such as malaise, myalgias, and headache. Abdominal pain may sometimes be significant, requiring in assessment for suspected acute abdomen (Tajiri et al., 2008).

Recurrent vomiting and diarrhea leading to dehydration in norovirus gastroenteritis are common. A study comparing the severity of illness in acute diarrhea caused by rotavirus and norovirus showed that the proportion of children with dehydrating illness, the number requiring hospital care, and the duration of hospital stay were similar between children with norovirus and those with rotavirus infection (Nakagomi et al., 2008). Other studies have shown more diarrhea, higher fever, and/or longer hospital stay in the rotavirus group (O'Ryan et al., 2010; Wu et al., 2008; Yang et al., 2010). A further study reported longer duration of vomiting and diarrhea in the norovirus group (Kawada et al., 2012). This suggests that symptoms of both norovirus and rotavirus may reflect the virulence of different circulating strains of the respective viruses. Although fatal illness secondary to severe dehydration appears to be uncommon in norovirus gastroenteritis (Sugata et al., 2014), there are relatively few reports from developing countries. The Global Enteric Multicenter Study (GEMS) study did not identify norovirus as a significant cause of morbidity or mortality (Kotloff et al., 2013). However, the multisite birth cohort study of pathogen-specific burdens of community diarrhea in developing countries (MAL-ED) study, which collected stools from eight sites in South America, Africa, and Asia, identified norovirus GII as the most common pathogen attributable to diarrhea in the first year of life and the second most common in the second year (Platts-Mills et al., 2015). Whether the high prevalence in this community setting translates to mortality is not clear. The MAL-ED study showed that bloody diarrhea was primarily associated with *Campylobacter* and *Shigella*, fever and vomiting with rotavirus, and vomiting with norovirus GII. Death due to necrotizing enterocolitis in premature infants related to norovirus has been reported (Trivedi et al., 2013).

6.2.3 LABORATORY FEATURES

The white cell count is generally normal or mildly elevated. Relative lymphopenia may be observed. One study comparing norovirus with rotavirus gastroenteritis reported a higher white cell count in the norovirus group but higher liver enzymes and C-reactive protein in the rotavirus group (Wu et al., 2008).

6.3 CLINICAL MANIFESTATIONS IN ADULTS

The incubation period of norovirus infection in adults is similar to the incubation period in children.

6.3.1 CLINICAL FEATURES

The clinical features of norovirus gastroenteritis in adults are also quite similar to those features observed in children. Fever, vomiting, and diarrhea are predominant symptoms. Diarrhea is the most predominant symptom, occurring in 90% of patients infected. Vomiting may affect up to 70% of infected individuals. A study prospectively assessing 60 outbreaks reported that vomiting, abdominal pain, and malaise were more common in children and adolescents, with diarrhea and myalgia being more common in adults (Arias et al., 2010). Another study noted abdominal pain in approximately 50% of adult patients with norovirus gastroenteritis (Tian et al., 2014). The majority of patients with norovirus gastroenteritis have between 3 and 10 episodes of diarrhea per day (Tian et al., 2014). As in children, the stools are usually watery with no blood or mucus.

6.3.2 LABORATORY FEATURES

A raised white cell count, predominantly neutrophils, may be seen. Relative lymphopenia may also be seen at the height of the illness. Renal function is generally normal unless there is severe dehydration.

6.4 CLINICAL MANIFESTATIONS IN IMMUNOSUPPRESSED PATIENTS

Norovirus can lead to persistent infection in immunocompromised hosts, resulting in prolonged virus shedding and gastrointestinal disease (Green, 2014).

6.4.1 AT-RISK GROUPS IN CHILDREN

Immunocompromised children at risk of developing persistent norovirus infection include those undergoing chemotherapy, those post-liver transplant, or those with congenital immunodeficiency (i.e., severe combined immunodeficiency) (Bok and Green, 2012; Green, 2014).

6.4.2 AT-RISK GROUPS IN ADULTS

Chronic norovirus infection has been documented in adults following hematopoietic stem cell transplant, solid organ transplant (heart and kidney), HIV infection, and malignancy or following chemotherapy for malignancy (Green, 2014).

6.4.3 CLINICAL FEATURES

It has been estimated that approximately one in six patients who are immunocompromised and who develop acute diarrhea has norovirus as the causative pathogen (Bok and Green, 2012). There is no seasonality in norovirus infection in immunocompromised hosts. In acute diarrhea, the onset of symptoms is usually acute, but the duration of diarrhea may be indefinite (Bok and Green, 2012). Complications include dehydration, malnutrition, and dysfunction of the intestinal barrier. All these may worsen the underlying illness (Bok and Green, 2012).

6.4.4 MORTALITY

Leading causes of death due to norovirus gastroenteritis in immunocompromised hosts include secondary bacterial sepsis, pneumonia, septic shock, severe gastroenteritis, and dehydration and malnutrition (Trivedi et al., 2013). Norovirus gastroenteritis is a major threat to patients with chemotherapy and hematopoietic stem cell transplant, emphasizing the need for meticulous infection control measures to prevent transmission of noroviruses to these patients (Schwartz et al., 2011).

6.5 ASSOCIATED EXTRAINTESTINAL MANIFESTATIONS

Norovirus infection has been associated with a number of extraintestinal manifestations.

6.5.1 CENTRAL NERVOUS SYSTEM

Comprehensive post-marketing surveillance was undertaken following the universal introduction of rotavirus vaccine in the United States to monitor for intussusception and other potential adverse events (Weinberg, 2014). Using information from the Vaccine Safety Data Link, an unexpected 18–21% reduction in afebrile and febrile seizures was identified following the introduction of rotavirus vaccines (Payne et al., 2014). This equated to more than $7 million in prevented health care costs per year. There is biological plausibility for this association with antigeniemia noted in 50% of rotavirus infections and viremia detected in the cerebrospinal fluid with polymerase chain reaction and electron microscopy. These rotavirus-related seizures may occur in clusters and may be afebrile. Similarly, seizures have been reported in children with norovirus infection (Kang and Kwon, 2014), and dissemination of norovirus to the bloodstream is not uncommon (Fumian et al., 2013). Benign convulsion with gastroenteritis (CwG) represents a distinct clinical entity defined as a convulsion in a previously healthy child with unknown central nervous system infection or encephalopathy, accompanying mild diarrhea without fever, electrolyte disturbance, or moderate to severe dehydration (Kang and Kwon, 2014). A number of studies have compared the rates and presentations of convulsions with both rotavirus and norovirus gastroenteritis. In some cases, seizures may be prolonged (Bartolini et al., 2011) and occur in clusters (Morioka et al., 2010; Ueda et al., 2015); in these cases, significant investigations, such as lumbar puncture, cerebral computed tomography, magnetic resonance imaging, and electroencephalogram, may be performed. Although transient splenial lesions have been reported on magnetic resonance imaging (Morioka et al., 2010), the outcome of these gastroenteritis-related seizures appears to be excellent and recognition of this association could reduce the need for extensive investigations and unnecessary medication (Chan et al., 2011). However, poor neurological outcome following suspected norovirus encephalopathy has been reported (Obinata et al., 2010). Several studies have reported that benign gastroenteritis-related seizures may be more common with norovirus than with rotavirus (Chan et al., 2011; Chen et al., 2009; Ueda et al., 2015). However, in the rotavirus group, seizures occurred earlier in the illness and were more likely to be associated with fever (Ueda et al., 2015).

6.5.2 LIVER INVOLVEMENT

In some young children, a mild elevation of transaminases (alanine transferase (ALT) and aspartate transferase (AST)) levels associated with norovirus infection has been observed (Tsuge et al., 2010). This occurred while the symptoms were severe. The transaminase levels significantly increased after gastroenteritis disappeared. The average period between the onset of gastroenteritis and peak transaminase levels was 2 weeks (Tsuge et al., 2010). These were young children, and the course of disease was similar to that of other causes of gastroenteritis. The clinical course was usually self-limiting, with the transaminases returning to normal limits (AST <50 IU/L and ALT <50 IU/L) 2 weeks after the peak increase in transaminase. Direct infiltration of the liver by norovirus has been postulated as the possible cause.

6.5.3 SKIN INVOLVEMENT

Both acute and chronic urticaria of the skin have been reported in association with norovirus infection (Leiste et al., 2008). Further study is required to determine whether this association is causal.

6.6 EFFECT OF GENOTYPE ON CLINICAL PRESENTATION

Emergence of a novel norovirus GII.4 has been associated with acute gastroenteritis with intestinal hemorrhage in children, suggesting greater virulence and pathogenicity (Chen et al., 2015b). Children infected with the novel strain were more likely to have fever, grossly bloody stool, and occult blood in the feces. Longer duration of diarrhea and vomiting, suggesting greater disease severity, has also been reported with GII.4 genotype (Huhti et al., 2011). Even within subtypes of GII.4, disease severity appears to differ, with more frequent diarrhea of longer duration, more hypoglycemia, and more electrolyte disturbances noted with the GII.4 2006b compared to the G11.4 2010 variant (Tsai et al., 2014). Convulsions were reported only in association with GII.4 2006b subtype.

6.7 CONCLUSIONS AND PERSPECTIVES

Norovirus infection is by far one of the most common causes of acute gastroenteritis seen in all age groups. Although the disease is perceived to be mild by most clinicians, the high transmissibility and prolonged persistence in a closed environment make it a top priority in infection control that often requires drastic actions involving disruption of service. The increased availability of sensitive molecular detection methods has improved our understanding of the clinical presentation and complications of norovirus infection, particularly the extraintestinal involvement. More vigorous search for and more intense investigation of the possible severe complications are needed to reveal the true disease impact associated with this ubiquitous virus.

REFERENCES

Arias, C., Sala, M.R., Dominguez, A., Torner, N., Ruiz, L., Martinez, A., et al., 2010. Epidemiological and clinical features of norovirus gastroenteritis in outbreaks: a population-based study. Clin. Microbiol. Infect.: Official publication of the Eur. Soc. Clin. Microbiol. Infect. Dis. 16 (1), 39−44.

Bartolini, L., Mardari, R., Toldo, I., Calderone, M., Battistella, P.A., Laverda, A.M., et al., 2011. Norovirus gastroenteritis and seizures: an atypical case with neuroradiological abnormalities. Neuropediatrics 42 (4), 167−169.

Bok, K., Green, K.Y., 2012. Norovirus gastroenteritis in immunocompromised patients. New Engl. J. Med. 367 (22), 2126−2132.

Chan, C.M.V., Chan, Cw.D., Ma, Ck, Chan, Hb, 2011. Norovirus as cause of benign convulsion associated with gastro-enteritis. J. Paediatr. Child Heal. 47 (6), 373−377.

Chen, S.Y., Tsai, C.N., Lai, M.W., Chen, C.Y., Lin, K.L., Lin, T.Y., et al., 2009. Norovirus infection as a cause of diarrhea-associated benign infantile seizures. Clin. Infect. Dis.: An official publication of the Infect. Dis. Soc. Am. 48 (7), 849−855.

Chen, C.J., Wu, F.T., Huang, Y.C., Chang, W.C., Wu, H.S., Wu, C.Y., et al., 2015. Clinical and epidemiologic features of severe viral gastroenteritis in children: a 3-year surveillance, multicentered study in Taiwan with partial rotavirus immunization. Medicine 94 (33), e1372. Available from: <http://www.ncbi.nlm.nih.gov/pmc/articles/PMC4616446/>.

Chen, S.Y., Feng, Y., Chao, H.C., Lai, M.W., Huang, W.L., Lin, C.Y., et al., 2015. Emergence in Taiwan of novel norovirus GII.4 variants causing acute gastroenteritis and intestinal haemorrhage in children. J. Med. Microbiol. 64 (Pt 5), 544−550.

Fumian, T.M., Justino, M.C., D'Arc Pereira Mascarenhas, J., Reymao, T.K.A., Abreu, E., Soares, L., et al., 2013. Quantitative and molecular analysis of noroviruses RNA in blood from children hospitalized for acute gastroenteritis in Belem, Brazil. J. Clin. Virol.: The official publication of the Pan Am. Soc. Clin. Virol. 58 (1), 31−35.

Green, K.Y., 2014. Norovirus infection in immunocompromised hosts. Clin. Microbiol. Infect. The official publication of the Eur. Soc. Clin. Microbiol. Infect. Dis. 20 (8), 717−723.

Huhti, L., Szakal, E.D., Puustinen, L., Salminen, M., Huhtala, H., Valve, O., et al., 2011. Norovirus GII-4 causes a more severe gastroenteritis than other noroviruses in young children. J. Infect. Dis. 203 (10), 1442−1444.

Kang, B., Kwon, Y.S., 2014. Benign convulsion with mild gastroenteritis. Kor. J. Pediatr. 57 (7), 304−309. Available from: <http://www.ncbi.nlm.nih.gov/pmc/articles/PMC4127392/>.

Kawada, J.I., Arai, N., Nishimura, N., Suzuki, M., Ohta, R., Ozaki, T., et al., 2012. Clinical characteristics of norovirus gastroenteritis among hospitalized children in Japan. Microbiol. Immunol. 56 (11), 756−759.

Kotloff, K.L., Nataro, J.P., Blackwelder, W.C., Nasrin, D., Farag, T.H., Panchalingam, S., et al., 2013. Burden and aetiology of diarrhoeal disease in infants and young children in developing countries (the Global Enteric Multicenter Study, GEMS): a prospective, case−control study. Lancet 382 (9888), 209−222.

Leiste, A., Skaletz-Rorowski, A., Venten, I., Altmeyer, P., Brockmeyer, N.H., 2008. Urticaria associated with norovirus infection: report of two cases. J. Germ. Soc. Dermatol. JDDG 6 (7), 563−565.

Morioka, S., Otabe, O., Uehara, H., Yokoi, K., Ohmizono, Y., Ishimaru, Y., et al., 2010. Recurrence of transient splenial lesions in a child with "benign convulsions with gastroenteritis". Brain Develop. 42 (6), 449−453.

Nakagomi, T., Correia, J.B., Nakagomi, O., Montenegro, F.M.U., Cuevas, L.E., Cunliffe, N.A., et al., 2008. Norovirus infection among children with acute gastroenteritis in Recife, Brazil: disease severity is comparable to rotavirus gastroenteritis. Arch. Virol. 153 (5), 957−960.

Obinata, K., Okumura, A., Nakazawa, T., Kamata, A., Niizuma, T., Kinoshita, K., et al., 2010. Norovirus encephalopathy in a previously healthy child. Pediatr. Infect. Dis. J. 29 (11), 1057−1059.

O'Ryan, M.L., Pena, A., Vergara, R., Diaz, J., Mamani, N., Cortes, H., et al., 2010. Prospective characterization of norovirus compared with rotavirus acute diarrhea episodes in Chilean children. Pediatr. Infect. Dis. J. 29 (9), 855−859.

Payne, D.C., Baggs, J., Zerr, D.M., Klein, N.P., Yih, K., Glanz, J., et al., 2014. Protective association between rotavirus vaccination and childhood seizures in the year following vaccination in US children. Clin. Infect. Dis.: An official publication of the Infect. Dis. Soc. Am. 58 (2), 173−177.

Platts-Mills, J.A., Babji, S., Bodhidatta, L., Gratz, J., Haque, R., Havt, A., et al., 2015. Pathogen-specific burdens of community diarrhoea in developing countries: a multisite birth cohort study (MAL-ED). Lancet Global Heal. 3 (9), e564−e575. Available from: <http://www.sciencedirect.com/science/article/pii/S2214109X15001515>.

Schwartz, S., Vergoulidou, M., Schreier, E., Loddenkemper, C., Reinwald, M., Schmidt-Hieber, M., et al., 2011. Norovirus gastroenteritis causes severe and lethal complications after chemotherapy and hematopoietic stem cell transplantation. Blood 117 (22), 5850−5856.

Sugata, K., Wakuda, M., Taniguchi, K., Asano, Y., Yoshikawa, T., 2014. Fatal case of norovirus gastroenteritis due to severe dehydration. J. Pediatr. Infect. Dis. Soc. 3 (4), 358−359. Available from: <http://jpids.oxfordjournals.org/content/3/4/358.short>.

Tajiri, H., Kiyohara, Y., Tanaka, T., Etani, Y., Mushiake, S., 2008. Abnormal computed tomography findings among children with viral gastroenteritis and symptoms mimicking acute appendicitis. Pediatr. Emerg. Care 24 (9), 601−604.

Tian, G., Jin, M., Li, H., Li, Q., Wang, J., Duan, Zj, 2014. Clinical characteristics and genetic diversity of noroviruses in adults with acute gastroenteritis in Beijing, China in 2008–2009. J. Med. Virol. 86 (7), 1235–1242.

Trivedi, T.K., Desai, R., Hall, A.J., Patel, M., Parashar, U.D., Lopman, B.A., 2013. Clinical characteristics of norovirus-associated deaths: a systematic literature review. Am. J. Infect. Cont. 41 (7), 654–657.

Tsai, C.N., Lin, C.Y., Lin, C.W., Shih, K.C., Chiu, C.H., Chen, S.Y., 2014. Clinical relevance and genotypes of circulating noroviruses in northern Taiwan, 2006–2011. J. Med. Virol. 86 (2), 335–346.

Tsuge, M., Goto, S., Kato, F., Morishima, T., 2010. Elevation of serum transaminases with norovirus infection. Clin. Pediatr. 49 (6), 574–578.

Ueda, H., Tajiri, H., Kimura, S., Etani, Y., Hosoi, G., Maruyama, T., et al., 2015. Clinical characteristics of seizures associated with viral gastroenteritis in children. Epilep. Res. 109, 146–154.

Weinberg, G.A., 2014. Editorial commentary: unexpected benefits of immunization: rotavirus vaccines reduce childhood seizures. Clin. Infect. Dis.: An official publication of the Infect. Dis. Soc. Am. 58 (2), 178–180.

Wu, T.C., Liu, H.H., Chen, Y.J., Tang, R.B., Hwang, B.T., Yuan, H.C., 2008. Comparison of clinical features of childhood norovirus and rotavirus gastroenteritis in Taiwan. J. Chin. Med. Assoc. 71 (11), 566–570.

Yang, S.Y., Hwang, K.P., Wu, F.T., Wu, H.S., Hsiung, C.A., Chang, W.C., et al., 2010. Epidemiology and clinical peculiarities of norovirus and rotavirus infection in hospitalized young children with acute diarrhea in Taiwan, 2009. J. Microbiol. Immunol. Infect. 43 (6), 506–514.

IMMUNE RESPONSE

Sasirekha Ramani, Mary K. Estes and Robert L. Atmar

Baylor College of Medicine, Houston, TX, United States

7.1 BACKGROUND

Human norovirus (HuNoV) infections are associated with nearly one-fifth of acute gastroenteritis cases worldwide (Ahmed et al., 2014). In the United States, HuNoVs are the leading cause of foodborne gastroenteritis across all age groups and have replaced rotavirus as the leading cause of diarrhea in young children (Gastanaduy et al., 2013; Payne et al., 2013; Scallan et al., 2011). The economic impact of norovirus illness is high, with billions of dollars spent in health care costs and due to loss of productivity each year (Bartsch et al., 2012). Understanding the mechanisms of immunity, particularly the correlates of protection from disease, is critical for the development and evaluation of therapeutics and vaccines. The lack of robust and reproducible cell culture systems to cultivate and study HuNoVs, or small animal models that recapitulate oral inoculation and gastrointestinal (GI) disease has impeded extensive studies on norovirus immunity. In this chapter, we discuss the different models used to understand norovirus immunity, findings on innate and adaptive responses following infection in these models, and correlates of protection from infection and disease in humans. We also provide a perspective on the current challenges and future directions for work on norovirus immunity.

7.2 MODELS TO STUDY NOROVIRUS IMMUNE RESPONSE

Most of the current knowledge on immune responses to norovirus in humans is derived from epidemiology studies, human volunteer challenge studies, and recently, vaccine trials using recombinant virus-like particle (VLP) vaccines. What is evident from these studies is that both host genetics and immune components contribute to protection from norovirus infection and disease. Genetically susceptible individuals acquire multiple HuNoV infections during their lifetime, and protective immune responses are likely short-lived (Johnson et al., 1990; Parrino et al., 1977). Norovirus illness in immunocompetent hosts is characterized by severe vomiting and diarrhea for a relatively short duration of time, and currently there are no small animal models that effectively mimic human disease. However, HuNoVs can infect some animal species, such as nonhuman primates, gnotobiotic pigs and calves, and immunocompromised mice. The routes of infection vary between different models and result in varying clinical outcomes (Table 7.1). Nonhuman primates infected

The Norovirus. DOI: http://dx.doi.org/10.1016/B978-0-12-804177-2.00007-5

orally or intravenously do not develop GI symptoms (Bok et al., 2011; Wyatt et al., 1978), whereas gnotobiotic pigs and calves develop mild GI symptoms following oral infection (Cheetham et al., 2006; Souza et al., 2008). Intraperitoneal injections of HuNoV in immunocompromised mice result in asymptomatic infections (Taube et al., 2013). Despite their limitations, these animal models provide insights into norovirus immunity. Noroviruses also cause infections in many animal species, such as cattle (bovine noroviruses), mice (murine noroviruses, MNVs), and dogs (canine noroviruses) (Bank-Wolf et al., 2010). Of these, many studies have been carried out on immune responses to MNVs. These viruses replicate primarily in macrophages, dendritic cells, and B cells (Jones et al., 2014; Wobus et al., 2004), and infections in wild-type mice result in the dissemination of viral RNA to multiple extraintestinal sites such as the spleen, liver, and lung. Although MNVs are shed in the feces of infected wild-type mice and have been used as a surrogate for HuNoVs, infections do not result in GI pathology in these animals. However, MNV infections in interferon (IFN) knockout mice result in some GI symptoms, such as gastric bloating and decreased water absorption in the colon (Karst et al., 2003; Mumphrey et al., 2007). Both innate and adaptive immune responses have been studied in humans and animal models; however, innate immunity is better characterized in animal models, whereas much of the work in humans involves studies on adaptive immune responses.

7.3 INNATE IMMUNE RESPONSES IN ANIMALS

The short duration of norovirus illness in immunocompetent individuals suggests a possible role for innate immune factors in controlling disease. Certainly, innate immunity plays a critical role in viral clearance in animal models. IFNs are the best studied innate immune effectors in animal models of norovirus infections. Intracerebral or intranasal inoculation of the MNV-1 strain in mice lacking both type I (IFN-α,β) and type II ((IFN-γ) receptors results in lethal infection compared to inoculation in wild-type mice, suggesting a role for IFNs in protection from disease (Karst et al., 2003). Lethality is primarily attributed to the development of encephalitis, meningitis, hepatitis, and pneumonia in this model. Following per oral infection of wild-type mice with MNV-1, viral RNA is rapidly disseminated to peripheral tissues but is cleared by 3 days postinfection. However, mice deficient in the transcription factor STAT-1 (signal transducer and activator of transcription-1) show significant pathology in the lung, liver, and spleen, and viral RNA is detected in multiple organs even at 7 days postinfection, indicating that STAT-1-dependent innate immune responses may be critical in clearing extraintestinal MNV infections (Karst et al., 2003). MNV can be detected in the feces of wild-type mice following oral inoculation but is not associated with significant GI symptoms. By contrast, STAT-1-deficient mice show weight loss and GI symptoms such as bloating and decreased water absorption in the colon, suggesting that clinical disease may also be prevented by STAT-1-mediated immune responses (Mumphrey et al., 2007). Recently, the type III IFN response (IFN-λ) has been identified as a critical component in the control of persistent MNV enteric infections. Some strains of MNV, such as CR6, are known to cause persistent enteric infections in mice. Intraperitoneal treatment with IFN-λ one day after oral inoculation with CR6 prevents persistent enteric infection, whereas exogenous treatment with IFN-λ results in viral clearance in persistently infected mice (Nice et al., 2015). When cured mice are challenged with CR6 after 2 weeks,

Table 7.1 Models to Study HuNoV Infections

System	Route of Infection	GI Symptoms	Studies on Innate and Adaptive Immunity	Challenges	References
Humans (experimental infection)	Oral	Diarrhea, vomiting	Yes	Ethical and logistical challenges	Atmar et al. (2008, 2014), Czako et al. (2012, 2015), Erdman et al. (1989), Graham et al. (1994), Johnson et al. (1990), Kavanagh et al. (2011), Lindesmith et al. (2003, 2005, 2010, 2015a), Newman et al. (2015, 2016), Parrino et al. (1977), Ponterio et al. (2013), Ramani et al. (2015)
Gnotobiotic pigs	Oral	Diarrhea	Yes	Expensive model systems; lack of microbiome confounds results	Cheetham et al. (2006), Jung et al. (2012)
Gnotobiotic calves	Oral	Diarrhea	Yes	Expensive model systems; lack of microbiome confounds results	Souza et al. (2008)
Chimpanzees	Intravenous	Asymptomatic	Yes	Route of infection does not mimic natural route of HuNoV infections; no clinical disease	Bok et al. (2011), Wyatt et al. (1978)
Immunocompromised mice	Intraperitoneal	Asymptomatic	Not described	Route of infection does not mimic natural route of HuNoV infections; no fecal shedding or clinical disease	Taube et al. (2013)

persistent infection is established, suggesting that IFN-λ-mediated protection may result from the stimulation of innate immunity rather than adaptive immune responses. Interestingly, treatment with antibiotics also prevents persistent MNV enteric infection and requires the presence of the IFN-λ receptor and the transcription factors STAT-1 and IRF3 (Baldridge et al., 2015). This suggests that the interplay between the gut microbiome and innate immune responses may be important in establishing persistent enteric norovirus infections, and this may be particularly relevant in the context of immunocompromised individuals in whom norovirus infection leads to chronic virus shedding. The elimination of persistent enteric MNV infections through exogenous treatment with IFN-λ offers a potential therapeutic for treatment of persons with persistent infections. However, it remains to be determined if IFN-λ administration will have a similar effect on HuNoVs, particularly when administered orally.

MNVs replicate primarily in macrophages and dendritic cells in wild-type mice (Wobus et al., 2004). Upon infection of cells, many proteins, such as Toll-like receptors (TLR), Rig-I-like helicases, and double-stranded RNA-activated protein kinase (PKR), are known to initiate IFN responses to viruses. In bone marrow-derived dendritic cells, melanoma differentiation associated protein-5 (MDA-5) acts as the predominant sensor of MNV-1 and initiates the production of type I IFN, interleukin-6 (IL-6), macrophage chemoattractant protein 1 (MCP-1), and tumor necrosis factor alpha (TNF-α) (McCartney et al., 2008). IFN regulatory factor-3 (IRF-3) and IRF-7 are required for the induction of IFN-α/β in macrophages but not in dendritic cells (Thackray et al., 2012). Translation of MNV-1 proteins is inhibited by both type I and type II IFNs through IFN-induced PKR-independent and PKR-dependent pathways, respectively (Changotra et al., 2009). IFN-γ mediates the inhibition of MNV replicase complex formation in macrophages through a complex formed by autophagy proteins (ATG) Atg5, Atg12, and Atg16L1 (Hwang et al., 2012). The process does not involve the formation of canonical autophagosomes, suggesting that specific components of the autophagy pathway can be used by host cells to induce an antiviral state. Interestingly, IFN-λ does not appear to directly act on immune cells because MNV infection of cultured bone marrow-derived dendritic cells was not inhibited by IFN-λ treatment (Nice et al., 2015). Microarray studies, quantitative polymerase chain reaction, and enzyme-linked immunosorbent assays (ELISA) following infection of macrophage cells (RAW264.7 cell line) with MNV-1 show upregulation of CCL2, CCL3, CCL4, CCL5, CXCL2, CXCL10, and CXCL11, suggesting a Th1-biased cytokine response to infection (Waugh et al., 2014).

Innate immune responses to HuNoVs have been studied in gnotobiotic pigs and calves that are susceptible to infection with some GII.4 strains and develop mild diarrhea (Cheetham et al., 2006; Souza et al., 2008). Unlike MNV infections, in which the virus replicates primarily in immune cells, HuNoV infections occur in the GI tract of gnotobiotic pigs and calves, as determined by the detection of virus antigens in intestinal epithelial cells. Contrary to the data from macrophage cell lines infected with MNV, the serum cytokine profile of pigs infected with HuNoV shows both Th1 and Th2 responses, with an early IFN-γ and delayed IFN-α response (Souza et al., 2007). Induction of the proinflammatory cytokine IL-6, the Th1 cytokine IL-12, the Th2 cytokine IL-4, and the Th2/T-regulatory cytokine IL-10 is seen in serum. Although this is suggestive of a balanced Th1/Th2 response, the numbers of IL-12 and IFN-γ (Th1) cytokine-secreting cells are higher than those of IL-4- and IL-6-secreting cells, both systemically and in intestinal contents. Whereas peak concentrations of IFN-γ and IL-6 are higher in intestinal contents than in serum, only IFN-α and IL-12 cytokine concentrations are significantly higher in the intestinal contents of infected pigs compared to controls. Cholesterol-lowering drugs such as simvastatin enhance the replication of HuNoV in gnotobiotic pigs, possibly through an effect on innate immunity (Jung et al., 2012). The induction of IFN-α in these animals is reduced after simvastatin treatment, which may contribute to increased virus shedding. Furthermore, oral administration of natural human IFN-α to gnotobiotic pigs reduces or even inhibits virus shedding. HuNoV infections in gnotobiotic calves result in more pronounced intestinal lesions compared to those in pigs, and in this model, early increases in IFN-γ and TNF-α in serum coincides with the onset of diarrhea. Cytokine levels in stool are elevated earlier than in serum (Souza et al., 2008). Innate immunity has also been studied in a few in vitro culture systems for HuNoVs. IFN-α and IFN-γ were effective inhibitors of Norwalk virus production in a replicon system (Chang and George, 2007; Chang et al., 2006). However, suppression of innate immunity did not result in enhanced replication following transfection of Norwalk virus RNA in cell lines deficient in IFN-β synthesis (Guix et al., 2007).

7.4 INNATE IMMUNE RESPONSES IN HUMANS

Much less is known about the mechanisms of protection through innate immune responses in humans. A Th1-biased cytokine response was observed in healthy adults who participated in a volunteer challenge study with the genogroup II, genotype 2 (GII.2) Snow Mountain virus. Significant increases in serum levels of IFN-γ and IL-2 were seen, but not other cytokines such as IL-6 and IL-10 at day 2 postchallenge (Lindesmith et al., 2005). Human volunteer challenge with GI.1 Norwalk virus also results in a predominantly Th1 response, although some Th2 cytokines and chemokines are also significantly elevated (Newman et al., 2015). IFN-γ, IL-2, IL-6, IL-8, IL-10, IL-12p70, MCP-1, and TNF-α were significantly higher in Norwalk virus-infected persons compared to uninfected persons. Persons who developed gastroenteritis had elevated levels of both Th1 and Th2 cytokines and IL-8 compared to those with asymptomatic infections. Furthermore, fecal virus titer correlated positively with IL-6 levels and negatively with IL-12p40 concentrations (Newman et al., 2016). Transient production of IFN-γ was also seen in dose-escalation studies with Norwalk virus VLPs (Tacket et al., 2003).

Whereas the bias toward Th1 response is evident from these experimental human infections and vaccination, there are only a few reports of cytokine responses following natural infections in adults and children. In adults hospitalized with acute gastroenteritis in Sweden, serum levels of IL-18, chemokines CXCL9 and CXCL10, soluble IL-2 receptor, and macrophage migration inhibitory factor (MIF) were higher in patients with norovirus infections compared to controls. Lower levels of CCL5 (or RANTES—regulated on activation, normal T cell expressed and secreted) were associated with longer duration of virus shedding (Gustavsson et al., 2015). Assessment of fecal cytokines in samples from US travelers to Mexico who developed norovirus gastroenteritis showed similar results as serum cytokine data from other studies, in which IL-2 and IFN-γ levels were significantly elevated following infection (Ko et al., 2006). Fecal cytokine levels determined in Mexican children showed genogroup-specific cytokine responses, with higher MCP-1 and IL-8 levels in children infected with GI and GII norovirus, respectively, compared to uninfected children (Long et al., 2006). IL-5 levels were higher following infections with both genogroups. In this randomized, double-blind, placebo-controlled, vitamin A supplementation trial, vitamin A showed genogroup-specific effects, with lower levels of MCP-1, IL-8, and IL-6 in cases of GII norovirus diarrhea compared to the placebo group, and increases in TNF-α and IL-4 levels in the GI group. These differences in the effect of vitamin A supplementation are unexpected and may be an outcome of genogroup-specific innate immune responses. Serum IL-6 and IL-8 levels together with clinical outcomes have been evaluated as diagnostic markers to distinguish bacterial and viral infections in children (Chen et al., 2012, 2014). Children infected with rotavirus have significantly higher levels of IL-8 compared to those infected with norovirus, whereas there are no differences in IL-6 levels. However, the diagnostic potential of these markers remains to be ascertained.

Additional studies are required to elucidate the mechanisms by which innate effector molecules mediate protection in humans, and whether and how the virus counters innate responses. The MNV genome codes for an additional open reading frame 4 (ORF-4), and the protein encoded by ORF-4 plays a critical role in antagonizing innate immune responses through interference of IFN pathways and apoptosis (McFadden et al., 2011). ORF-4 has not been described in any HuNoV strain to date. Whether cytokines are a mediator of severe symptoms experienced by individuals infected with HuNoV is another important unanswered question.

7.5 ADAPTIVE IMMUNE RESPONSES IN ANIMALS

Adaptive immune responses to noroviruses have been studied in animal models and following infections in humans. B cell-mediated antibody responses, $CD8^+$ T cells, and $CD4^+$ T cells all appear to play important roles in the control of primary MNV infections. Mice deficient in recombination activation gene (RAG) and that do not produce mature B and T lymphocytes are persistently infected with MNV (Karst et al., 2003; Mumphrey et al., 2007). Although MNV infections are not lethal in $RAG1^{-/-}$ and $RAG2^{-/-}$ mice, viral RNA can be detected in feces and in multiple organs even at 90 days postinfection, indicating that B and T cell responses are critical for virus clearance. MNV replicates to higher titers in B cell-deficient mice early in infection compared to wild-type control mice. Interestingly, B cells have been reported as a site of MNV and HuNoV replication (Jones et al., 2014). Transfer of B cells alone, from mice incapable of producing anti-MNV antibodies, does not result in virus clearance in $RAG1^{-/-}$ mice. However, intraperitoneal injection of MNV immune polyclonal sera results in significant reduction in virus titers systemically and in different segments of the intestine (Chachu et al., 2008b). Similar results are seen with IgG neutralizing monoclonal antibodies made against the MNV capsid protein, suggesting that antibody responses mediated by B cells are important in controlling MNV infections. Depletion of $CD4^+$ and/or $CD8^+$ T cells before adoptive transfer of splenocytes from MNV immune wild-type mice to $RAG1^{-/-}$ recipients results in significant increases in MNV titers in intestinal segments, demonstrating that both immune $CD4^+$ and $CD8^+$ T cells are required for clearance of persistent enteric MNV infection (Chachu et al., 2008a). Importantly, oral infection with MNV induces T cell responses at mucosal sites (Tomov et al., 2013). The relative contributions of each of these cells in adaptive immune responses to MNV are not completely understood. Adaptive responses to MNV, however, appear to be strain-dependent; infections with the CR6 strain that induces chronic infection result in suboptimal $CD8^+$ T cells compared to infections with the CW3 strain that induces an acute infection that is subsequently cleared (Tomov et al., 2013). Primary infection with the virulent MNV-1 strain does not result in protection from homotypic secondary infection, whereas primary infection with the more attenuated and persistent MNV-3 results in protection from the same strain on secondary exposure, as well as providing heterotypic protection against MNV-1 infection (Liu et al., 2009; Zhu et al., 2013). The magnitude of IgA and IgG antibody responses elicited to MNV-1 is lower than that for MNV-3. Notably, divergent MNV strains belong to the same serotype but show strain-specific differences in immune response (Thackray et al., 2007). This may be in part due to strain-specific differences in the induction of innate immune responses or in engaging antigen-presenting cells. Together, these data suggest roles for both host-specific and virus-specific determinants in resistance to and clearance of MNV infections.

Humoral, mucosal, and cellular immune responses to HuNoVs have been determined in gnotobiotic pigs and calves. Infection of gnotobiotic pigs with HuNoV GII.4 strain resulted in the induction of IgM, IgA, and IgG antibodies in sera and intestinal contents with varying kinetics (Souza et al., 2007). In serum, IgM responses peaked on day 4, whereas IgA and IgG responses peaked on day 28. IgM and IgA responses in intestinal contents peaked on day 6, whereas IgG peaked on day 28. Seroconversion occurred in approximately 65% of infected pigs 28 days after infection. Severity of diarrhea correlated with convalescent-phase IgA and IgG levels in serum and intestinal contents. Low numbers of IgA and IgG antibody-secreting cells (ASCs) were detected both systemically and in the intestines of infected animals. Infection of gnotobiotic calves with GII.4 resulted in similar adaptive responses as those of gnotobiotic pigs (Souza et al., 2008). Seroconversion was seen in all infected calves compared to 67% of gnotobiotic pigs. The numbers of intestinal IgA and IgG ASCs were higher in the calf model and correlate with more extensive intestinal lesions in this model compared to pigs.

Antibody responses have also been reported in chimpanzees following oral or intravenous experimental infection of Norwalk virus (Wyatt et al., 1978; Bok et al., 2011). Serum antibody responses following intravenous inoculation were mainly IgM and IgG isotypes, whereas IgA was almost undetectable in stool and serum. Norwalk virus-specific serum antibody levels correlated with protection against challenge in this model, in which virus was inoculated intravenously (Bok et al., 2011). HuNoVs bind histo-blood group antigens (HBGAs) as putative receptors, and antibodies that block the binding of VLPs to HBGAs have been shown to correlate with protection from infection and disease in humans (discussed later) (Atmar et al., 2011, 2015; Reeck et al., 2010). Similar HBGA-blocking activity is seen in chimpanzees. Sera from animals susceptible to infection after challenge did not inhibit VLP binding to H type 3 (H3) HBGA, whereas sera from chimpanzees that were protected could block binding to H3 HBGA. Rhesus macaques also appear to be susceptible to HuNoVs because Norwalk virus-specific IgG and IgM have been detected 2 weeks postinfection in one out of four infected macaques. Seroconversion was not detected in other nonhuman primates, such as marmosets, tamarins, or cynomolgus macaques, when infected with HuNoVs (Rockx et al., 2005b).

7.6 ADAPTIVE IMMUNE RESPONSES IN HUMANS

Adaptive immune responses in humans have been studied in epidemiological studies, volunteer challenge studies, and clinical trials with VLP vaccines. Seroprevalence studies show that the majority of adults worldwide have antibodies to HuNoVs, with higher seroprevalence rates in developing countries (Gray et al., 1993; Greenberg et al., 1979; Menon et al., 2013; Smit et al.,

1999; Carmona-Vicente et al., 2015; O'Ryan et al., 1998; Steinberg et al., 2004; Mesquita and Nascimento, 2014). Early volunteer challenge studies suggest that experimental infection does not confer long-term protection, and protection from disease following exposure to the same strain lasts only for a duration of 6 months to 2 years (Johnson et al., 1990; Parrino et al., 1977; Wyatt et al., 1974). However, recent studies found that only a fraction of genetically susceptible persons were infected after challenge with Norwalk virus, suggesting acquired resistance to infection (Lindesmith et al., 2003). In addition, a mathematical model based on epidemiological observations of norovirus illness frequency estimated that immunity following natural infection lasts 4–9 years (Simmons et al., 2013) (Table 7.2).

The kinetics of antibody responses have been determined through experimental human infections. Following infection with Norwalk virus, serum IgA responses are detected as early as 7 days and peak at approximately 14 days postinfection, whereas IgG responses peak at 4 weeks postinfection (Kavanagh et al., 2011; Erdman et al., 1989). IgM response serves as a marker of recent infection (Brinker et al., 1999; Gray et al., 1994; Erdman et al., 1989). Similar to serum IgA responses, Norwalk virus-specific IgA levels in saliva and fecal samples peak at day 14 after challenge in infected persons (Ramani et al., 2015). Infection with Norwalk virus induces the production of functional antibodies that can block the binding to Norwalk virus VLPs to HBGA (Reeck et al., 2010).

Table 7.2 Immune Correlates of Protection Against HuNoV Infection, Illness, or Virus Shedding

Time Point	Study Type	Immune Correlate of Protection	Outcome	References
Preexposure	Experimental infection	Serum histo-blood antigen (HBGA) group blocking antibody	Infection, gastroenteritis	Reeck et al. (2010)
		Serum hemagglutination inhibition	Gastroenteritis	Czako et al. (2012)
		Virus-specific salivary IgA	Gastroenteritis	Ramani et al. (2015)
		Virus-specific IgG memory B cells	Gastroenteritis	Ramani et al. (2015)
		Virus-specific fecal IgA	Peak virus shedding	Ramani et al. (2015)
	Infectious virus challenge after vaccination	Serum HBGA group blocking antibody	Infection, gastroenteritis	Atmar et al. (2011, 2015)
		Serum IgA	Infection, gastroenteritis	Atmar et al. (2015)
	Natural infection (in children)	Serum IgG	Gastroenteritis	Malm et al. (2014)
		Serum HBGA group blocking antibody	Gastroenteritis	Malm et al. (2014)
Postexposure	Experimental infection	Rapid salivary IgA response (day 5)	Infection	Lindesmith et al. (2003)
		Rapid fecal IgA response (day 7)	Duration of virus shedding	Ramani et al. (2015)

The isotype of "blocking antibodies" has not been well characterized to date, but peak-blocking anti-body titers are seen 4 weeks postinfection, suggesting that at least some of these antibodies may be IgG. On the other hand, IgA purified from serum collected on day 14 from Norwalk virus-infected individuals has also been shown to have HBGA-blocking activity (Lindesmith et al., 2015a). Infection with Norwalk virus induces the production of heterotypic-blocking antibody responses, including to virus genotypes not detected at the time of Norwalk virus challenge (Czako et al., 2015; Lindesmith et al., 2010). This is important because early cross-challenge studies in human volunteers did not demonstrate protective immunity to heterotypic virus strains, although it is possible that some of these results may be due to the high inoculum dosages used (Wyatt et al., 1974). The peak titers and fold increases in cross-blocking antibody levels were modest in comparison to those of the homologous response, but blocking activity was seen against other GI viruses as well as GII.4 variants. Humoral immunity has also been measured following challenge with genogroup II Snow Mountain strain (GII.2) (Lindesmith et al., 2005). Seroconversion, as defined by a greater than four-fold increase in antibody titer from prechallenge levels, occurred in 100% of infected persons by day 14 postinfection. The serum IgG response cross-reacted with VLPs from other genogroup II strains but not with any genogroup I strains tested. A greater than four-fold change in salivary IgA levels was seen in 67% of volunteers and was less cross-reactive compared to serum IgG.

Heterotypic ELISA antibody responses have also been examined in serum samples collected after HuNoV outbreaks. In general, IgG responses were higher to VLPs more closely related to the outbreak strain than to other strains. However, there were genogroup-specific differences in response, with greater frequency of anti-Norwalk VLP antibodies seen when the outbreak strain showed less than 30% amino acid variability from Norwalk virus versus for GII viruses, for which responses were seen only to VLPs that showed less than 6.5% variability from the outbreak strain (Noel et al., 1997). Interestingly, the avidity of antibodies was not found to be different between homologous and heterologous responses in serum samples collected from outbreaks with four different GII HuNoV strains (Rockx et al., 2005a).

The experimental challenge studies were all performed in adults who likely had been primed by multiple previous norovirus infections. There are far fewer studies on immune responses in children. Humoral immune responses were examined in two children presenting with HuNoV gastroenteritis in Japan (Iritani et al., 2007). Kinetics of IgM, IgA, and IgG responses were similar to those of adults, with an early IgM response, peak IgA response approximately 2 weeks after infection, and peak IgG response more than 18 days after infection. Similar to most studies in adults, seroresponses were stronger to homologous VLPs and weaker to VLPs from heterologous strains. Similar results were obtained in another study examining homologous and heterologous IgG and HBGA-blocking antibody responses in five children infected with a GII.4 HuNoV in Finland in which the magnitude of responses was higher to homologous VLPs than to VLPs made from other GII.4 strains (Blazevic et al., 2015c). Follow-up studies have provided insight into the course of development of HuNoV antibodies in children (Blazevic et al., 2015a,b). Multiple HuNoV infections were seen in two Finnish children followed up from birth to 8 years of age (Blazevic et al., 2015a). The level of maternal antibodies, avidity, and HBGA-blocking activity appeared to determine susceptibility to HuNoV infections in infancy. Low-avidity IgG responses were seen in the first year of life, whereas antibodies with high blocking potential and avidity were developed after 2 years.

Much less is known about cellular immune responses in humans following natural or experimental infection. Following experimental challenge with Norwalk virus, IgA and IgG ASC responses peak on day 7 and are biased toward IgA, whereas memory B cell responses peak on day 14 postchallenge and are biased toward IgG. Peak IgA ASC levels correlate with serum and mucosal IgA responses. Virus-specific memory B cells, but not ASCs, persist 180 days after infection. Stimulation of peripheral blood mononuclear cells (PBMCs) from Norwalk virus-infected persons with other GI VLPs shows induction of a broadly reactive T cell response as measured by IFN-γ secretion (Lindesmith et al., 2010). Stimulation of PBMCs collected from Snow Mountain virus-challenged persons on days 8 and 21 postchallenge with VLPs shows a predominant, but not exclusive, Th1 cellular response (Lindesmith et al., 2005). As with serological responses, the cross-reactive Th1 response is seen on stimulation with VLPs from the same genogroup but not other genogroups. Depletion of CD4$^+$ T cells, but not CD8$^+$ T cells, from PBMCs prior to stimulation with VLPs results in decreased IFN-γ production, indicating that this response is dependent on CD4$^+$ T cells. Stimulation of PBMCs from 5 adult volunteer donors with GII.4 VLPs and analysis for activation/maturation markers shows increases in expression of CD80, CD40, and HLADR markers in CD14$^+$ monocytes and CD40, CD86, and HLADR activation markers in CD11c$^+$ myeloid dendritic cells (Ponterio et al., 2013). Upregulation of these markers is known to prime T cells and provides signals for T cell activation and survival. In this case, PBMC stimulation results in increases in production of cytokines, such as TNF-α, IL-6, and IFN-γ. T cell responses appear to be important for clearance of chronic HuNoV infections in immunocompromised persons. In a case series of 13 pediatric hematopoietic stem cell transplant patients with prolonged HuNoV shedding, viral clearance was associated with T cell recovery following immune reconstitution (Saif et al., 2011).

Findings on humoral, mucosal, and cellular immune responses from natural or experimental infection have been confirmed by data obtained from clinical trials with recombinant VLP vaccines (reviewed in Ramani et al., 2016a). Oral immunization with increasing doses of recombinant Norwalk virus VLPs in healthy adults resulted in serum antibody responses in 90% of vaccinees receiving two doses of VLPs (250 μg) administered 3 weeks apart, with no further increase in the higher dosage groups (Tacket et al., 2003). All vaccinees developed significant increases in IgA ASCs. Mucosal IgA responses occurred in less than 50% of vaccinees. Transient lymphoproliferative and IFN-γ responses were seen in lower dosage groups. Significant increases in IgA ASCs were seen in 95% of persons consuming transgenic potatoes expressing the Norwalk virus capsid protein, although IgG and IgA antibody responses were only modest (Tacket et al., 2000). Intranasal administration of Norwalk virus VLP vaccines with monophosphoryl lipid A (MPL) as adjuvant, chitosan as a mucoadherent, and sucrose and mannitol excipients resulted in dose-dependent increases in serum IgA and IgG antibodies, and induction of functional antibodies as measured by hemagglutination inhibition assay (El-Kamary et al., 2010). Immunization by this mucosal route elicited virus-specific IgA ASCs with homing potential to the gut mucosa and peripheral lymphoid tissues and IgG ASCs with homing receptors to peripheral lymphoid tissues. Furthermore, functional memory B cell responses were also induced in response to intranasal immunization, and the frequency of antigen-specific memory B cells correlated with serum antibody and mucosally primed ASCs (Ramirez et al., 2012). Immune responses have also been analyzed following intramuscular immunization with bivalent VLP formulations including GI.1 VLPs and a "consensus" GII.4 VLP designed by aligning the VP1 sequence from three human GII.4 viruses (Parra et al., 2012). Although this route of immunization does not mimic natural infection, robust antibody and cellular responses were seen following vaccination, with a greater magnitude of response to GI.1 VLP compared to GII.4 consensus VLP (Sundararajan et al., 2015; Treanor et al., 2014). Similar to recent experimental infection studies with Norwalk virus,

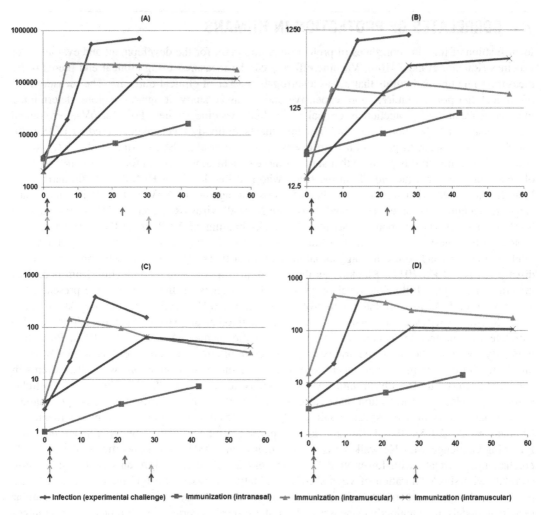

FIGURE 7.1

Kinetics of antibody responses following experimental infection with Norwalk virus or immunization with VLP vaccines. Panels represent serum (A) total ELISA antibody (Ab), (B) histo-blood group (HBGA)-blocking Ab, (C) immunoglobulin A (IgA), and (D) immunoglobulin G (IgG) responses. The time points (days) for infection or immunization are indicated below the X-axis for each graph. Data are collated from studies on norovirus experimental challenge (Atmar et al., 2014) and intranasal (Atmar et al., 2011) and intramuscular immunization (Bernstein et al., 2015; Treanor et al., 2014) with VLP vaccines.

vaccination induced a rapid increase in IgG- and HBGA-blocking antibodies to diverse strains, including those not in circulation at the time of vaccination (Lindesmith et al., 2015b). Serological responses to vaccination occur more rapidly than those to infection, with peak responses by day 7 (Atmar et al., 2015; Treanor et al., 2014); however, the antibody titers post-vaccination are lower compared to natural infection (Fig. 7.1).

7.7 CORRELATES OF PROTECTION IN HUMANS

Identification of immune correlates of protection is important for the development and evaluation of vaccines (Ramani et al., 2016b). Vaccine efficacy can be measured using clinical end points or by measuring immune end points that act as a surrogate marker of clinical outcome. The measurement of clinical end points requires more expensive and intensive study designs; therefore, determining immune correlates of protection is critical to facilitate vaccine studies. For HuNoVs, serological responses appear to be short-lived, and in many studies, antibody levels as measured by ELISA did not always correlate with protection from disease (Johnson et al., 1990; Parrino et al., 1977; Reeck et al., 2010), although it is possible that some of these conclusions were confounded by the inclusion of genetically resistant individuals in the study who had low levels of HuNoV-specific antibodies. Identification of the first immune correlate of protection against HuNoV gastroenteritis in humans came from a human volunteer challenge study with Norwalk virus (Reeck et al., 2010). Prechallenge levels of a functional antibody in serum that blocks binding of VLPs to HBGAs correlate with protection from gastroenteritis. The blocking response can also be measured using hemagglutination inhibition assays, and serum hemagglutination inhibition titers also correlate with protection from disease (Czako et al., 2012). Blocking antibodies are also a correlate of protection from norovirus infection and disease following vaccination with VLP vaccines. In these studies, the presence and levels of serum IgA also correlated with protection from HuNoV infection and disease (Atmar et al., 2011, 2015). Norovirus genotype-specific serum IgG antibodies and HBGA-blocking antibodies also correlate with protection in children in a strain-specific manner (Malm et al., 2014). Protective immunity appears to be strain-specific because induction of strong antibody responses after primary infection with one strain did not appear to protect from subsequent infections with other strains in one child followed up from birth until 2 years of age (Blazevic et al., 2015b). Mucosal and cellular immune correlates of protection have also been identified in experimental challenge studies. Prechallenge levels of virus-specific salivary IgA correlated with protection from gastroenteritis (Ramani et al., 2015). Rapid salivary IgA response correlated with protection from infection following challenge with Norwalk virus (Lindesmith et al., 2003). Virus-specific fecal IgA levels prechallenge correlate with lower viral load, whereas levels of fecal IgA on day 7 postinfection correlate with shorter duration of virus shedding. Finally, virus-specific IgG memory B cell levels prior to challenge also correlate with protection from disease (Ramani et al., 2015). Thus, similar to animal models, both antibody responses and cellular responses correlate with protection from infection and/or disease. The identification of multiple immune correlates of protection raises important questions regarding the mechanisms of protective immunity to HuNoVs. It is likely that some of these immune effector responses covary, and therefore changes in one immune correlate may be reflective of changes in other immune effectors. This makes it difficult to determine the best predictor of protection.

7.8 CONCLUSIONS AND PERSPECTIVES

A comprehensive picture of immune response to noroviruses remains incomplete. MNV infections in wild-type mice do not mimic human disease and thus only serve as infection models for HuNoVs. Given that the cellular tropism for HuNoVs is still unclear, and the possibility that the replication sites for MNVs and HuNoVs are different, it remains to be determined whether findings on innate immune responses to MNVs will be applicable to human strains. Nonetheless, studies with MNV have provided insights into norovirus immune responses. Infections in gnotobiotic pigs and calves mimic human disease to a greater extent and are physiologically closer models to the human gut. However, these pigs and calves lack a functional microbiome, which may confound results on protective immune responses. Although there are a significant number of studies on humoral responses to HuNoVs in humans, there are few data on other aspects of immunity, such as mucosal, T cell, and cytokine responses. Moreover, most of the current data on immune responses are from studies of healthy adults. Data on how these responses vary in children and in immuno-compromised persons are limited and remain to be clearly understood. The development of robust and reproducible cell culture systems for HuNoVs will facilitate quicker progress in understanding immune responses and pathogenesis. A better understanding of immune responses to HuNoVs, particularly the correlates of protection from infection and disease, is critical for vaccine studies and the development of therapeutics.

REFERENCES

Ahmed, S.M., Hall, A.J., Robinson, A.E., Verhoef, L., Premkumar, P., Parashar, U.D., et al., 2014. Global prevalence of norovirus in cases of gastroenteritis: a systematic review and meta-analysis. Lancet Infect. Dis. 14, 725–730.

Atmar, R.L., Opekun, A.R., Gilger, M.A., Estes, M.K., Crawford, S.E., Neill, F.H., et al., 2008. Norwalk virus shedding after experimental human infection. Emerg. Infect. Dis. 14, 1553–1557.

Atmar, R.L., Bernstein, D.I., Harro, C.D., Al-Ibrahim, M.S., Chen, W.H., Ferreira, J., et al., 2011. Norovirus vaccine against experimental human Norwalk Virus illness. New Engl. J. Med. 365, 2178–2187.

Atmar, R.L., Opekun, A.R., Gilger, M.A., Estes, M.K., Crawford, S.E., Neill, F.H., et al., 2014. Determination of the 50% human infectious dose for Norwalk virus. J. Infect. Dis. 209, 1016–1022.

Atmar, R.L., Bernstein, D.I., Lyon, G.M., Treanor, J.J., Al-Ibrahim, M.S., Graham, D.Y., et al., 2015. Serological correlates of protection against a GII.4 norovirus. Clin. Vaccine Immunol. 22, 923–929.

Baldridge, M.T., Nice, T.J., Mccune, B.T., Yokoyama, C.C., Kambal, A., Wheadon, M., et al., 2015. Commensal microbes and interferon-lambda determine persistence of enteric murine norovirus infection. Science 347, 266–269.

Bank-Wolf, B.R., Konig, M., Thiel, H.J., 2010. Zoonotic aspects of infections with noroviruses and sapo-viruses. Vet. Microbiol. 140, 204–212.

Bartsch, S.M., Lopman, B.A., Hall, A.J., Parashar, U.D., Lee, B.Y., 2012. The potential economic value of a human norovirus vaccine for the United States. Vaccine 30, 7097–7104.

Bernstein, D.I., Atmar, R.L., Lyon, G.M., Treanor, J.J., Chen, W.H., Jiang, X., et al., 2015. Norovirus vaccine against experimental human GII.4 virus illness: a challenge study in healthy adults. J. Infect. Dis. 211, 870–878.

Blazevic, V., Malm, M., Honkanen, H., Knip, M., Hyoty, H., Vesikari, T., 2015a. Development and maturation of norovirus antibodies in childhood. Microbes Infect 18, 263–269.

Blazevic, V., Malm, M., Salminen, M., Oikarinen, S., Hyoty, H., Veijola, R., et al., 2015b. Multiple consecu-tive norovirus infections in the first 2 years of life. Eur. J. Pediatr. 174, 1679–1683.

Blazevic, V., Malm, M., Vesikari, T., 2015c. Induction of homologous and cross-reactive GII.4-specific block-ing antibodies in children after GII.4 New Orleans norovirus infection. J. Med. Virol. 87, 1656–1661.

Bok, K., Parra, G.I., Mitra, T., Abente, E., Shaver, C., et al., 2011. Chimpanzees as an animal model for human norovirus infection and vaccine development. Proc. Natl. Acad. Sci. USA 108, 325–330.

Brinker, J.P., Blacklow, N.R., Jiang, X., Estes, M.K., Moe, C.L., Herrmann, J.E., 1999. Immunoglobulin M antibody test to detect genogroup II Norwalk-like virus infection. J. Clin. Microbiol. 37, 2983–2986.

Carmona-Vicente, N., Fernandez-Jimenez, M., Ribes, J.M., Tellez-Castillo, C.J., Khodayar-Pardo, P., Rodriguez-Diaz, J., et al., 2015. Norovirus infections and seroprevalence of genotype GII.4-specific antibodies in a Spanish population. J. Med. Virol. 87, 675–682.

Chachu, K.A., Lobue, A.D., Strong, D.W., Baric, R.S., Virgin, H.W., 2008a. Immune mechanisms responsible for vaccination against and clearance of mucosal and lymphatic norovirus infection. PLoS Pathog. 4, e1000236.

Chachu, K.A., Strong, D.W., Lobue, A.D., Wobus, C.E., Baric, R.S., Virgin, H.W.T., 2008b. Antibody is critical for the clearance of murine norovirus infection. J. Virol. 82, 6610–6617.

Chang, K.O., George, D.W., 2007. Interferons and ribavirin effectively inhibit Norwalk virus replication in replicon-bearing cells. J. Virol. 81, 12111–12118.

Chang, K.O., Sosnovtsev, S.V., Belliot, G., King, A.D., Green, K.Y., 2006. Stable expression of a Norwalk virus RNA replicon in a human hepatoma cell line. Virology 353, 463–473.

Changotra, H., Jia, Y., Moore, T.N., Liu, G., Kahan, S.M., Sosnovtsev, S.V., et al., 2009. Type I and type II interferons inhibit the translation of murine norovirus proteins. J. Virol. 83, 5683–5692.

Cheetham, S., Souza, M., Meulia, T., Grimes, S., Han, M.G., Saif, L.J., 2006. Pathogenesis of a genogroup II human norovirus in gnotobiotic pigs. J. Virol. 80, 10372–10381.

Chen, S.M., Ku, M.S., Lee, M.Y., Tsai, J.D., Sheu, J.N., 2012. Diagnostic performance of serum interleukin-6 and interleukin-10 levels and clinical predictors in children with rotavirus and norovirus gastroenteritis. Cytokine 59, 299–304.

Chen, S.M., Lin, C.P., Tsai, J.D., Chao, Y.H., Sheu, J.N., 2014. The significance of serum and fecal levels of interleukin-6 and interleukin-8 in hospitalized children with acute rotavirus and norovirus gastroenteritis. Pediatr. Neonatol. 55, 120–126.

Czako, R., Atmar, R.L., Opekun, A.R., Gilger, M.A., Graham, D.Y., Estes, M.K., 2012. Serum hemagglutination inhibition activity correlates with protection from gastroenteritis in persons infected with Norwalk virus. Clin. Vaccine Immunol. 19, 284–287.

Czako, R., Atmar, R.L., Opekun, A.R., Gilger, M.A., Graham, D.Y., Estes, M.K., 2015. Experimental human infection with Norwalk virus elicits a surrogate neutralizing antibody response with cross-genogroup activity. Clin. Vaccine Immunol. 22, 221–228.

El-Kamary, S.S., Pasetti, M.F., Mendelman, P.M., Frey, S.E., Bernstein, D.I., Treanor, J.J., et al., 2010. Adjuvanted intranasal Norwalk virus-like particle vaccine elicits antibodies and antibody-secreting cells that express homing receptors for mucosal and peripheral lymphoid tissues. J. Infect. Dis. 202, 1649–1658.

Erdman, D.D., Gary, G.W., Anderson, L.J., 1989. Serum immunoglobulin A response to Norwalk virus infection. J. Clin. Microbiol. 27, 1417–1418.

Gastanaduy, P.A., Hall, A.J., Curns, A.T., Parashar, U.D., Lopman, B.A., 2013. Burden of norovirus gastroenteritis in the ambulatory setting—United States, 2001–2009. J. Infect. Dis. 207, 1058–1065.

Graham, D.Y., Jiang, X., Tanaka, T., Opekun, A.R., Madore, H.P., Estes, M.K., 1994. Norwalk virus infection of volunteers: new insights based on improved assays. J. Infect. Dis. 170, 34–43.

Gray, J.J., Jiang, X., Morgan-Capner, P., Desselberger, U., Estes, M.K., 1993. Prevalence of antibodies to Norwalk virus in England: detection by enzyme-linked immunosorbent assay using baculovirus-expressed Norwalk virus capsid antigen. J. Clin. Microbiol. 31, 1022–1025.

Gray, J.J., Cunliffe, C., Ball, J., Graham, D.Y., Desselberger, U., Estes, M.K., 1994. Detection of immunoglobulin M (IgM), IgA, and IgG Norwalk virus-specific antibodies by indirect enzyme-linked immunosorbent assay with baculovirus-expressed Norwalk virus capsid antigen in adult volunteers challenged with Norwalk virus. J. Clin. Microbiol. 32, 3059–3063.

Greenberg, H.B., Valdesuso, J., Kapikian, A.Z., Chanock, R.M., Wyatt, R.G., Szmuness, W., et al., 1979. Prevalence of antibody to the Norwalk virus in various countries. Infect. Immun. 26, 270–273.

Guix, S., Asanaka, M., Katayama, K., Crawford, S.E., Neill, F.H., Atmar, R.L., et al., 2007. Norwalk virus RNA is infectious in mammalian cells. J. Virol. 81, 12238–12248.

Gustavsson, L., Skovbjerg, S., Lindh, M., Westin, J., Andersson, L.M., 2015. Low serum levels of CCL5 are associated with longer duration of viral shedding in norovirus infection. J. Clin. Virol. 69, 133–137.

Hwang, S., Maloney, N.S., Bruinsma, M.W., Goel, G., Duan, E., Zhang, L., et al., 2012. Nondegradative role of Atg5–Atg12/Atg16L1 autophagy protein complex in antiviral activity of interferon gamma. Cell. Host Microb. 11, 397–409.

Iritani, N., Seto, T., Hattori, H., Natori, K., Takeda, N., Kubo, H., et al., 2007. Humoral immune responses against norovirus infections of children. J. Med. Virol. 79, 1187–1193.

Johnson, P.C., Mathewson, J.J., Dupont, H.L., Greenberg, H.B., 1990. Multiple-challenge study of host susceptibility to Norwalk gastroenteritis in US adults. J. Infect. Dis. 161, 18–21.

Jones, M.K., Watanabe, M., Zhu, S., Graves, C.L., Keyes, L.R., et al., 2014. Enteric bacteria promote human and mouse norovirus infection of B cells. Science 346, 755–759.

Jung, K., Wang, Q., Kim, Y., Scheuer, K., Zhang, Z., Shen, Q., et al., 2012. The effects of simvastatin or interferon-alpha on infectivity of human norovirus using a gnotobiotic pig model for the study of antivirals. PLoS ONE 7, e41619.

Karst, S.M., Wobus, C.E., Lay, M., Davidson, J., Virgin, H.W.T., 2003. STAT1-dependent innate immunity to a Norwalk-like virus. Science 299, 1575–1578.

Kavanagh, O., Estes, M.K., Reeck, A., Raju, R.M., Opekun, A.R., Gilger, M.A., et al., 2011. Serological responses to experimental Norwalk virus infection measured using a quantitative duplex time-resolved fluorescence immunoassay. Clin. Vaccine Immunol. 18, 1187–1190.

Ko, G., Jiang, Z.D., Okhuysen, P.C., Dupont, H.L., 2006. Fecal cytokines and markers of intestinal inflammation in international travelers with diarrhea due to Noroviruses. J. Med. Virol. 78, 825–828.

Lindesmith, L., Moe, C., Marionneau, S., Ruvoen, N., Jiang, X., Lindblad, L., et al., 2003. Human susceptibility and resistance to Norwalk virus infection. Nat. Med. 9, 548–553.

Lindesmith, L., Moe, C., Lependu, J., Frelinger, J.A., Treanor, J., Baric, R.S., 2005. Cellular and humoral immunity following Snow Mountain virus challenge. J. Virol. 79, 2900–2909.

Lindesmith, L.C., Donaldson, E., Leon, J., Moe, C.L., Frelinger, J.A., Johnston, R.E., et al., 2010. Heterotypic humoral and cellular immune responses following Norwalk virus infection. J. Virol. 84, 1800–1815.

Lindesmith, L.C., Beltramello, M., Swanstrom, J., Jones, T.A., Corti, D., Lanzavecchia, A., et al., 2015a. Serum immunoglobulin A cross-strain blockade of human noroviruses. Open Forum Infect. Dis. 2, ofv084.

Lindesmith, L.C., Ferris, M.T., Mullan, C.W., Ferreira, J., Debbink, K., Swanstrom, J., et al., 2015b. Broad blockade antibody responses in human volunteers after immunization with a multivalent norovirus VLP candidate vaccine: immunological analyses from a phase I clinical trial. PLoS Med. 12, e1001807.

Liu, G., Kahan, S.M., Jia, Y., Karst, S.M., 2009. Primary high-dose murine norovirus 1 infection fails to protect from secondary challenge with homologous virus. J. Virol. 83, 6963–6968.

Long, K.Z., Santos, J.I., Estrada Garcia, T., Haas, M., Firestone, M., Bhagwat, J., et al., 2006. Vitamin A supplementation reduces the monocyte chemoattractant protein-1 intestinal immune response of Mexican children. J. Nutr. 136, 2600–2605.

Malm, M., Uusi-Kerttula, H., Vesikari, T., Blazevic, V., 2014. High serum levels of norovirus genotype-specific blocking antibodies correlate with protection from infection in children. J. Infect. Dis. 210, 1755–1762.

Mccartney, S.A., Thackray, L.B., Gitlin, L., Gilfillan, S., Virgin, H.W., Colonna, M., 2008. MDA-5 recognition of a murine norovirus. PLoS Pathog. 4, e1000108.

Mcfadden, N., Bailey, D., Carrara, G., Benson, A., Chaudhry, Y., Shortland, A., et al., 2011. Norovirus regulation of the innate immune response and apoptosis occurs via the product of the alternative open reading frame 4. PLoS Pathog. 7, e1002413.

Menon, V.K., George, S., Aladin, F., Nawaz, S., Sarkar, R., Lopman, B., et al., 2013. Comparison of age-stratified seroprevalence of antibodies against norovirus GII in India and the United Kingdom. PLoS ONE 8, e56239.

Mesquita, J.R., Nascimento, M.S., 2014. Norovirus GII.4 antibodies in the Portuguese population. J. Infect. Dev. Countr. 8, 1201–1204.

Mumphrey, S.M., Changotra, H., Moore, T.N., Heimann-Nichols, E.R., Wobus, C.E., Reilly, M.J., et al., 2007. Murine norovirus 1 infection is associated with histopathological changes in immunocompetent hosts, but clinical disease is prevented by STAT1-dependent interferon responses. J. Virol. 81, 3251–3263.

Newman, K.L., Moe, C.L., Kirby, A.E., Flanders, W.D., Parkos, C.A., Leon, J.S., 2015. Human norovirus infection and the acute serum cytokine response. Clin. Exp. Immunol. 182, 195–203.

Newman, K.L., Moe, C.L., Kirby, A.E., Flanders, W.D., Parkos, C.A., Leon, J.S., 2016. Norovirus in symptomatic and asymptomatic individuals: cytokines and viral shedding. Clin. Exp. Immunol 41, 227–232.

Nice, T.J., Baldridge, M.T., Mccune, B.T., Norman, J.M., Lazear, H.M., Artyomov, M., et al., 2015. Interferon-lambda cures persistent murine norovirus infection in the absence of adaptive immunity. Science 347, 269–273.

Noel, J.S., Ando, T., Leite, J.P., Green, K.Y., Dingle, K.E., Estes, M.K., et al., 1997. Correlation of patient immune responses with genetically characterized small round-structured viruses involved in outbreaks of nonbacterial acute gastroenteritis in the United States, 1990 to 1995. J. Med. Virol. 53, 372–383.

O'ryan, M.L., Vial, P.A., Mamani, N., Jiang, X., Estes, M.K., Ferrecio, C., et al., 1998. Seroprevalence of Norwalk virus and Mexico virus in Chilean individuals: assessment of independent risk factors for antibody acquisition. Clin. Infect. Dis. 27, 789–795.

Parra, G.I., Bok, K., Taylor, R., Haynes, J.R., Sosnovtsev, S.V., Richardson, C., et al., 2012. Immunogenicity and specificity of norovirus consensus GII.4 virus-like particles in monovalent and bivalent vaccine formulations. Vaccine 30, 3580–3586.

Parrino, T.A., Schreiber, D.S., Trier, J.S., Kapikian, A.Z., Blacklow, N.R., 1977. Clinical immunity in acute gastroenteritis caused by Norwalk agent. New Engl. J. Med. 297, 86–89.

Payne, D.C., Vinje, J., Szilagyi, P.G., Edwards, K.M., Staat, M.A., Weinberg, G.A., et al., 2013. Norovirus and medically attended gastroenteritis in U.S. children. New Engl. J. Med. 368, 1121–1130.

Ponterio, E., Petrizzo, A., DI Bartolo, I., Buonaguro, F.M., Buonaguro, L., Ruggeri, F.M., 2013. Pattern of activation of human antigen presenting cells by genotype GII.4 norovirus virus-like particles. J. Transl. Med. 11, 127.

Ramani, S., Estes, M.K., Atmar, R.L., 2016a. Norovirus vaccine development. In: Svensson, L., Desselberger, U., Estes, M.K., Greenberg, H.B. (Eds.), Viral Gastroenteritis. Elsevier, Amsterdam.

Ramani, S., Estes, M.K., Atmar, R.L., 2016b. Correlates of protection against norovirus infection and disease—where are we now, where do we go? PloS Pathog. 12 (4), e1005334.

Ramani, S., Neill, F.H., Opekun, A.R., Gilger, M.A., Graham, D.Y., Estes, M.K., et al., 2015. Mucosal and cellular immune responses to Norwalk virus. J Infect Dis. 212, 397–405.

Ramirez, K., Wahid, R., Richardson, C., Bargatze, R.F., El-Kamary, S.S., Sztein, M.B., et al., 2012. Intranasal vaccination with an adjuvanted Norwalk virus-like particle vaccine elicits antigen-specific B memory responses in human adult volunteers. Clin. Immunol. 144, 98–108.

Reeck, A., Kavanagh, O., Estes, M.K., Opekun, A.R., Gilger, M.A., Graham, D.Y., et al., 2010. Serological correlate of protection against norovirus-induced gastroenteritis. J. Infect. Dis. 202, 1212–1218.

Rockx, B., Baric, R.S., DE Grijs, I., Duizer, E., Koopmans, M.P., 2005a. Characterization of the homo- and heterotypic immune responses after natural norovirus infection. J. Med. Virol. 77, 439–446.

Rockx, B.H., Bogers, W.M., Heeney, J.L., Van Amerongen, G., Koopmans, M.P., 2005b. Experimental norovirus infections in non-human primates. J. Med. Virol. 75, 313–320.

Saif, M.A., Bonney, D.K., Bigger, B., Forsythe, L., Williams, N., Page, J., et al., 2011. Chronic norovirus infection in pediatric hematopoietic stem cell transplant recipients: a cause of prolonged intestinal failure requiring intensive nutritional support. Pediatr. Transplant. 15, 505–509.

Scallan, E., Hoekstra, R.M., Angulo, F.J., Tauxe, R.V., Widdowson, M.A., Roy, S.L., et al., 2011. Foodborne illness acquired in the United States—major pathogens. Emerg. Infect. Dis. 17, 7–15.

Simmons, K., Gambhir, M., Leon, J., Lopman, B., 2013. Duration of immunity to norovirus gastroenteritis. Emerg. Infect. Dis. 19, 1260–1267.

Smit, T.K., Bos, P., Peenze, I., Jiang, X., Estes, M.K., Steele, A.D., 1999. Seroepidemiological study of genogroup I and II calicivirus infections in South and southern Africa. J. Med. Virol. 59, 227–231.

Souza, M., Cheetham, S.M., Azevedo, M.S., Costantini, V., Saif, L.J., 2007. Cytokine and antibody responses in gnotobiotic pigs after infection with human norovirus genogroup II.4 (HS66 strain). J. Virol. 81, 9183–9192.

Souza, M., Azevedo, M.S., Jung, K., Cheetham, S., Saif, L.J., 2008. Pathogenesis and immune responses in gnotobiotic calves after infection with the genogroup II.4-HS66 strain of human norovirus. J. Virol. 82, 1777–1786.

Steinberg, E.B., Mendoza, C.E., Glass, R., Arana, B., Lopez, M.B., Mejia, M., et al., 2004. Prevalence of infection with waterborne pathogens: a seroepidemiologic study in children 6–36 months old in San Juan Sacatepequez, Guatemala. Am. J. Trop. Med. Hyg. 70, 83–88.

Sundararajan, A., Sangster, M.Y., Frey, S., Atmar, R.L., Chen, W.H., Ferreira, J., et al., 2015. Robust mucosal-homing antibody-secreting B cell responses induced by intramuscular administration of adjuvanted bivalent human norovirus-like particle vaccine. Vaccine 33, 568–576.

Tacket, C.O., Mason, H.S., Losonsky, G., Estes, M.K., Levine, M.M., Arntzen, C.J., 2000. Human immune responses to a novel Norwalk virus vaccine delivered in transgenic potatoes. J. Infect. Dis. 182, 302–305.

Tacket, C.O., Sztein, M.B., Losonsky, G.A., Wasserman, S.S., Estes, M.K., 2003. Humoral, mucosal, and cellular immune responses to oral Norwalk virus-like particles in volunteers. Clin. Immunol. 108, 241–247.

Taube, S., Kolawole, A.O., Hohne, M., Wilkinson, J.E., Handley, S.A., Perry, J.W., et al., 2013. A mouse model for human norovirus. MBio 4, e00450–13.

Thackray, L.B., Wobus, C.E., Chachu, K.A., Liu, B., Alegre, E.R., Henderson, K.S., et al., 2007. Murine noroviruses comprising a single genogroup exhibit biological diversity despite limited sequence divergence. J. Virol. 81, 10460–10473.

Thackray, L.B., Duan, E., Lazear, H.M., Kambal, A., Schreiber, R.D., Diamond, M.S., et al., 2012. Critical role for interferon regulatory factor 3 (IRF-3) and IRF-7 in type I interferon-mediated control of murine norovirus replication. J. Virol. 86, 13515–13523.

Tomov, V.T., Osborne, L.C., Dolfi, D.V., Sonnenberg, G.F., Monticelli, L.A., Mansfield, K., et al., 2013. Persistent enteric murine norovirus infection is associated with functionally suboptimal virus-specific CD8 T cell responses. J. Virol. 87, 7015–7031.

Treanor, J.J., Atmar, R.L., Frey, S.E., Gormley, R., Chen, W.H., Ferreira, J., et al., 2014. A novel intramuscular bivalent norovirus virus-like particle vaccine candidate—reactogenicity, safety, and immunogenicity in a phase 1 trial in healthy adults. J. Infect. Dis. 210, 1763–1771.

Waugh, E., Chen, A., Baird, M.A., Brown, C.M., Ward, V.K., 2014. Characterization of the chemokine response of RAW264.7 cells to infection by murine norovirus. Virus Res. 181, 27–34.

Wobus, C.E., Karst, S.M., Thackray, L.B., Chang, K.O., Sosnovtsev, S.V., Belliot, G., et al., 2004. Replication of norovirus in cell culture reveals a tropism for dendritic cells and macrophages. PLoS Biol. 2, e432.

Wyatt, R.G., Dolin, R., Blacklow, N.R., Dupont, H.L., Buscho, R.F., Thornhill, T.S., et al., 1974. Comparison of three agents of acute infectious nonbacterial gastroenteritis by cross-challenge in volunteers. J. Infect. Dis. 129, 709−714.

Wyatt, R.G., Greenberg, H.B., Dalgard, D.W., Allen, W.P., Sly, D.L., Thornhill, T.S., et al., 1978. Experimental infection of chimpanzees with the Norwalk agent of epidemic viral gastroenteritis. J. Med. Virol. 2, 89−96.

Zhu, S., Regev, D., Watanabe, M., Hickman, D., Moussatche, N., Jesus, D.M., et al., 2013. Identification of immune and viral correlates of norovirus protective immunity through comparative study of intra-cluster norovirus strains. PLoS Pathog. 9, e1003592.

DETECTION AND DIAGNOSIS

IV

CHAPTER

DETECTION AND LABORATORY DIAGNOSIS OF NOROVIRUSES

Xiaoli Pang

University of Alberta, Edmonton, Alberta, Canada

8.1 INTRODUCTION

As a result of the development and application of advanced molecular tools in diagnostics, surveillance, and research, norovirus has been recognized as the most important pathogen of sporadic gastroenteritis and global epidemics of gastroenteritis outbreaks (Siebenga et al., 2009; Ahmed et al., 2014). Norovirus has caused at least six global epidemics of gastroenteritis outbreaks and 50–70% of institutional outbreaks worldwide since 1996 (Siebenga et al., 2009; Vinjé, 2015). With the administration of rotavirus vaccine in many countries, norovirus is quickly becoming the leading cause of sporadic gastroenteritis in both pediatric and adult populations (Ahmed et al., 2014; Payne et al., 2013; Koo et al., 2013; Hemming et al., 2013). Based on a systematic review of 31 studies in both developed and developing countries, it was estimated that norovirus accounted for 10–15% of severe gastroenteritis cases in children younger than age 5 years and 9–15% of mild and moderate diarrheal disorders in populations of various ages, leading to 1.7–1.9 million outpatient visits and 19–21 million total illnesses per year in the United States (Payne et al., 2013). Clinically, severe norovirus-associated diseases could lead to hospitalization, increased morbidity, and even death among infants, children, the elderly, and immunocompromised persons. Thus, rapid and accurate identification of causative viral agents is critical for the management of ill patients and the prevention and control of hospital-acquired infections and community outbreaks. Noroviruses are also common causative agents of foodborne, waterborne, and even airborne infectious diseases (Tung-Thompson et al., 2015). Norovirus is readily transmitted by eating or drinking contaminated food or beverages, which usually results in outbreaks in social gatherings. A large waterborne outbreak caused by drinking water contaminated with norovirus was recently reported in Prague; it involved approximately 32,000 people with virus exposure, 12,000 illnesses, and 33 hospital admissions (Kozisek, 2015).

Noroviruses are a group of small (30–38 nm in diameter), round, nonenveloped, single-stranded, positive-sense RNA viruses classified into the genus *Norovirus* of the family *Caliciviridae*. Norovirus is classified into seven genogroups (GI–GVII) and more than 40 genotypes based on viral protein 1 (VP1) nucleotide sequences. The GI, GII, and GIV genogroups are mainly involved in human infections. Nine genotypes of GI, 22 genotypes of GII, and 2 genotypes of GIV have been identified (Zheng et al., 2006; Vinjé, 2015). Up to 85% of global epidemics of

The Norovirus. DOI: http://dx.doi.org/10.1016/B978-0-12-804177-2.00008-7

norovirus infections have been dominated by different GII genotype 4 (GII.4) variants, which are also important for sporadic gastroenteritis (Hoa Tran et al., 2013; Lee et al., 2008). Norovirus GII.4 was found to have a higher mutation rate and a faster pace of evolution than other norovirus strains, increasing its epidemiological fitness and diagnostic challenges (Bull et al., 2010). A novel strain, GII.P17_GII.17 strain (GII.17 Kawasaki 2014), emerged in 2014 and surpassed GII.4 as the predominant strain in outbreak settings in the winter of 2014−15 in China (Fu et al., 2015; Lu et al., 2015; Han et al., 2015). Norovirus GII.17 strains have been sporadically detected in Africa, Asia, Europe, North America, and South America (de Graaf et al., 2015). Recent analysis of 81 complete VP1 sequences of GII.17 Kawasaki 2014 suggested that this strain has mutated faster than GII.4 Sydney 2012 (Chan et al., 2015).

Laboratory testing for norovirus has undergone significant development during the past four decades since the virus was discovered by Dr. Kapikian using immune electron microscopy (EM) (Kapikian et al., 1972). Although research laboratories can produce recombinant P particles and virus-like particles (VLPs) that share similar morphological and antigenic characteristics with native norovirus and can be used as a vehicle for vaccine development, the inability to produce a large volume of naturally occurring viral particles in in vitro culture and the absence of small animal models hamper the development of serological diagnostic assays (Aliabadi et al., 2015; Yi et al., 2015). Currently, quantitative reverse transcription−polymerase chain reaction (RT-qPCR) is considered the most sensitive assay to detect norovirus in both research and clinical settings (Vinjé, 2015; Pang and Lee, 2015). However, there are still limitations with this approach, including the need for a multistep procedure, relatively high cost, need for special instruments, and being "too sensitive" to provide results relevant to clinical situations. Simple, affordable, and rapid testing methods such as enzyme immunoassay (EIA) or enzyme-linked immunosorbent assay (ELISA) for norovirus have been developed but generally have low sensitivity and thus limited utility. Novel nanotechnology array-based assays for norovirus are in development and/or being validated. A major breakthrough with nanotechnology-based assays will be the development of point-of-care tests featuring rapidity, affordability, and potential use in many settings, including resource-limited regions and in the field. Some of these prototypes still require validation before their implementation in clinical diagnostics. The future direction of technology development for norovirus detection will likely focus on method simplification, cost-effectiveness, analytic precision, and accuracy. This chapter discusses methods used in the detection of norovirus and the evolution of laboratory diagnostic technologies in this regard.

8.2 LABORATORY TESTING METHODS FOR NOROVIRUSES

8.2.1 DIRECT DETECTION

8.2.1.1 Electron microscopy

Norovirus can be identified using EM by visualizing the shape and size of intact viral particles during examination of a very small amount of stool sample. This traditional method offers the advantages of simple preparation of sample and the ability to detect norovirus and other viruses with different morphologies, if present. However, EM has low sensitivity for small round-structured viruses and cannot differentiate norovirus, sapovirus, and astrovirus due to similar shape and size. In a prospective study, EM missed all 403 norovirus-positive samples out of 2486 stool samples as detected by RT-qPCR (Pang et al., 2014). There is also a high cost associated with the maintenance of the EM instrument and the requirement for specialized technical expertise; thus, EM is usually performed only in public health or large hospital laboratories. EM with its low sensitivity and specificity has largely been replaced by molecular methods for the detection of norovirus (Pang and Lee, 2015).

8.2.1.2 Immunoassays for norovirus antigen detection

Since 2003, numerous antigenic detection assays have been developed for direct detection of norovirus antigen due to its rapid, relatively inexpensive, simple protocol and the fact that it is highly adoptable for use (Richards et al., 2003; Burton-MacLeod et al., 2004; Gray et al., 2007; Takanashi et al., 2008; Khamrin et al., 2008; Derrington et al., 2009; Bruins et al., 2010; Kirby et al., 2010a; Bruggink et al., 2011; Geginat et al., 2012; Ambert-Balay and Pothier, 2013; Shigemoto et al., 2014). Common formats of antigen detection assays include the conventional 96-well microplate EIA, rapid membrane-based immunochromatographic assays, and, recently, bioluminescent EIA (Shigemoto et al., 2014). However, the number of antigen detection assays remains limited for norovirus because of the absence of broadly recognizing antibodies that can capture and detect conserved viral antigens in this highly diversified virus. Due to the high degree of antigenic diversity of norovirus, the sensitivity of many antigen detection assays is still low, even though their test performance is better than that of EM. Further improvement in the sensitivity of existing antigen detection assays is needed.

Although a number of norovirus antigen detection assays have been commercialized, most of these assays are only CE marked in Europe for in vitro diagnostic use and are not yet available in North America. Only one norovirus assay (RIDASCREEN Norovirus 3rd Generation EIA from R-Biopharm AG, Darmstadt, Germany) has been licensed by the US Food and Drug Administration and used for preliminary identification of norovirus in outbreak screening. Norovirus antigen detection assays have been used mainly in research settings and are not recommended for routine clinical diagnostic applications (Dunbar et al., 2013). Several evaluation studies on commercial EIA and immunochromatographic kits for norovirus showed much lower sensitivity compared to RT-PCR, with significantly lower detection of norovirus GI and GII (Duizer et al., 2007).

8.2.2 NUCLEI ACID-BASED DETECTION

Nucleic acid testing (NAT) methods based on RT-PCR, available since the 1990s with the cloning of norovirus, are currently considered the gold standard for norovirus diagnostics (Pang and Lee, 2015; Jiang et al., 1993) (Fig. 8.1). These NAT amplification methods are very sensitive and have become increasingly important for accurate detection of norovirus in clinical samples (Dunbar et al., 2013). On the other hand, the clinical interpretation of a positive result of norovirus NAT in patients who might have prolonged, probably asymptomatic, shedding (e.g., solid organ or bone marrow transplant patients) is complicated. Moreover, the inability to assess infectiousness of human norovirus also presents unanswered questions for infection control for these patients.

8.2.2.1 Extraction and preparation of norovirus RNA for amplification testing

One of the major challenges of virus detection in stool specimens by NAT is the presence of PCR/RT-PCR inhibitors, which can lead to false-negative results. Different approaches have been

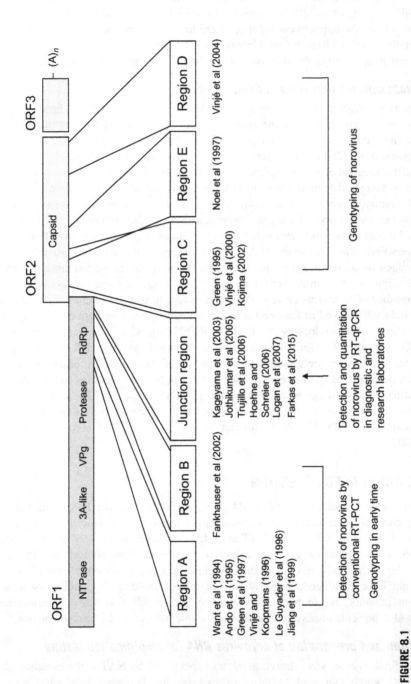

FIGURE 8.1

Schematic of norovirus genome and position of the primers and probes that are commonly used in the detection and genotyping of norovirus.

developed and undertaken to reduce inhibitory substances and their effects—for example, dilution of stool samples and/or extracted total nucleic acid (TNA); adding chelating agents, detergents, or denaturing chemicals during RNA extraction; and inclusion of amplification facilitators such as bovine serum albumin and betaine during PCR (Rasool et al., 2002; Al-Soud and Radstrom, 2001). An inhibitory effect on PCR can be monitored by adding known exogenous DNA/RNA to the sample as an internal control during TNA extraction. Most commercial TNA extraction protocols now use silica- or magnetic bead-based extraction technologies that are simple, efficient, and provide an adequate amount of high-quality TNA. Establishment of an efficient extraction method is essential for the removal of contaminants from cellular proteins, carbohydrates, and lipids to eliminate inhibitors or interference in the downstream amplification step.

TNA extracts from stool specimens usually contain large amounts of nonviral RNA from different microorganisms and host cells that can be nonspecifically amplified by primers specifically designed for norovirus. These nonspecific RT-PCR products cannot be eliminated even under the high-stringency conditions of the reactions. Thus, hybridization with norovirus-specific probes or amplicon sequencing is usually required as part of the process to confirm the results.

8.2.2.2 Quantitative real-time RT-PCR

Currently, real-time RT-qPCR is commonly used by clinical laboratories to detect norovirus with a variety of primers, probes, and amplification conditions (Table 8.1). RT-qPCR detects norovirus RNA in a "real-time" manner (at each PCR cycle) using either nonspecific intercalating dyes or fluorescent dyes bound to target-specific probes. Advantages of this technology include preoptimized universal reagents and conditions for amplification, simplified assay platform and software for designing primers and probes, multiple detection chemistries, high-throughput capabilities, enhanced reproducibility, flexibility to develop multiplex assays for different norovirus genogroups in a single reaction, low risk of contamination, increased sensitivity and specificity in comparison with conventional RT-PCR (cRT-PCR), and automation with software-driven operation.

The open reading frame (ORF)1−ORF2 junction region is the most conserved region of the norovirus genome, with a high level of nucleotide sequence identity across the strains within genogroup (Kageyama et al., 2003). This feature makes this region ideal for designing primers for RT-qPCR assays to achieve high analytical sensitivity as well as broad detection of many norovirus genotypes, even recent emerging strains such as the GII.17 Kawasaki 2014 variant (Kageyama et al., 2003; Lee and Pang, 2015). However, the primers and probes designed from conserved sequence may not secure the sensitivity of RT-qPCR because the mutation even with single nucleotide polymorphism could occur unpredictably (Zhuo et al., 2015). Thus, monitoring sequence changes in the primer and probe binding sites should be performed regularly. With primers specific to individual genogroups (GI and GII), a multiplex RT-qPCR was developed to detect and differentiate norovirus by genogroup (Pang et al., 2005). The multiplex assay increases testing efficiency by decreasing testing time more than 50% and reduces reagent costs significantly. An RT-qPCR assay with additional primers and probes targeting GIV norovirus was also developed using the LightCycler instrument (Trujillo et al., 2006). The multiplex assay platforms are widely used in clinical laboratories worldwide, especially in Europe and North America (Hoehne and Schreier, 2006; Jothikumar et al., 2005; Logan et al., 2007; Stals et al., 2009; Neesanant et al., 2013; Farkas et al., 2015). In recent years, a number of norovirus RT-qPCR commercial kits have become available, although few studies have evaluated the efficacy of these kits. The NoV Type I and Type II

Table 8.1 Current Application of Real-Time RT-PCR Assays for the Detection of Norovirus

Genogroup	Primer/Probe[a]	Sequence (5′ → 3′)[b]	Probe/Dye[c]	Length (bp)	Type/Platform	References
GI	COG1-F	CGYTGGATGCGNTTYCATGA	TaqMan	85	Multiplex RT-qPCR ABI 7700/7000/7300/7500	Kageyama et al. (2003), Pang et al. (2005)
	COG1-R	CTTAGACGCCATCATCATTYAC				
	Probe (a)-R	AGATYGCGATCYCCGTCCA	VIC/TAMRA			
	Probe (b)-R	AGATCGCGGTCTCCGTCCA	FAM/TAMRA			
GII	COG2-F	CARGARBCNATGTTYAGRTGGATGAG	TaqMan	98		
	COG2-R	TCGACGCCATCTTCATTCACA				
	Probe-F	TGGGAGGGCGATCGCAATCT	FAM/TAMRA			
GI	NV192-F	GCYATGTTCCGCTGGATGC	MGB	98	Multiplex RT-qPCR ABI 7700	Hoehne and Schreier (2006)
	NV193-R	CGTCCTTAGACGCCATCATCA				
	Probe-F	TGGGAGGGCGATCGCAATCTGGC	VIC/NFQ			
GII	NV107(a)-F	AGCCAATGTTCAGATGGATG	TaqMan	94		
	NV107(b)-F	AICCIATGTTYAGITGGATG				
	NV119-R	TCGACGCCATCTTCATTCAC				
	Probe-F	TGGGAGGGCGATCGCAATCTGGC	FAM/NFQ			
GI	JJV1-F	GCCATGTTCCGITGGATG	TaqMan	96	Multiplex RT-qPCR Bio-Rad iCycler, Cepheid SmartCycler, and ABI 5700	Jothikumar et al. (2005)
	JJV1-R	TCCTTAGACGCCATCATCAT				
	Probe-F	TGTGGACAGGAGATCGCA ATCTC	FAM/BHQ			
GII	JJV2-F	CAAGAGTCA ATGTTTAGGTGGATGAG	TaqMan	98		
	COG2-R	TCGACGCCATCTTCATTCACA				
	Probe-F	TGGGAGGGCGATCGCAATCT	JOE /BHQ			
GI	COG1-F	CGYTGGATGCGNTTYCATGA	TaqMan	85	Monoplex RT-qPCR for GI, GII, and GIV Roche LightCycler	Trujillo et al. (2006)
	COG1-R	CTTAGACGCCATCATCATTYAC				
	Probe (a)-R	AGATYGCGATCYCCTGTCCA	FAM/ BHQ			
	Probe (b)-R	AGATCGCGGTCTCCGTCCA	FAM/ BHQ			
GII	COG2-F	CARGARBCNATGTTYAGRTGGATGAG	TaqMan	98		
	COG2-R	TCGACGCCATCTTCATTCACA				
	Probe-F	TGGGAGGGCGATCGCAATCT	FAM/ BHQ			

Group	Name	Sequence	Dye/Quencher	Efficiency (%)	Method/Platform	Reference
GIV	Mon 4-F	TTTGAGTCYATGTACAAGTGGATGC		98		
	Mon 4-R	TCGACGCCATCTTCATTCACA				
GI	Probe-F	TGGGAGGGGATGCGGATCT	FAM/ BHQ MGB	87	Monoplex RT-qPCR for GI	Logan et al. (2007)
	COG1-F	CGYTGGATGCGNTTYCATGA			Multiplex RT-qPCR for GII and GIV ABI 7000	
	GI-R	TCCTTAGACGCCATCATCATTYAC		97		
	Probe (a)-R	AGATYGCGATCYCCTGTCCA	VIC/NFQ			
	Probe (b)-R	AGATCGCGGTCTCCTGTCCA	VIC/NFQ			
GII	GII-F	CARGARBCNATGTTYAGRTGGATGAG	MGB			
	Probe-R	ATTGCGATCGCCCTC	FAM/NFQ			
GIV	GIV-F	CCAAAGTTTGAGTCYATGTACAAGTG	MGB	103		
	Probe-F	CGATCTCGCTCCCG	VIC/NFQ			
GII/GIV[d]	GII/GIV-R	CGACGCCATCTTCATTCACA				
GI	QNIF4-F	CGCTGGATGCGNTTCCAT	TaqMan	86	Multiplex RT-qPCR Roche LightCycler 480	Stals et al. (2009)
	NV1LC-R	CCTTAGACGCCATCATCATTTAC				
	Probe-F	TGGACAGGAGAYCGCRATCT	FAM/BHQ			
GII	QNIF2-F	ATGTTCAGRTGGATGAGRTTCTCWGA	TaqMan	89		
	COG2-R	TCGACGCCATCTTCATTCACA				
	Probe-F	AGCACGTGGGAGGGCGATCG	Texas Red/ BHQ			
GI	GI1-F	ATGTTCCGYTGGATGCGIT	TaqMan	Variable	Multiplex RT-qPCR ABI 7900	Neesanant et al. (2013)
	GI2-F	TTGGATGCGITTYCATGA				
	GI1-R	GGTCAGAAGCATTAACCTCCG				
	GI2-R	GGTCAGCTGTATTAACCTCCG				
	GI3-R	AGCTGRCCGGCACCACT				
	GI4-R	CACTRGTGCCATCCATGTTT				
	Probe-R	GCGTCCTTAGACGCCATCTTCATTTAC	VIC/?			
GII	GII-F	BCIATGTTYAGRTGGATGAG	TaqMan	91		
	GII-R	CGACGCCATCTTCATTCAC				
	Probe-R	AGATTGCGATCGCCCTCCA	FAM/?			

(Continued)

Table 8.1 Current Application of Real-Time RT-PCR Assays for the Detection of Norovirus *Continued*

Genogroup	Primer/Probe[a]	Sequence (5′ → 3′)[b]	Probe/Dye[c]	Length (bp)	Type/Platform	References
GI	Cog1F	CGY TGG ATG CGI TTY CAT GA			Multiplex RT-qPCR ABI 7500	Farkas et al. (2015)
	Cog1R	CTT AGA CGC CAT CAT CAT TYA C				
GII	Ring1C	AGA TYG CGI TCI CCT GTC CA	FAM/BHQ	85		
	Cog2F	CAR GAR BCN ATG TTY AGR TGG ATG AG				
	Cog2R	TCG ACG CCA TCT TCA TTC ACA				
GIV	Ring2	TGG GAG GGC GAT CGC AAT CT	CY5/BHQ	98		
	Mon4F	TTT GAG TCY ATR TAC AAG TGG ATG C				
	TF4F	CCA TGT ACC GST GGA TGC				
	Mon4R	TCG ACG CCA TCT TCA TTC ACA				
	TF4R	TAG ACG CCA TCT TCA TTC ACR				
	Ring4TFh	ATC GCG ATC TCG CTC CCG ATT T	TAMRA/BHQ	92/98		
	Ring4TFa	ATC GCA ATC TCG CTC CCG AST A	TAMRA/BHQ			

[a]F, forward (virus sense); R, reverse (antivirus sense).

[b]Mixed bases in degenerate primers and probes are indicated as follows: Y, C or T; R, A or G; I, inosin; B, not A; N, any.

[c]VIC, proprietary fluorescent reporter; FAM, 6-carboxyfluorescein reporter; TAMRA, 6-carboxy-tetramethylrhodamine quencher; MGB, minor groove binder; NFQ, nonfluorescent quencher; BHQ, Black Hole quencher.

[d]GII and GIV sharing same reverse primer.

kits (Generon, Castelnuovo Rangone, Italy) and the AnDiaTec NoV real-time RT-PCR kit (AnDiaTec, Kornwestheim, Germany) failed to detect the most common norovirus GI strains in a validation study (Butot et al., 2010). The RIDAGENE (R-Biopharm, Darmstadt, Germany) NoV genogroup I and II real-time PCR assay can detect a broad array of genotype with good sensitivity and specificity (Dunbar et al., 2014). The assays Xpert NoV kit (Cepheid, Sunnyvale, CA) and RoboGene Norovirus RNA Detection Kit (Analytik Jena, Jena, Germany) obtained clearance for use in Europe and are commercially available for norovirus detection. There is no feedback yet in terms of their clinical applicability and analytic precision.

Current detection methods (e.g., RT-qPCR) are also applied to detect norovirus RNA in water, food, and environmental specimens. Detection of norovirus in food requires appropriate elution and concentration techniques that need to be tailored for each type of food before RT-qPCR is performed. Currently, these methods are not routinely available. In addition to detecting norovirus RNA in clinical samples, relatively small optimizations of the primers and probes have resulted in sensitive assays to detect norovirus RNA in environmental samples (e.g., food and water) (Loisy et al., 2005; da Silva et al., 2007; Pang et al., 2012; Qiu et al., 2015). Recently, a few commercial RT-qPCR kits, such as the Norovirus GI and GII Detection Kit (CEERAM S.A.S., La Chapelle sur Erdre, France), have become available for detection of norovirus from environmental samples, including water, wastewater, seawater, sludge, air, surface, and food (e.g., shellfish, fruits, vegetables, and processed food). The foodproof Norovirus Detection Kit (GI, GII, and GIV (BIOTECON Diagnostics, Potsdam, Germany) is also available for detection of norovirus in food samples. However, there are no reports on the validation and assessment of these kits.

The extreme analytical sensitivity of norovirus RT-qPCR assays allows the detection of a very low quantity of virus that might be present in samples from persons without disease caused by norovirus (i.e., asymptomatic infection) (Phillips et al., 2009). For this reason, low viral load results obtained by the NAT assays should be interpreted with caution (Vinjé, 2015; Corcoran et al., 2014).

8.2.2.3 Conventional RT-PCR

cRT-PCR refers to the traditional amplification process in which amplified product is allowed to accumulate as the thermal cycling continues to an end point and the reaction reaches a plateau before detection or analysis steps are conducted. Amplified PCR products are usually detected by size fractionation using agarose or polyacrylamide gel electrophoresis. Jiang et al. (1992) first used cRT-PCR to detect human norovirus using specific primers targeting Norwalk virus, the prototype of norovirus. As a detection method, cRT-PCR has the disadvantages of being a complex multistep procedure that is associated with high variability, has low throughput, is labor-intensive and time-consuming, and poses a significant risk of contamination by manipulating postamplified products in an open-air environment. Although cRT-PCR is still commonly used to detect norovirus in epidemiological studies of gastroenteritis, it has not been widely adopted by diagnostic laboratories. Different primer sets targeting various genetic regions were developed to study the evolution and molecular epidemiology of norovirus. The combination of cRT-PCR and DNA sequencing of the amplicons has been used to study the genetic variations among norovirus strains (Zheng et al., 2006; Mattison et al., 2009).

8.2.2.4 Isothermal amplification assays

In contrast to thermal cycle-based amplification, which uses a constant temperature for nucleic acid amplification with analytical sensitivity similar to that of RT-qPCR, nucleic acid sequence-based amplification (NASBA) and loop-mediated isothermal amplification (LAMP) have been developed for detection of norovirus from stool specimens. However, NASBA assay is unappealing for diagnostic laboratory use due to concerns with regard to specificity when amplifying norovirus RNA at relatively low temperatures ($\sim 40°C$) (Moore et al., 2004). LAMP technology has the advantages of speed and simplicity, with the reaction being performed in a single tube and requiring no more than 1 hour to complete (Notomi et al., 2000). Reactions normally show a high tolerance to biological products, so extensive TNA preparation is not needed. LAMP does not require sophisticated equipment, and a simple heat block or water bath can be used because amplification occurs at low and constant temperatures, ranging from 60° to 65°C. When there is a positive reaction using LAMP, magnesium pyrophosphate precipitates out of the solution, causing turbidity, which can be easily visualized by eye or measured using a turbidity meter. A fluorescent indicator can also be added to enhance readability. Due to the simplicity of the LAMP platform, it is a superior choice for laboratories with limited resources and experiences in performing NAT. Laboratory-developed LAMP assays have been used to detect norovirus GI and GII and demonstrated compatible results with RT-qPCR (Iturriza-Gómara et al., 2008; Yoda et al., 2009; Suzuki et al., 2011; Luo et al., 2014). Recently, a commercial LAMP kit for norovirus GI and GII was developed by Eiken Chemical (Tokyo) that showed assay sensitivity as good as that of laboratory-developed LAMP assay (Yoda et al., 2009). However, LAMP is still not widely used because of specific requirements for primer design. In the near future, LAMP may provide an alternate method for fast and reliable detection of norovirus in diagnostic laboratories and point-of-care application.

8.2.2.5 Nanotechnology for norovirus detection

Nanotechnology has been intensively developed to create commercial medical devices. Advances in microelectronics, microfluidics, and microfabrication have paved the way for novel and miniature technologies to reach the ultimate goal of creating simple, affordable, point-of-care molecular diagnostic devices. Nanotechnology is being used to develop sample-in/answer-out testing for laboratories regardless of size, resources, or capacity with the use of the smallest quantities of reagents and samples. It also supports multiplex diagnostics testing for comprehensive syndrome-specific assessment of various diseases.

Zhang et al. (2015) reviewed two commercial syndrome-specific multiplex tests, Luminex xTAG Gastrointestinal Pathogen Panel (GPP) (Luminex, Austin, TX) and FilmArray gastrointestinal panel (BioFire Diagnostics, Salt Lake City, UT), and reported that the multiplex PCR tests have shown superior sensitivity to conventional methods for detection of most pathogens. The xTAG GPP and FilmArray Gastrointestinal norovirus GI and GII were compared in a recent study (Khare et al., 2014). These fully closed and automated systems show great potential for use in identifying enteric pathogens associated with sporadic gastroenteritis and outbreaks while saving significant time in terms of assay processing (total hands-on time of 2–5 minutes) and turnaround report time (~1 hour). These improvements will provide physicians with prompt clinical intervention and disease control. Similar devices being developed include Verigene Enteric Pathogens Nucleic Acid Test (Nanosphere, Northbrook, IL) and Allplex Gastrointestinal Panel (Seegene, Toronto). A summary of these commercial robotic assay platforms is provided in Table 8.2.

Table 8.2 Update of Commercial Molecular Assays for the Detection of Norovirus

Assay	License/ Approval Information	Principle of the Test	Instrument	Vendor	Reference With Validation/Evaluation Data
AndiaTee Norovirus real RT-PCR kit	CE-IVD	Real-time RT-PCR Taqman	ABI system and a comparable instrument (e.g., Roche 480, Stratagene and Qiagen/ Corbett)	AndiaTee GmbH (Komvesthein, Germany)	Butot et al. (2010)
RealStar Norovirus RT-PCR kit	CE-IVD	Real-time RT-PCR Taqman	m2000rt, Mx 3005P VERSANT kPCR ABI 7500 /7500 Fast LightCycler 480 Rotor-Gene 3000/6000, Rotor-Gene Q 5/6 plex	Altona Diagnostics GmbH (Hamburg, Germany)	http://www.altona-diagnostics.com
Xpert Norovirus kit	CE-IVD	Real-time RT-PCR	Xpert system	Cepheid (Sunnyvale, CA)	http://www.cepheid.com
Luminex xTAG GPP	FDA-cleared/ Health Canada- approved IVD	Multiplex RT-PCR and Liquid Array for 15 pathogens	Luminex system	Luminex (Austin, TX)	Khare et al. (2014)
FilmArray GI panel	FDA cleared-IVD	Nested RT-PCR and FilmArray for 24 pathogens	FilmArray platform	BioFire Diagnostics (Salt Lake City, UT)	Khare et al. (2014)
Verigen Enteric Pathogens Necleic Acide Test (EP)	FDA cleared-IVD	Multiplex RT-PCR and array hybridization	Verigene platform	Nanosphere (Northbrook, IL)	http://www.nanosphere.us
Allplex Gastrointestinal Full Panel Assay	CE-IVD	Multiplex real-time RT-PCR for 25 pathogens in four multiplex qPCR panels	CFX96 real-time PCR detection system (Bio-Rad)	Seegene (Toronto)	http://www.seegene.com/neo/en/products/Gastrointestinal/allplex_GI_fp.php

IVD, *in vitro diagnostic use.*

8.2.3 GENOTYPING OF NOROVIRUSES

Genetic typing provides essential information to further our understanding of norovirus genetic evolution, classification, and molecular epidemiology. The information on genetic traits of norovirus causing regional gastroenteritis outbreaks in a spatiotemporal manner can be exchanged nationally and internationally to map the trend of norovirus strains causing endemic, epidemic, or pandemic events. Genetic information of norovirus is also critical for the development of preventive strategies against norovirus infections such as vaccines.

Norovirus genotyping is performed largely in research and public health laboratories because it usually has no direct impact on clinical decision-making and patient management except in special outbreak investigations or clinical settings. Human noroviruses are classified into genogroups, genotypes, and variants. With the highly diversified genome of noroviruses, genotyping may require sequencing of postamplified RT-PCR products. Five different regions (designated A–E) of the genome have been used successfully for genotyping of noroviruses (Vinjé et al., 2004; Kojima et al., 2002; Pang et al., 2010). In recent years, primers targeting to the norovirus viral capsid gene (regions C–E) have been preferred for genotyping because viral capsid is directly involved in host–receptor interaction and immune response and contains relevant genetic variations. Although the sequences of regions C and E have been used widely for genotyping strains by clinical diagnostic laboratories in the United States, Canada, Europe, and Japan, the resolution of these regions is not sufficient to distinguish differences between certain GII.4 variants, which are the predominant strains associated with outbreaks (Zheng et al., 2010; Mattison et al., 2009). The gold standard for genotyping norovirus strains is full capsid sequencing. However, for clinical samples with lower norovirus viral load, amplifying partial capsid sequences is more practical and has only slightly less discriminatory power than full capsid sequencing (Vinjé et al., 2004). Hasing et al. (2014) reported that the primers in the ORF1/2 junction region worked better for identifying norovirus antigenic drift than recombination events. Sequence alignment followed by phylogenetic analysis is being used to classify norovirus. More than 40 genotypes associated with NoV gastroenteritis have been categorized into the two major norovirus genogroups (GI and GII).

Recently, next-generation sequencing (NGS), a fundamentally different approach to gene sequencing, has triggered numerous groundbreaking discoveries and will likely revolutionize genomic science. The principle of NGS is similar to that of capillary electrophoresis-based Sanger sequencing: The bases of a small DNA fragment are sequentially identified from signals emitted as each fragment is resynthesized from a DNA template strand. NGS extends this process across millions of reactions in a massively parallel manner. This technological advancement enables rapid sequencing of large stretches of DNA spanning entire genomes, with the latest instruments capable of producing hundreds of gigabases of data in a single sequencing run (Srivatsan et al., 2008; Rasmussen et al., 2010). NGS has advantageous features such as high throughput, powerful scalability, tunable resolution, increasingly fast speed, and wide dynamic range and sensitivity. Because norovirus has a relatively small genome size of approximately 7500 nucleotides, characterization using NGS may become a new approach to studying norovirus. The latest NGS amplicon library preparation kits allow researchers to perform rapid amplification of custom-targeted regions from norovirus genome. Using this approach, thousands of amplicons spanning multiple samples can be simultaneously prepared and indexed. NGS enables researchers to simultaneously analyze all genomic content of interest in a single experiment (Lo and Chiu, 2009). With sufficient depth of coverage, NGS can identify common and rare sequence variations of norovirus in clinical samples (Hasing et al., 2016). This application is particularly useful for tracking the genetic evolution of norovirus and the discovery of emerging variants, which may potentially cause outbreaks of NoV gastroenteritis. NGS has increasingly been used in research laboratories and is anticipated to be incorporated into clinical diagnostic workflows with further development of standard reagents and targeting kits in the near future (Wong et al., 2013; Batty et al., 2013; Kundu et al., 2013; Cotten et al., 2014; Bavelaar et al., 2015).

8.2.4 **CELL CULTURE**

Regardless of the clinical and public health importance of norovirus in sporadic and outbreak gastroenteritis, the pathogenic mechanism is still largely unknown because norovirus is difficult to grow in cell culture. The extensive efforts during the past two decades to culture human norovirus have been not successful until very recently. In considering the enteric nature of human norovirus, the intestinal epithelial cells were selected to establish a cell culture system at an early stage and the efforts were unsuccessful (Duizer et al., 2004; Papafragkou et al., 2013; Takanashi et al., 2014; Herbst-Kralovetz et al., 2013). A hypothesis that human norovirus might replicate in such human cell types similar to murine macrophages and dendritic cells in which murine norovirus established tropism did not lead to a promising outcome (Wobus et al., 2004; Changotra et al., 2009; Lay et al., 2010). Subsequently, there was a report of human norovirus replication in a three-dimensional culture model using human intestinal epithelial cell lines INT-407 and Caco-2 in vitro, but the methods could not be replicated by others (Takanashi et al., 2014; Straub et al., 2007, 2011; Straub et al., 2013). Jones et al. (2015) published an in vitro culture model for human norovirus through joint multiinstitutional efforts. In their protocol, human norovirus has been successfully replicated in human B cells (BJAB and Raji cell lines) with the presence of bacteria that expressed histo-blood group antigens (HBGAs), although the increase in norovirus RNA was modest ($<2 \log_{10}$). Several key differences from previous failed trials were illustrated in the protocol: (1) Human B cell line was used rather than epithelial cell lines and macrophages; (2) unfiltered, unprocessed stool was directly used as an inoculum, which ensures the presence of commensal HBGA-expressing bacteria as a cofactor for infection (facilitating viral entry via B cell receptor), whereas others used filtered virus-positive stool sample or further purified virions as inoculum; and (3) GII.4 Sydney 2012 strain with high viral load in the inoculum was selected instead of GI.1 Norwalk virus, which had less pathogenic virulence. The preliminary success of human norovirus cell culture provides a breakthrough for the future study of the norovirus pathogenic mechanism, immunology, disinfection, and vaccine development, even though there is still a modest level of viral replication and output in the system and many unknowns with regard to the inconsistency of the B cell model to natural norovirus infection. Human norovirus cell culture has its most significant impacts on research and development fields rather than direct benefits and application for clinical diagnosis because in vitro cell culture is labor-intensive, lacks sensitivity, and is time-consuming at this stage.

8.3 SAMPLE COLLECTION AND REQUIREMENTS FOR NOROVIRUS TESTING

8.3.1 CLINICAL SAMPLES

8.3.1.1 Stool

Stool is the standard specimen type for laboratory testing of norovirus. A few grams (pea-size) of stool sample is sufficient for norovirus detection by EM, antigen testing, or NAT. It is advised to urinate before stool samples are collected. For patients in a health care setting, a bed pan, catching device, or portable commode is often used to collect the stool, from which a small amount can be transferred to nonleak plastic containers usually equipped with a screw top and small scoop. However, very often stool samples need to be collected from outpatients at home. For adults or toilet-trained children, a catching device that is provided by clinics or a piece of plastic (e.g., Saran Wrap) can be placed over the toilet seat with a dip in the center. After defecation, a small amount of stool can be collected into the nonleak container labeled with patient identification. For babies and infants, stool samples can be obtained from a diaper using either a wooden tongue depressor or the scoop of the nonleak container. It is preferable to collect stool sample within the first 48 hours of illness because viral shedding is at its maximal level. If this is not possible, specimens collected later or after resolution (i.e., up to 7–10 days after onset) might still provide an opportunity to confirm norovirus infection in a suspected source case-patient (e.g., a food handler with a recent history of diarrhea). If specimens are collected late in the illness, their adequacy for diagnosis and result interpretation should be discussed with laboratory personnel before proceeding with a test.

8.3.1.2 Rectal swab

Obtaining bulk stool specimens is challenging, especially at home. Recent evidence supports the use of rectal swabs, which provide equivalent results of norovirus detection as RT-qPCR (Arvelo et al., 2013; Sidler et al., 2014; Goldfarb et al., 2014). However, rectal swabs are not recommended for EM examination and antigen detection test (EIA/ELISA). It is easy and convenient to collect a rectal swab, but further validation is needed to support its use as a routine diagnostic specimen type.

8.3.1.3 Serum

Serum samples can be tested for norovirus viremia in patients with severe illness or complications (e.g., extraintestinal symptoms such as seizures and encephalopathy) (Ito et al., 2006; Turcios-Ruiz et al., 2008; Takanashi et al., 2009; Medici et al., 2010; Fumian et al., 2013). Serum samples are also used to detect acute and convalescent antibodies against norovirus, which has limited value for acute phase diagnostics of norovirus gastroenteritis but is informative for seroprevalence studies. Acute phase serum sample should be collected as soon as possible after illness onset, whereas the acute and convalescent serum samples should be tested simultaneously if available.

8.3.1.4 Oral swab

Norovirus can be found in the vomitus of infected persons (Kirby et al., 2010b, 2011; Makison Booth, 2014). However, it is difficult to collect and test vomitus. The oral swab has been used as an alternate specimen type for the detection of norovirus infections, especially in patients with vomiting only. Oral swab is not routinely accepted for diagnostic testing, and further studies are needed.

8.3.2 ENVIRONMENTAL SAMPLES

Drinking water, food, beverages, and other environmental specimens are sometimes collected for the investigation of outbreaks associated with norovirus. However, validated methods are available only at limited laboratories (e.g., water at the Centers for Disease Control and Prevention and shellfish at the US Food and Drug Administration's Gulf Coast Seafood Laboratory). If a food or water is suspected to be the source of an outbreak, specimens should be obtained as early as possible and stored under appropriate conditions. Environmental surface swabs are used to detect norovirus RNA in specific outbreak settings (Boxman et al., 2009). Because testing of these types of specimen is not routinely performed in most diagnostic laboratories and they often require special handling and processing, a reference laboratory with the capability to perform these specialized tasks should be contacted to obtain appropriate instructions before specimen collection.

8.3.3 STORAGE AND TRANSPORTATION

Adequate storage, shipment, and preparation of samples can minimize degradation of virus particles, proteins, and/or nucleic acids and cross-contamination. In principle, fresh stool sample is best for obtaining reliable testing results, especially when EM is used to identify norovirus. Stool samples should be stored at 4°C immediately after collection and promptly transported to the laboratory for processing and EM examination. If repeat testing is expected for the sample, single-use aliquots of the sample should be prepared and stored for future testing. The ideal storage temperature for aliquots, especially in terms of preserving nucleic acids, is $-70°C$. With our working experience, norovirus could be detected using NAT in stool samples after storage at $-20°C$ for 3 years. Stool samples can be shipped on wet or dry ice, depending on their storage requirements (e.g., short- or long-term storage). Repeat freezing and thawing should be avoided. Processed serum specimens can be stored at $2-8°C$ up to several days and then stored at $-20°C$ or colder for prolonged period.

8.3.4 TESTING FREQUENCY

For investigation of norovirus outbreak, it is recommended to test up to six stool samples per outbreak in order to confirm or rule out norovirus as the causative agent (Duizer et al., 2007). Once two stool samples from the same outbreak test positive, norovirus can be confirmed as a causative agent. If all six samples are negative, an outbreak can be defined as non-norovirus-associated, and further investigation for other pathogens may be required (Kojima et al., 2002). Repeat testing of norovirus from the same patient by NAT should not be performed except for special clinical reasons because norovirus can be shed from weeks to months in immunosuppressed patients (Krones and Högenauer, 2012; Bok and Green, 2012).

8.4 CONCLUSIONS AND PERSPECTIVES

The current assays used to detect norovirus all have advantages and disadvantages; as such, none is perfect. Each laboratory needs to select an adequate detection platform that meet its needs and objectives (diagnostic vs research), laboratory setting (reference vs regional diagnostic laboratories), test volume and throughput, instrument availability, and technical expertise. Immunoassays for norovirus can be used as preliminary tests for suspected norovirus gastroenteritis outbreaks, but they are not recommended for routine diagnostic use due to their low analytical sensitivity. RT-qPCR is considered to be an excellent method for norovirus detection in stool, food, and environmental samples. However, it must be remembered that due to diverse norovirus genotypes and continuous genetic evolution, false-negative results can still be obtained, especially when a single pair of specific primers is used. Utilization of multiple primer sets targeting different regions of norovirus genome or degenerated primers based on sequence variations of known norovirus references has been used to improve the sensitivity and accuracy of norovirus detection. Other technologies, such as LAMP, nanotechnology array-based multiplex panel, and NGS, have been developed and used to detect norovirus mostly in research settings. It is anticipated that these new technologies will be used in the routine diagnosis of norovirus infections in clinical laboratories in the future.

REFERENCES

Ahmed, S.M., Hall, A.J., Robinson, A.E., et al., 2014. Global prevalence of norovirus in cases of gastroenteritis: a systematic review and meta-analysis. Lancet Infect. Dis. 14, 725–730.

Aliabadi, N., Lopman, B.A., Parashar, U.D., Hall, A.J., 2015. Progress toward norovirus vaccines: considerations for further development and implementation in potential target populations. Expert Rev. Vaccines 14, 1241–1253.

Al-Soud, W.A., Radstrom, P., 2001. Purification and characterization of PCR-inhibitory components in blood cells. J. Clin. Microbiol. 39, 485–493.

Ambert-Balay, K., Pothier, P., 2013. Evaluation of 4 immunochromatographic tests for rapid detection of norovirus in faecal samples. J. Clin. Virol. 56, 194–198.

Ando, T., Monroe, S.S., Gentsch, J.R., Jin, Q., Lewis, D.C., Glass, R.I., 1995. Detection and differentiation of antigenically distinct small round-structured viruses (Norwalk-like viruses) by reverse transcription-PCR and southern hybridization. J. Clin. Microbiol 33 (1), 64–71.

Arvelo, W., Hall, A.J., Estevez, A., et al., 2013. Diagnostic performance of rectal swab versus bulk stool specimens for the detection of rotavirus and norovirus: implications for outbreak investigations. J. Clin. Virol. 58, 678–682.

Batty, E.M., Wong, T.H., Trebes, A., et al., 2013. A modified RNA-Seq approach for whole genome sequencing of RNA viruses from faecal and blood samples. PLoS 8, e66129.

Bavelaar, H.H., Rahamat-Langendoen, J., Niesters, H.G., Zoll, J., Melchers, W.J., 2015. Whole genome sequencing of fecal samples as a tool for the diagnosis and genetic characterization of norovirus. J. Clin. Virol. 72, 122–125.

Bok, K., Green, K.Y., 2012. Norovirus gastroenteritis in immunocompromised patients. New Engl. J. Med. 367, 2126–2132.

Boxman, I.L., Dijkman, R., te Loeke, N.A., et al., 2009. Environmental swabs as a tool in norovirus outbreak investigation, including outbreaks on cruise ships. J. Food Prot. 72, 111–119.

Bruggink, L.D., Witlox, K.J., Sameer, R., et al., 2011. Evaluation of the RIDA®QUICK immunochromatographic norovirus detection assay using specimens from Australian gastroenteritis incidents. J. Virol. Methods 173, 121–126.

Bruins, M.J., Wolfhagen, M.J., Schirm, J., et al., 2010. Evaluation of a rapid immunochromatographic test for the detection of norovirus in stool samples. Eur. J. Clin. Microbiol. Infect. Dis. 29, 741—743.

Bull, R.A., Eden, J.S., Rawlinson, W.D., et al., 2010. Rapid evolution of pandemic noroviruses of the GII.4 lineage. PLoS Pathog. 6, e1000831.

Burton-MacLeod, J.A., Kane, E.M., Beard, R.S., et al., 2004. Evaluation and comparison of two commercial enzyme-linked immunosorbent assay kits for detection of antigenically diverse human noroviruses in stool samples. J. Clin. Microbiol. 42, 2587—2595.

Butot, S., Le Guyader, F.S., et al., 2010. Evaluation of various real-time RT-PCR assays for the detection and quantitation of human norovirus. J. Virol. Methods 167, 90—94.

Chan, M.C., Lee, N., Hung, T.N., et al., 2015. Rapid emergence and predominance of a broadly recognizing and fast-evolving norovirus GII.17 variant in late 2014. Nat. Commun. 6, 10061.

Changotra, H., Jia, Y., Moore, T.N., et al., 2009. Type I and type II interferons inhibit the translation of murine norovirus proteins. J. Virol. 83, 5683—5692.

Corcoran, M.S., van Well, G.T., van Loo, I.H., 2014. Diagnosis of viral gastroenteritis in children: interpretation of real-time PCR results and relation to clinical symptoms. Eur. J. Clin. Microbiol. Infect. Dis. 33, 1663—1673.

Cotten, M., Petrova, V., Phan, M.V., et al., 2014. Deep sequencing of norovirus genomes defines evolutionary patterns in an urban tropical setting. J. Virol. 88, 11056—11069.

da Silva, A.K., Le Saux, J.C., Parnaudeau, S., Pommepuy, M., Elimelech, M., Le Guyader, F.S., 2007. Evaluation of removal of noroviruses during wastewater treatment, using real-time reverse transcription-PCR: different behaviors of genogroups I and II. Appl. Environ. Microbiol. 73, 7891—7897.

de Graaf, M., van Beek, J., Vennema, H., et al., 2015. Emergence of a novel GII.17 norovirus—end of the GII.4 era? Euro. Surveill. 20, 26.

Derrington, P., Schreiber, F., Day, S., et al., 2009. Norovirus Ridaquick: a new test for rapid diagnosis of norovirus. Pathology 41, 687—688.

Duizer, E., Schwab, K.J., Neill, F.H., Atmar, R.L., Koopmans, M.P., Estes, M.K., 2004. Laboratory efforts to cultivate noroviruses. J. Gen. Virol. 85, 79—87.

Duizer, E., Pielaat, A., Vennema, H., et al., 2007. Probabilities in norovirus outbreak diagnosis. J. Clin. Virol. 40, 38—42.

Dunbar, S.A., Zhang, H., Tang, Y.W., 2013. Advanced techniques for detection and identification of microbial agents of gastroenteritis. Clin. Lab. Med. 33, 527—552.

Dunbar, N.L., Bruggink, L.D., Marshall, J.A., 2014. Evaluation of the RIDAGENE real-time PCR assay for the detection of GI and GII norovirus. Diagn. Microbiol. Infect. Dis. 79, 317—321.

Fankhauser, R.L., Monroe, S.S., Noel, J.S., Humphrey, C.D., Bresee, J.S., Parashar, U.D., et al., 2002. Epidemiologic and molecular trends of "Norwalk-like viruses" associated with outbreaks of gastroenteritis in the United States. J. Infect. Dis. 186 (1), 1—7.

Farkas, T., Singh, A., Le Guyader, F.S., La Rosa, G., Saif, L., McNeal, M., 2015. Multiplex real-time RT-PCR for the simultaneous detection and quantification of GI, GII and GIV noroviruses. J. Virol. Methods 223, 109—114.

Fu, J., Ai, J., Jin, M., Jiang, C., et al., 2015. Emergence of a new GII.17 norovirus variant in patients with acute gastroenteritis in Jiangsu, China, September 2014 to March 2015. Euro. Surveill. 20, 24.

Fumian, T.M., Justino, M.C., D'Arc Pereira Mascarenhas, J., et al., 2013. Quantitative and molecular analysis of noroviruses RNA in blood from children hospitalized for acute gastroenteritis in Belém, Brazil. J. Clin. Virol. 58, 31—35.

Geginat, G., Kaiser, D., Schrempf, S., 2012. Evaluation of third-generation ELISA and a rapid immunochromatographic assay for the detection of norovirus infection in fecal samples from inpatients of a German tertiary care hospital. Eur. J. Clin. Microbiol. Infect. Dis. 31, 733—737.

Goldfarb, D.M., Steenhoff, A.P., Pernica, J.M., et al., 2014. Evaluation of anatomically designed flocked rectal swabs for molecular detection of enteric pathogens in children admitted to hospital with severe gastroenteritis in Botswana. J. Clin. Microbiol. 52, 3922–3927.

Gray, J.J., Kohli, E., Ruggeri, F.M., et al., 2007. European multicenter evaluation of commercial enzyme immunoassays for detecting norovirus antigen in fecal samples. Clin. Vaccine Immunol. 14, 1349–1355.

Green, J., Gallimore, C.I., Norcott, J.P., Lewis, D., Brown, D.W., 1995. Broadly reactive reverse transcriptase polymerase chain reaction for the diagnosis of SRSV-associated gastroenteritis. J. Med. Virol 47 (4), 392–398.

Green, S.M., Lambden, P.R., Caul, E.O., Clarke, I.N., 1997. Capsid sequence diversity in small round structured viruses from recent UK outbreaks of gastroenteritis. J. Med. Virol 52 (1), 14–19.

Han, J., Ji, L., Shen, Y., Wu, X., Xu, D., Chen, L., 2015. Emergence and predominance of norovirus GII.17 in Huzhou, China, 2014–2015. Virol. J. 12, 139.

Hasing, M.E., Hazes, B., Lee, B.E., Preiksaitis, J.K., Pang, X.L., 2014. Detection and analysis of recombination in GII.4 norovirus strains causing gastroenteritis outbreaks in Alberta. Infect. Genet. Evol. 27, 181–192.

Hasing, M.E., Hazes, B., Lee, B.E., Preiksaitis, J.K., Pang, X.L., 2016. A next generation sequencing-based method to study the intra-host genetic diversity of norovirus in patients with acute and chronic infection. BMC Genomics 17 (1), 480. Available from: http://dx.doi.org/10.1186/s12864-016-2831-y.

Hemming, M., Räsänen, S., Huhti, L., Paloniemi, M., Salminen, M., Vesikari, T., 2013. Major reduction of rotavirus, but not norovirus, gastroenteritis in children seen in hospital after the introduction of RotaTeq vaccine into the National Immunization Programme in Finland. Eur. J. Pediatr. 172, 739–746.

Herbst-Kralovetz, M.M., Radtke, A.L., Lay, M.K., et al., 2013. Lack of norovirus replication and histo-blood group antigen expression in 3-dimensional intestinal epithelial cells. Emerg. Infect. Dis. 19, 431–438.

Hoa Tran, T.N., Trainor, E., Nakagomi, T., Cunliffe, N.A., Nakagomi, O., 2013. Molecular epidemiology of noroviruses associated with acute sporadic gastroenteritis in children: global distribution of genogroups, genotypes and GII.4 variants. J. Clin. Virol. 56, 185–193.

Hoehne, M., Schreier, E., 2006. Detection of norovirus genogroup I and II by multiplex real-time RT-PCR using a 3′-minor groove binder-DNA probe. BMC Infect. Dis. 6, 69.

Ito, S., Takeshita, S., Nezu, A., et al., 2006. Norovirus-associated encephalopathy. Pediatr. Infect. Dis. J. 25, 651–652.

Iturriza-Gómara, M., Xerry, J., Gallimore, C.I., et al., 2008. Evaluation of the Loopamp (loop-mediated isothermal amplification) kit for detecting norovirus RNA in faecal samples. J. Clin. Virol. 42, 389–393.

Jiang, X., Huang, P.W., Zhong, W.M., Farkas, T., Cubitt, D.W., Matson, D.O., 1999. Design and evaluation of a primer pair that detects both Norwalk- and Sapporo-like caliciviruses by RT-PCR. J. Virol. Methods 83 (1–2), 145–154.

Jiang, X., Wang, J., Graham, D.Y., Estes, M.K., 1992. Detection of Norwalk virus in stool by polymerase chain reaction. J. Clin. Microbiol. 30, 2529–2534.

Jiang, X., Wang, M., Wang, K., Estes, M.K., 1993. Sequence and genomic organization of norwalk virus. Virology 195, 51–61.

Jones, M.K., Grau, K.R., Costantini, V., et al., 2015. Human norovirus culture in B cells. Nat. Protoc. 10, 1939–1947.

Jothikumar, N., Lowther, J.A., Henshilwood, K., Lees, D.N., Hill, V.R., Vinjé, J., 2005. Rapid and sensitive detection of noroviruses by using TaqMan-based one-step reverse transcription-PCR assays and application to naturally contaminated shellfish samples. Appl. Environ. Microbiol. 71, 1870–1875.

Kageyama, T., Kojima, S., Shinohara, M., et al., 2003. Broadly reactive and highly sensitive assay for norwalk-like viruses based on real-time quantitative reverse transcription-PCR. J. Clin. Microbiol. 41, 1548–1557.

Kapikian, A.Z., Wyatt, R.G., Dolin, R., Thornhill, T.S., Kalica, A.R., Chanock, R.M., 1972. Visualization by immune electron microscopy of a 27-nm particle associated with acute infectious nonbacterial gastroenteritis. J. Virol. 10, 1075–1081.

Khamrin, P., Nguyen, T.A., Phan, T.G., et al., 2008. Evaluation of immunochromatography and commercial enzyme-linked immunosorbent assay for rapid detection of norovirus antigen in stool samples. J. Virol. Methods 147, 360−363.

Khare, R., Espy, M.J., Cebelinski, E., et al., 2014. Comparative evaluation of two commercial multiplex panels for detection of gastrointestinal pathogens by use of clinical stool specimens. J. Clin. Microbiol. 52, 3667−3673.

Kirby, A., Gurgel, R.Q., Dove, W., et al., 2010a. An evaluation of the RIDASCREEN and IDEIA enzyme immunoassays and the RIDAQUICK immunochromatographic test for the detection of norovirus in faecal specimens. J. Clin. Virol. 49, 254−257.

Kirby, A., Dove, W., Ashton, L., Hopkins, M., Cunliffe, N.A., 2010b. Detection of norovirus in mouthwash samples from patients with acute gastroenteritis. J. Clin. Virol. 48, 285−287.

Kirby, A., Ashton, L., Hart, I.J., 2011. Detection of norovirus infection in the hospital setting using vomit samples. J. Clin. Virol. 51, 86−87.

Kojima, S., Kageyama, T., Fukushi, S., et al., 2002. Genogroup-specific PCR primers for detection of Norwalk-like viruses. J. Virol. Methods 100, 107−114.

Koo, H.L., Neill, F.H., Estes, M.K., et al., 2013. Noroviruses: the most common pediatric viral enteric pathogen at a large university hospital after introduction of rotavirus vaccination. J. Pediatr. Infect. Dis. Soc. 2, 57−60.

Kozisek, F., 2015. Waterborne outbreak in Prague. Water research Australia. The 18th International Symposium on Health-Related Water Microbiology 80, 4−6. Available from: http://www.waterra.com.au/publications/latest-news/2015/health-stream.

Krones, E., Högenauer, C., 2012. Diarrhea in the immunocompromised patient. Gastroenterol. Clin. North Am. 41, 677−701.

Kundu, S., Lockwood, J., Depledge, D.P., et al., 2013. Next-generation whole genome sequencing identifies the direction of norovirus transmission in linked patients. Clin. Infect. Dis. 57, 407−414.

Lay, M.K., Atmar, R.L., Guix, S., et al., 2010. Norwalk virus does not replicate in human macrophages or dendritic cells derived from the peripheral blood of susceptible humans. Virology 406, 1−11.

Le Guyader, F., Estes, M.K., Hardy, M.E., Neill, F.H., Green, J., Brown, D.W., et al., 1996. Evaluation of a degenerate primer for the PCR detection of human caliciviruses. Arch. Virol. 141 (11), 2225−2235.

Lee, B.E., Preiksaitis, J.K., Chui, N., Chui, L., Pang, X.L., 2008. Genetic relatedness of noroviruses identified in sporadic gastroenteritis in children and gastroenteritis outbreaks in northern Alberta. J. Med. Virol. 80, 330−337.

Lee, E.B., Pang, X.L., 2015. The amazing race of norovirus. Can. J. Infect. Dis. Med. Microbiol. (in press).

Lo, Y.M., Chiu, R.W., 2009. Next-generation sequencing of plasma/serum DNA: an emerging research and molecular diagnostic tool. Clin. Chem. 55, 607−608.

Logan, C.L., O'Leary, J.J., O'Sullivan, N., 2007. Real-time reverse transcription PCR detection of norovirus, sapovirus and astrovirus as causative agents of acute viral gastroenteritis. J. Virol. Methods 146, 36−44.

Loisy, F., Atmar, R.L., Guillon, P., Le Cann, P., Pommepuy, M., Le Guyader, F.S., 2005. Real-time RT-PCR for norovirus screening in shellfish. J. Virol. Methods 123, 1−7.

Lu, J., Sun, L., Fang, L., et al., 2015. Gastroenteritis outbreaks caused by norovirus GII.17, Guangdong Province, China, 2014−2015. Emerg. Infect. Dis. 21, 1240−1242.

Luo, J., Xu, Z., Nie, K., et al., 2014. Visual detection of norovirus genogroup II by reverse transcription loop-mediated isothermal amplification with hydroxynaphthol blue dye. Food Environ. Virol. 6, 196−201.

Makison Booth, C., 2014. Vomiting Larry: a simulated vomiting system for assessing environmental contamination from projectile vomiting related to norovirus infection. J. Infect. Prev. 15, 176−180.

Mattison, K., Grudeski, E., Auk, B., et al., 2009. A multi-center comparison of two norovirus ORF2-based genotyping protocols. J. Clin. Microbiol. 47, 3927−3932.

Medici, M.C., Abelli, L.A., Dodi, I., Dettori, G., Chezzi, C., 2010. Norovirus RNA in the blood of a child with gastroenteritis and convulsions—a case report. J. Clin. Virol. 48, 147−149.

Moore, C., Clark, E.M., Gallimore, C.I., et al., 2004. Evaluation of a broadly reactive nucleic acid sequence based amplification assay for the detection of noroviruses in faecal material. J. Clin. Virol. 29, 290–296.

Neesanant, P., Sirinarumitr, T., Chantakru, S., et al., 2013. Optimization of one-step real-time reverse transcription-polymerase chain reaction assays for norovirus detection and molecular epidemiology of noroviruses in Thailand. J. Virol. Methods 194, 317–325.

Noel, J.S., Ando, T., Leite, J.P., Green, K.Y., Dingle, K.E., Estes, M.K., et al., 1997. Correlation of patient immune responses with genetically characterized small in the United States, 1990 to 1995. J. Med. Virol. 53 (4), 372–383.

Notomi, T., Okayama, H., Masubuchi, H., et al., 2000. Loop-mediated isothermal amplification of DNA. Nucleic Acids Res. 28, E63.

Pang, X., Lee, B.E., 2015. Laboratory diagnosis of noroviruses: present and future. Clin. Lab. Med. 35, 345–362.

Pang, X.L., Preiksaitis, J.K., Lee, B., 2005. Multiplex real time RT-PCR for the detection and quantitation of norovirus genogroups I and II in patients with acute gastroenteritis. J. Clin. Virol. 33, 168–171.

Pang, X.L., Preiksaitis, J.K., Wong, S., et al., 2010. Influence of novel norovirus GII.4 variants on gastroenteritis outbreak dynamics in Alberta and the Northern Territories, Canada between 2000 and 2008. PLoS ONE 5, e11599.

Pang, X.L., Lee, B.E., Pabbaraju, K., et al., 2012. Pre-analytical and analytical procedures for the detection of enteric viruses and enterovirus in water samples. J. Virol. Methods 184, 77–83.

Pang, X.L., Preiksaitis, J.K., Lee, B.E., 2014. Enhanced enteric virus detection in sporadic gastroenteritis using a multi-target real-time PCR panel—a one-year study. J. Med. Virol. 86, 1594–1601.

Papafragkou, E., Hewitt, J., Park, G.W., Greening, G., Vinje, J., 2013. Challenges of culturing human norovirus in three-dimensional organoid intestinal cell culture models. PLoS ONE 8, e63485.

Payne, D.C., Vinjé, J., Szilagyi, P.G., et al., 2013. Norovirus and medically attended gastroenteritis in U.S. children. New Engl. J. Med. 368, 1121–1130.

Phillips, G., Lopman, B., Tam, C.C., Iturriza-Gomara, M., Brown, D., Gray, J., 2009. Diagnosing norovirus-associated infectious intestinal disease using viral load. BMC Infect. Dis. 9, 63.

Qiu, Y., Lee, B.E., Neumann, N., et al., 2015. Assessment of human virus removal during municipal wastewater treatment in Edmonton, Canada. J. Appl. Microbiol. 6, 1729–1739.

Rasmussen, M., Li, Y., Lindgreen, S., et al., 2010. Ancient human genome sequence of an extinct Palaeo-Eskimo. Nature 463, 757–762.

Rasool, N.B., Monroe, S.S., Glass, R.I., 2002. Determination of a universal nucleic acid extraction procedure for PCR detection of gastroenteritis viruses in faecal specimens. J. Virol. Methods 100, 1–16.

Richards, A.F., Lopman, B., Gunn, A., et al., 2003. Evaluation of a commercial ELISA for detecting Norwalk-like virus antigen in faeces. J. Clin. Virol. 26, 109–115.

Shigemoto, N., Tanizawa, Y., Matsuo, T., et al., 2014. Clinical evaluation of a bioluminescent enzyme immunoassay for detecting norovirus in fecal specimens from patients with acute gastroenteritis. J. Med. Virol. 86, 1219–1225.

Sidler, J.A., Käch, R., Noppen, C., et al., 2014. Rectal swab for detection of norovirus by real time PCR: similar sensitivity compared to faecal specimens. Clin. Microbiol. Infect. 20, O1017–O1019.

Siebenga, J.J., Vennema, H., Zheng, D.P., et al., 2009. Norovirus illness is a global problem: emergence and spread of norovirus GII.4 variants, 2001–2007. J. Infect. Dis. 200, 802–812.

Srivatsan, A., Han, Y., Peng, J., Tehranchi, A.K., et al., 2008. High-precision, whole-genome sequencing of laboratory strains facilitates genetic studies. PLoS Genet. 4, e1000139.

Stals, A., Baert, L., Botteldoorn, N., et al., 2009. Multiplex real-time RT-PCR for simultaneous detection of GI/GII noroviruses and murine norovirus 1. J. Virol. Methods 161, 247–253.

Straub, T.M., Honer zu Bentrup, K., Orosz-Coghlan, P., et al., 2007. In vitro cell culture infectivity assay for human noroviruses. Emerg. Infect. Dis. 13, 396–403.

Straub, T.M., Bartholomew, R.A., Valdez, C.O., et al., 2011. Human norovirus infection of caco-2 cells grown as a threedimensional tissue structure. J. Water Health 9, 225–240.

Straub, T.M., Hutchison, J.R., Bartholomew, R.A., et al., 2013. Defining cell culture conditions to improve human norovirus infectivity assays. Water Sci. Technol. 67, 863−868.

Suzuki, Y., Narimatsu, S., Furukawa, T., et al., 2011. Comparison of real-time reverse-transcription loop-mediated isothermal amplification and real-time reverse-transcription polymerase chain reaction for detection of noroviruses in municipal wastewater. J. Biosci. Bioeng. 112, 369−372.

Takanashi, S., Okame, M., Shiota, T., et al., 2008. Development of a rapid immunochromatographic test for noroviruses genogroups I and II. J. Virol. Methods 148, 1−8.

Takanashi, S., Hashira, S., Matsunaga, T., et al., 2009. Detection, genetic characterization, and quantification of norovirus RNA from sera of children with gastroenteritis. J. Clin. Virol. 44, 161−163.

Takanashi, S., Saif, L.J., Hughes, J.H., et al., 2014. Failure of propagation of human norovirus in intestinal epithelial cells with microvilli grown in three-dimensional cultures. Arch. Virol. 159, 257−266.

Trujillo, A.A., McCaustland, K.A., Zheng, D.P., et al., 2006. Use of TaqMan real-time reverse transcription-PCR for rapid detection, quantification, and typing of norovirus. J. Clin. Microbiol. 44, 1405−1412.

Tung-Thompson, G., Libera, D.A., Koch, K.L., de Los Reyes, F.L., Jaykus, L.A., 2015. Aerosolization of a human norovirus surrogate, bacteriophage MS2, during simulated vomiting. PLoS One 10, e0134277.

Turcios-Ruiz, R.M., Axelrod, P., St John, K., et al., 2008. Outbreak of necrotizing enterocolitis caused by norovirus in a neonatal intensive care unit. J. Pediatr. 153, 339−344.

Vinjé, J., 2015. Advances in laboratory methods for detection and typing of norovirus. J. Clin. Microbiol. 53, 373−381.

Vinjé, J., Green, J., Lewis, D.C., Gallimore, C.I., Brown, D.W., Koopmans, M.P., 2000. Genetic polymorphism across regions of the three open reading frames of "Norwalk-like viruses". Arch. Virol 145 (2), 223−241.

Vinjé, J., Koopmans, M.P., 1996. Molecular detection and epidemiology of small round-structured viruses in outbreaks of gastroenteritis in the Netherlands. J. Infect. Dis. 174 (3), 610−615.

Vinjé, J., Hamidjaja, R.A., Sobsey, M.D., 2004. Development and application of a capsid VP1 (region D) based reverse transcription PCR assay for genotyping of genogroup I and II noroviruses. J. Virol. Methods 116, 109−117.

Wang, J., Jiang, X., Madore, H.P., Gray, J., Desselberger, U., Ando, T., et al., 1994. Sequence diversity of small, round-structured viruses in the Norwalk virus group. J. Virol 68 (9), 5982−5990.

Wobus, C.E., Karst, S.M., Thackray, L.B., et al., 2004. Replication of norovirus in cell culture reveals a tropism for dendritic cells and macrophages. PLoS Biol. 2, e432.

Wong, T.H., Dearlove, B.L., Hedge, J., et al., 2013. Whole genome sequencing and de novo assembly identifies Sydney-like variant noroviruses and recombinants during the winter 2012/2013 outbreak in England. Virol. J. 10, 335.

Yi, J., Wahl, K., Sederdahl, B.K., et al., 2015. Molecular epidemiology of norovirus in children and the elderly in Atlanta, Georgia, United States. J. Med. Virol. (Epubished ahead of print).

Yoda, T., Suzuki, Y., Yamazaki, Y., et al., 2009. Application of a modified loop-mediated isothermal amplification kit for detecting norovirus genogroups I and II. J. Med. Virol. 81, 2072−2078.

Zhang, H., Morrison, S., Tang, Y.T., 2015. Multiplex polymerase chain reaction tests for detection of pathogens associated with gastroenteritis. Clin. Lab. Med. 35, 461−466.

Zheng, D.P., Ando, T., Fankhauser, R.L., et al., 2006. Norovirus classification and proposed strain nomenclature. Virology 346, 312−323.

Zheng, D.P., Widdowson, M.A., Glass, R.I., Vinjé, J., 2010. Molecular epidemiology of genogroup II-genotype 4 noroviruses in the United States between 1994 and 2006. J. Clin. Microbiol. 48, 168−177.

Zhuo, R., Hasing, M.E., Team of Molecular Diagnostics, Pang, X.L., 2015. A single nucleotide polymorphism at the TaqMan probe-binding site impedes real-time reverse transcription-PCR-based detection of norovirus GII.4 Sydney. J. Clin. Microbiol. 53, 3353−3354.

PCR ASSAYS FOR DIAGNOSIS

Hong Kai Lee and Evelyn Siew-Chuan Koay
National University Health System, Singapore

9.1 BACKGROUND

Norovirus is the most common viral causative agent in both localized outbreaks and sporadic gastroenteritis in all age groups (Gu et al., 2015; Khare et al., 2014). Of the seven current genetically classified norovirus genogroups, only genogroup I (GI), GII, and GIV viruses cause disease in humans (Vinje, 2015), with the GI and GII viruses being responsible for the majority of human infections. Norovirus outbreaks are frequently reported in semicontained communities, such as long-term care facilities, schools, hospitals, cruise ships, and restaurants (Bert et al., 2014; Vega et al., 2014; Bitler et al., 2013). In urban areas of Southeast Asia and some other Asian countries, where hawker centers or cooked food centers are commonly found, norovirus-infected food handlers from these centers could be the vectors spreading the norovirus in the community. An efficient laboratory diagnostic facility with rapid turnaround time is essential for reducing the speed and magnitude of the disease spreading in the community.

To date, human noroviruses remain noncultivable in most of the culture systems available (Papafragkou et al., 2014; Herbst-Kralovetz et al., 2013; Duizer et al., 2004). Although successful human norovirus replication in human B cells, with commensal bacteria acting as a cofactor in the culture, has been demonstrated recently (Jones et al., 2015), the modest level of viral replication achieved still prohibits its use for clinical viral culture testing. A molecular polymerase chain reaction (PCR)-based test can function as a rapid and accurate clinical diagnostic and/or surveillance tool, especially when other alternatives, such as immunochromatographic lateral flow assays and enzyme immunoassays, are not sufficiently sensitive for detecting the multiple antigenically distinct human norovirus genotypes and the rapid antigenic drift of certain genotypes (e.g., GII.4) over time (Vinje, 2015; Ambert-Balay and Pothier, 2013; Costantini et al., 2010; Vega et al., 2011).

9.1.1 COMMERCIAL PCR ASSAYS

Currently, there is no US Food and Drug Administration (FDA)-approved stand-alone norovirus quantitative reverse transcription–PCR (RT-qPCR) commercial assay. However, two gastrointestinal diagnostic assays that can simultaneously detect pathogenic enteric viruses, bacteria, and parasites have been FDA-approved—the xTAG Gastrointestinal Pathogen Panel (GPP; Luminex, Austin, TX) and the FilmArray Gastrointestinal Panel (GI Panel; BioFire Diagnostic, Salt Lake

The Norovirus. DOI: http://dx.doi.org/10.1016/B978-0-12-804177-2.00009-9

City, UT). Both assays can simultaneously detect and distinguish between norovirus GI and GII viruses (Buss et al., 2015; Gu et al., 2015; Khare et al., 2014; Navidad et al., 2013). Similar to the laboratory-developed assay described later, both assays have included internal controls (IC) for nucleic acid extraction and PCR inhibition (Buss et al., 2015; Navidad et al., 2013).

Gu et al. (2015) and Khare et al. (2014) reported a slightly higher sensitivity of the xTAG GPP (100%) to detect noroviruses compared to the FilmArray GI Panel (92%). The significant differences in overall test turnaround times and throughputs between both assays could be used appropriately for outbreak screening or for sporadic clinical testing. The xTag GPP can complete 24-sample testing within 5 hours (excluding sample extraction), which is more suitable for outbreak screening compared to the FilmArray GI Panel, which can process only 1-sample testing on the instrument at one time, although the overall FilmArray GI Panel testing from unprocessed sample to results can be completed within 1 hour (Vinje, 2015). However, the FilmArray GI Panel with rapid turnaround time and minimal hands-on time could function as a suitable platform for processing sporadic clinical testing that requires much lower throughput compared to outbreak screening.

9.1.2 STAND-ALONE NOROVIRUS QUANTITATIVE PCR ASSAYS

Several stand-alone norovirus RT-qPCR assays that have been developed for simultaneous detection of norovirus GI and GII viruses in single-tube format may fit the requirements for both sporadic clinical testing and outbreak screening (Miura et al., 2013; Rolfe et al., 2007; Vega et al., 2011; Trujillo et al., 2006). However, the robustness of these assays has not been characterized extensively on routine clinical samples or proficiency testing materials. Here, a sensitive and specific, high-throughput, triplex, universal norovirus GI and GII RT-qPCR, with MS2 gene amplification acting as an IC, is described. This assay was tested on 2158 clinical samples and validated on 58 proficiency-testing samples from the Quality Control for Molecular Diagnostics (QCMD) external quality assurance program (Scotland, UK). Several precautionary measures and useful practical notes when performing clinical PCR testing on stool samples, which are not limited to diagnosis for norovirus only, are discussed in detail.

9.2 METHODOLOGY

9.2.1 PRIMERS AND PROBES

All genome sequences of norovirus GI and GII were downloaded from Virus Pathogen Resource (last accessed: November 10, 2015). All sequences were aligned using MUSCLE software (Edgar, 2004) according to genogroups I and II. Overlapping regions of the open reading frames I and II in both genogroups' genomes were confirmed to be the most conserved and suitable regions for design of PCR primers. Primers and probes for norovirus GI, GII, and MS2 were designed to minimize the formation of secondary structures during PCR amplification. The probes were labeled with different fluorophores—namely YAK, 6FAM, and Cy5, respectively—to allow simultaneous detections of both genogroups and IC in single-tube format.

9.2.2 MS2 BACTERIOPHAGE PREPARATION

A live MS2 bacteriophage (15597-B1) stock was commercially obtained from American Type Culture Collection, USA. The lyophilized stock was first resuspended in 1 mL of carrier RNA (cRNA) solution, followed by a 10^5-fold dilution using the cRNA solution. The cRNA solution was prepared from the Qiagen EZ1 Virus Mini Kit v2.0 (Qiagen, Valencia, CA) according to the manufacturer's instructions.

9.2.3 RNA EXTRACTION WITH INCLUSION OF MS2 VIRUS AS AN IC

All stool samples were pretreated with 1X phosphate-buffered saline (1X-PBS) or 0.9% saline to a final concentration of 10−20% (mass/volume). The samples were vortexed vigorously for 10 seconds, followed by a centrifugation at 3400 relative centrifugal force (*g*) for 10 minutes. A total of 200 μL of the supernatant was used for extraction, with either the Qiagen EZ1 Virus Mini Kit v2.0 or the QIAsymphony Virus/Bacteria mini kit, using the proprietary Bio Robot EZ1 and QIAsymphony automated platforms (Qiagen), respectively. For rectal swabs, samples were pretreated in 500 μL of 1X-PBS or 0.9% saline prior to extraction. For vomitus, sample was pretreated with 1X-PBS or 0.9% saline to a final concentration of 10−20% (volume/volume).

Prior to the extraction, 10 μL of 10^5-fold diluted MS2 virus was spiked into 60 μL of the cRNA solution mentioned previously. The viral RNA extracted from 200 μL of treated specimens was eluted with 60 μL of elution buffer. For each batch of sample extraction, a blank 1X-PBS or 0.9% saline was included for separate extraction with the inclusion of MS2 IC in cRNA solution as described previously.

9.2.4 RT-PCR

Amplification and detection of norovirus GI, GII, and MS2 target regions were performed in single-tube format using 5′ exonuclease probe-based RT-qPCR. The RT-qPCR was performed with the SuperScript III Platinum One-Step qRT-PCR reagents (Invitrogen, Carlsbad, CA) using the LightCycler 480 II System (Roche Molecular Diagnostics, Pleasanton, CA). The 20-μL PCR consisted of 2 μL of extracted RNA template, 0.5 μL of enzyme mix, 10 μL of 2X reaction mix, and appropriate amounts of primers/probes as summarized in Table 9.1. All primers and probes were obtained from Eurogentec AIT (Seraing, Belgium) and TIB MOLBIOL (Berlin, Germany), respectively. The RT-qPCR was initiated with reverse transcription (55°C, 8 minutes) and initial denaturation (95°C, 2.5 minutes), followed by 45 amplification cycles at 95°C for 22 seconds, 58°C for 25 seconds, and 68°C for 20 seconds. Fluorescence signals were collected at every 68°C stage of each cycle. The GI, GII, and MS2 amplification signal curves were analyzed at the emission wavelength of 560 nm for YAK, 530 nm for 6FAM, and 610 nm for Cy5 fluorophores, respectively. All fluorescence signals were color-compensated at the LightCycler 480 II system according to the manufacturer's manual.

The clinical samples were subjected to neat and/or 10-fold diluted testing. A blank sample with MS2 IC included during sample extraction, a positive control, and a nontemplate control were included in all test runs.

Table 9.1 Primer and Probe Sequences Used

Primers/ Probes	Sequence	Working Concentration (μmol/L)	Forward or Reverse Orientation	Nucleotide Position
GI	5′-GCCATGTTCCGCTGGATGC-3′	0.175	Forward	5278–5296[a]
	5′-GCCATGTTCCGTTGGATGC-3′	0.175	Forward	5278–5296[a]
	5′-GTCCTTAGACGCCATCATCAT-3′	0.35	Reverse	5374–5354[a]
	5′-YAK-ACAGGAGATCGCGATCTTCTGCC CGA-BHQ1-3′	0.125	Forward	5320–5345[a]
	5′-YAK-ACAGGAGATCGCAATCTCCTGCC CGA-BHQ1-3′	0.125	Forward	5320–5345[a]
GII	5′-GGATTTTTACGTGCCCAGGCAAGA-3′	0.175	Forward	4980–5003[b]
	5′-GGANTTTTATGTGCCCAGACAAGA-3′	0.175	Forward	4980–5003[b]
	5′-TCATTCGACGCCATCTTCATTCAC-3′	0.35	Reverse	5100–5077[b]
	5′-6FAM-CCAGATTGCGATCGCCCTCCC A-BHQ1-3′	0.25	Reverse	5065–5045[b]
MS2 IC	5′-TCGCTGAACAAGCAACCGTTAC-3′	0.3	Forward	2203–2224[c]
	5′-TGTAAACACTCCGTTCCCTACAAC-3′	0.3	Reverse	2345–2322[c]
	5′-Cy5-TCCACGGCGCACATTGGTCTCGG A-BBQ-3′	0.25	Reverse	2277–2254[c]

[a]*Based on Norovirus Hu/GI.1/CHA5A010/2009/USA GenBank accession number KF039732.*
[b]*Based on Norovirus Hu/GII.4/Aomori7/2011/JP GenBank accession number AB933713.*
[c]*Based on phage MS2 genome GenBank accession number V00642.*

9.2.5 RNA STANDARDS

Norovirus GI- and GII-positive clinical samples with high viral loads were selected for absolute quantifications with the QX200 Droplet Digital PCR (ddPCR) system (Bio-Rad Laboratories, Hercules, CA) using the RT-qPCR assays mentioned previously. Briefly, 10^3- to 10^8-fold dilutions of both neat samples were subjected to the absolute quantifications using the ddPCR platform. Subsequently, eight 10-fold serial dilutions from the quantified neat RNAs were prepared according to Table 9.2. The standard dilutions were subsequently tested in triplicate to determine the linear dynamic ranges of the RT-qPCR assays. All the sample dilutions were performed using RNase-free water.

Separately, the lower detection limit of the GI RT-qPCR assay was tested with eight 2-fold serial dilutions ranging from 0.78 to 100 copies per PCR in eight replicates of each 2-fold serial dilution and repeated for three separate runs. The lower detection limit of the GII RT-qPCR assay was tested with eight 2-fold serial dilutions ranging from 0.20 to 25 copies per PCR in eight replicates for three separate runs. All the sample dilutions were performed using 10-fold diluted negative RNA extract.

9.2.6 CLINICAL AND QUALITY CONTROL SAMPLES

A total of 2158 clinical samples were collected between August 20, 2011 and October 22, 2015, at the National University Hospital (NUH), Singapore. Of these, 2155 (99.9%) were collected as stool

Table 9.2 Summary of the Cycle Threshold Values (From Triplicates) of 10-Fold Serially Diluted RNAs of Norovirus GI and GII Viruses, at Concentrations of $2-2 \times 10^7$ Copies/PCR

Log (Copies/PCR)	Norovirus GI		Norovirus GII	
	Mean	SD	Mean	SD
7.3	18.49	0.06	–	–
6.3	21.90	0.05	18.63	0.08
5.3	25.48	0.04	22.10	0.05
4.3	28.98	0.10	25.68	0.01
3.3	32.46	0.13	29.14	0.02
2.3	36.18	0.10	32.62	0.08
1.3	39.15	0.77	35.97	0.11
0.3	–	–	39.55[a]	0.63[a]

[a]Value derived from only two replicates.

samples. The remaining 3 (0.1%) consisted of 2 rectal swabs and 1 vomitus. Of the 2158 samples, 1929 (89.4%) were collected from persons suspected of causing (i.e., index cases) or involved in localized outbreaks, including food handlers and workers from nursing and child care centers. The remaining 229 (10.6%) were received as sporadic cases collected from in- or outpatients with gastroenteritis. Separately, a total of 58 proficiency samples of 5 consecutive years between 2011 and 2015 from the QCMD External Quality Assurance program were also tested using the same assay. The diagnostic sensitivity and specificity of the assay were based on test data generated from these quality control samples.

9.2.7 STATISTICAL ANALYSES

All categorical and nonparametric continuous variables were compared using two-tailed Fisher's exact and Mann−Whitney U tests, respectively. Two-tailed p values <0.05 were considered to be statistically significant. The limit of detection at the 95% confidence level was determined by probit analysis. All the statistical analyses and 95% confidence intervals (CIs) were performed using the IBM SPSS Statistics software for Mac version 22 (SPSS, Chicago, IL).

9.3 RESULTS

9.3.1 ANALYTICAL SENSITIVITY AND SPECIFICITY

In silico comparison of the sequences of the primers and probes against 31 norovirus GI genome sequences showed 100% matching for GI forward and reverse primers. Only 4 (13%) GI genomes have single or dual mismatches found on the GI probe target region. Comparison of the primers and probe sequences against 623 norovirus GII genome sequences found single or dual mismatches near the 5′ end of the GII reverse primer region of 214 (34%) virus strains and near the 5′ or the 3′ end of the GII probe region of 29 (5%) virus strains, but these were not expected to significantly affect the performance of the assay. Single base-pair mismatches were found near the 3′ end region of the GII forward primer in 31 (5%) GII strains. Such mismatches could affect the GII assay sensitivity.

Using the standard dilutions, linear dynamic ranges of GI and GII assays were determined as 2×10^2 to 2×10^7 copies/PCR ($r^2 = 0.9997$) and 2×10^1 to 2×10^6 copies/PCR ($r^2 = 0.9998$), respectively (Table 9.2). Both slopes of standard curves for GI and GII PCRs were 3.48, thus producing an amplification factor of 1.94 and PCR efficiency of 93.8% in both PCRs. The estimates of detection limit at the 95% CI for the GI and GII targets were 79.3 (95% CI, 48.1−169.4) and 1.5 (95% CI, 1.1−2.7) copies per PCR, respectively.

The testing of the 58 QCMD proficiency samples detected 19 GI-positive(s), 29 GII-positive(s), 1 GI and GII coinfection, and 9 negative(s). The coinfection that was detected was confirmed as a norovirus GIV.1 strain, according to the QCMD survey feedback. The diagnostic sensitivity and specificity of the GI assay were found to be 100% (95% CI, 82.35−100.00%) and 97.44% (95% CI, 86.52−99.94%), respectively. On the other hand, GII assay has a diagnostic sensitivity of 100% (95% CI, 88.06−100.00%) and diagnostic specificity of 96.55% (95% CI, 82.24−99.91%).

9.3.2 CLINICAL DIAGNOSIS

Of the 2158 samples collected between August 20, 2011 and October 22, 2015, 277 (12.8%) samples were detected as norovirus-positive using the RT-qPCR assay. The 277 positive samples included samples submitted for new cases as well as for follow-up testing of positive cases. Of these, 70 (25.3%) norovirus GI, 203 (73.3%) norovirus GII, and 4 (1.4%) norovirus GI and GII coinfections were detected. Of the 70 norovirus GI cases, 69 (98.6%) were detected from the outbreak-suspected clusters. The remaining 1 (1.4%) was collected from an inpatient. On the other hand, 175 of the 203 (86.2%) norovirus GII cases were detected from the outbreak-suspected clusters, and the remaining 28 (13.8%) were detected from the in-/outpatient clinics. The 4 norovirus GI and GII coinfections were detected from the outbreak-related individuals.

Only 68 out of the 70 GI-positive samples were tested with both neat and 10-fold diluted samples. Of the 68 samples, 52 (76%), 13 (19%), and 3 (4%) were detected in the three subcategories: (1) both neat and 10-fold diluted sample testing, (2) neat sample testing only, and (3) 10-fold diluted sample testing only, respectively. The median of cycle threshold (Ct) values obtained from the 13 neat samples only tested (subcategory 2) was 37.82 (values ranged between 31.82 and 40). The Ct values obtained from the three 10-fold diluted samples only tested (subcategory 3) were 35.96, 38.19, and >40, respectively.

Only 168 of the 203 GII-positive samples were tested with both neat and 10-fold diluted samples. Of the 168 samples, 120 (71%), 18 (11%), and 30 (18%) were detected in the three subcategories: (1) both neat and 10-fold diluted sample testing, (2) neat sample testing only, and (3) 10-fold diluted sample testing only, respectively. The median of Ct values obtained from the 18 neat samples only tested (subcategory 2) was 40 (values ranged between 31.73 and 40). The median of Ct values obtained from the 30 10-fold diluted samples only tested (subcategory 3) was 35.27 (values ranged between 24.38 and 40).

9.3.3 VIRAL LOADS OF POSITIVE SAMPLES

There were 27 (20%) GI-positive and 109 (80%) GII-positive samples after removal of duplicated or serial samples received from the same individual for follow-up testing. Viral loads of the GI- and GII-positive neat samples were extrapolated from the GI and GII standard curves derived from 10-fold serial dilutions of the quantified RNAs, respectively (Table 9.2). Interestingly, we found significant differences in viral loads between norovirus GI and GII viruses in outbreak-related samples (Table 9.3). The viral loads of GI-positive samples (median = 4.9 log viral copies/PCR) were found to be significantly higher than those of GII-positive samples (median = 2.8 log viral copies/PCR, $p < 0.00005$). Separately, we found significantly higher viral loads in GII-positive samples collected from in-/outpatients (median = 5.5 log viral copies/PCR) compared to those collected from outbreak cases (median = 2.8 log viral copies/PCR; $p < 0.000001$). The

Table 9.3 Summary of Viral Loads Derived From Neat Sample Testing and Patients' Demographic Information, According to Norovirus Genogroups and Sample Origins[a]

	Norovirus GI	Norovirus GII	*p* value
Outbreak causals			
Total positive	26	82	
Viral load in log(copies)/PCR (neat)			
Median	4.88	2.81	< 0.00005
Min−max	1.19−8.05	0.17−5.88	
Age			
Median	40	41	0.577
Min−max	21−63	21−75	
Gender			
Male	17	42	0.260
Female	9	40	
In-/outpatients			
Total positive	1	27	
Viral load in log(copies)/PCR (neat)			
Median	−[b]	5.53	−[b]
Min−max	−[b]	1.16−7.09	
Age			
Median	4	27	−[b]
Min−max	−[b]	1−92	
Gender			
Male	1	18	1
Female	0	9	

[a]*All the follow-up or repeated tests were removed from this table. Ct values of some samples were not available for the analyses due to PCR inhibitions occurring during neat sample testing.*
[b]*Statistic was not computed due to insufficient/no data available for analysis.*

Table 9.4 PCR Inhibition Status Observed in 1889 Neat and 1638 10-Fold Diluted Negative Samples, According to Years of Collection

Collection Period	Neat Samples		10-Fold Diluted Samples	
	Total	PCR Inhibition	Total	PCR Inhibition
2015	314	56 (17.8%)	314	3 (1.0%)
2014	481	70 (14.6%)	435	2 (0.5%)
2013	699	101 (14.4%)	498	6 (1.2%)
2012	225	82 (36.4%)	219	2 (0.9%)
2011, August–December	170	69 (40.6%)	172	2 (1.2%)
Total	1889	378 (20.0%)	1638	15 (0.9%)

Mann–Whitney U test could not be performed in GI-positive samples collected from both groups because there was only one GI-positive detected from the in-/outpatients group.

9.3.4 PCR INHIBITION

A total of 1879 samples tested as norovirus GI- and GII-negative. Another 2 samples were reported as indeterminate due to "overwhelming" PCR inhibition. Both these stool samples were extracted twice, and the extracted RNAs from both extractions were subjected to neat and 10-fold dilution sample testing; both gave negative readings.

All but 240 norovirus-negative samples were subjected to pairwise neat and 10-fold diluted testing; of the remaining 240 norovirus-negative samples, 222 and 18 samples were tested with neat only and 10-fold dilution only, respectively. The 222 samples tested as neat only were performed in six runs, and this testing mode was adopted when occasional large sample volumes were received. The 18 samples tested with 10-fold dilution only were performed in a single run, during the assay evaluation stage in 2011.

All the neat and 10-fold diluted samples that tested negative for norovirus GI and GII targets were included for PCR inhibition analysis. These negative samples included those that tested negative for both neat and 10-fold diluted samples, those that tested negative only for neat samples, and those that tested negative only for 10-fold diluted samples. Of the 1889 neat samples that tested negative for norovirus GI and GII targets, 378 (20.0%) failed to amplify the MS2 IC target (Table 9.4). In comparison, of the 1638 10-fold diluted samples that tested negative for norovirus GI and GII targets, only 15 (0.9%) failed in MS2 IC amplification.

9.4 DISCUSSION

9.4.1 MONITORING PCR INHIBITIONS AND EXTRACTION EFFICIENCY

Norovirus can be detected from stool, rectal swab, or vomitus collected from an infected patient (Vinje, 2015). Of these sample types, the stool sample is preferred as it contains higher viral titers compared to the other two types (Vinje, 2015). However, using stool samples for PCR diagnosis can be problematic because they are associated with higher PCR inhibition compared to other specimen types (Frickmann et al., 2015; Scipioni et al., 2008). Most of the clinical samples (99.9%) received for PCR testing at NUH were stools. A careful paradigm for norovirus PCR testing was implemented from RNA extraction until PCR setup to minimize false-negative and false-positive results. An IC, which consisted of live MS2 bacteriophage, was added during sample extraction (Rolfe et al., 2007). The MS2 bacteriophage, an RNA virus similar to norovirus, functions as an ideal medium for monitoring extraction efficiency and PCR inhibition status, both of which will impact the validity of the diagnostic results.

Between August 20, 2011 and October 22, 2015, a total of 2158 clinical samples were tested in a total of 207 runs, thus producing 207 IC Ct values for blank samples (Fig. 9.1A). The IC spiked into cRNA during the sample extraction was optimally set at a concentration that registered a Ct value of approximately 31 during RT-qPCR (Fig. 9.1A) in order to provide consistent interrun readings (standard deviation (SD) of 1.21) and to minimize PCR interference (i.e., competing for the essential PCR components) that could affect the sensitivity for detecting norovirus GI and GII targets (Stals et al., 2012).

9.4.2 PCR INHIBITION

An apparent right skew of the frequency histogram of IC Ct values was found when the extracted RNAs were tested neat, without dilution (Fig. 9.1B). This indicated that varying degrees of PCR inhibition could be present in the stool samples. This problem was resolved with 10-fold dilutions of the neat RNAs (Fig. 9.1C). Because the IC was spiked during the sample extraction, the higher Ct value of the IC during RT-qPCR could also be caused by suboptimal RNA extraction efficiency due to different matrices of stool resuspension. When no IC amplification was found in both neat and 10-fold diluted samples, an RNA reextraction from the stool sample was performed for repeat testing.

In this study, only negative samples were included for PCR inhibition analyses in order to avoid interference from norovirus GI-/GII-positive gene amplification that will compete for the essential PCR components. Such competition can result in delayed/biased Ct values for IC gene amplification. Scipioni et al. (2008) found complete PCR inhibition in 15.2% of the 86 stool samples extracted for norovirus PCR testing. In our study, complete PCR inhibition was detected in 378 (20.0%) of the 1889 norovirus-negative stool samples collected between 2011 and 2015 (Table 9.4). However, the overall 20% is the average during the 5-year period; notably, up to 36.4% and 40.6% of the extracted stool samples were found to encounter complete PCR inhibition in 2011 and 2012, respectively.

A 10-fold dilution of the extracted RNA is often effective to resolve PCR inhibition because the PCR inhibitors can usually be diluted out. However, the target nucleic acid must be in sufficient quantities in order to be detected after dilution. For the 236 norovirus-positive samples tested with both neat and 10-fold diluted samples, it was shown that performing the testing only on neat samples or on 10-fold dilution caused 33 (14%) and 31 (13%) false-negative results, respectively. Furthermore, the false-negative results of the 31 samples detected positive with neat sample testing only but not with 10-fold diluted samples were likely caused by insufficient quantities of the target nucleic acid to be detected after the 10-fold dilution (Ct values ranged between 31.73 and 40.00 during neat sample testing). Therefore, it is crucial to perform both neat and 10-fold dilution testing

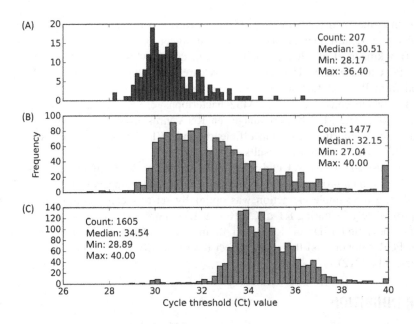

FIGURE 9.1

(A) Frequency histogram of IC cycle threshold (Ct) values for blank(s) with IC included during sample extraction ($n = 207$). A blank was included alongside a new batch of clinical sample testing. (B) Frequency histogram of IC Ct values for clinical samples with IC included during sample extraction ($n = 1477$). All the 1477 samples tested negative in both norovirus GI and GII targets. (C) Frequency histogram of IC Ct values for 10-fold diluted clinical samples with IC included during sample extraction ($n = 1605$). All the 1605 samples tested negative in both norovirus GI and GII targets.

to minimize false-negative results caused by PCR inhibition and insufficient quantities of the target nucleic acid after the dilution, respectively. Scipioni et al. (2008) showed that an alternative way to remove the PCR inhibition is to add bovine serum albumin in the RT-PCR mix. However, the assay performance of such an approach in terms of sensitivity and specificity in detecting gene target should be evaluated.

9.4.3 LABOR- AND COST-EFFECTIVE MODE

When unexpectedly large numbers of samples are received for screening during a major outbreak, the limited throughput of the 96-well real-time PCR machine to allow simultaneous testing of both neat and 10-fold diluted samples could constrain timely reporting of results. In light of the 10–20% PCR inhibition rate observed in testing neat samples, it is more economical and appropriate to perform neat sample testing only as the first-line screening. This eliminates the additional time spent on sample dilutions and reduces reagent costs. If PCR inhibition is detected during the first-line neat sample screening of a sample, a 10-fold dilution of the specific sample can be performed in the subsequent run to dilute out the PCR inhibitors. Such a practice would allow more timely reporting for most of the samples submitted for disease outbreak testing. Between 2011 and 2015, this algorithm of first-line screening was used in six runs involving 222 samples in order to process the high sample volumes received during four norovirus outbreaks.

9.4.4 COINFECTION OR NONSPECIFIC DETECTION

We detected four norovirus GI and GII coinfections from four outbreak-related individuals. Although the use of 5′ exonuclease probe in the RT-qPCR should have high specificity (Vinje, 2015), the possibility of nonspecific detections cannot be excluded because the coinfection found in one of the QCMD proficiency samples tested in this study was actually from a GIV.1-positive sample.

9.4.5 ANALYSES OF NOROVIRUS VIRAL LOAD

In addition to detecting the presence of a virus, RT-qPCR can provide relative/absolute quantification for viral loads. A recent study reported that a higher norovirus GII viral load was present in individuals with clinical symptoms compared to those without clinical symptoms, and it defined a clinically significant Ct cutoff value of 31 for patients of all ages (Phillips et al., 2009). Similarly, this study found higher norovirus GII viral loads ($p < 0.000001$) in the samples collected from in- or outpatients with gastroenteritis (median = 5.5 log viral copies/PCR) compared to the samples collected from outbreak-related cases (median = 2.8 log viral copies/PCR). The outbreak cases are more likely to have minimal or no clinical symptoms because most of them would have resumed their work, enabled by the lack of symptomatic disease burden, thus causing spread of the virus in the community.

In this study, all the norovirus-positive workers detected from the outbreak clusters (usually food handlers and healthcare workers) were required to submit stool samples for follow-up testing every week until two consecutive samples submitted for testing were found to be norovirus-negative. This testing algorithm ensured total viral clearance from the infected individuals before they resumed their work. From the positive samples detected from these outbreak-linked cases, we found no statistical difference in the time of the viral shedding period between GI-infected (median, 18 days (range, 2−48 days); $n = 21$) and GII-infected individuals (median, 12 days (range, 6−83 days); $n = 48$). A separate study reported that the median viral load of norovirus GII was at least 100-fold higher than that of GI in stool samples collected from symptomatic patients (Chan et al., 2006). Our study suggests that GII viruses may be shed off in higher magnitude compared to the GI viruses, although higher viral loads can be observed in GII patients during early infection.

However, comparison of norovirus GI and GII viral loads using multiplex RT-qPCRs should be interpreted with care because the PCR efficiency targeting different viruses and the Ct values registered by different fluorophores or by different PCR instruments could bias the viral load derivatives/estimations. In this study, we adopted a ddPCR platform to quantify the absolute copy numbers of norovirus GI- and GII-positive clinical samples used for RNA standard dilutions. Such an approach is expected to provide more accurate and unbiased viral load estimations (Dong et al., 2015; Bharuthram et al., 2014).

9.5 CONCLUSIONS AND PERSPECTIVES

Rapid laboratory diagnosis for norovirus is important to support disease containment of a norovirus outbreak. RT-qPCR assays for norovirus diagnosis are currently the most suitable methods to provide both highly sensitive and specific results and fast test turnaround time. However, because norovirus diagnosis is frequently performed on stool samples, extraction efficiency and PCR inhibitions should be monitored closely to minimize false-negative results.

Additional factors to consider when choosing a suitable diagnostic kit for viral testing are the test volume (including both expected and unexpected) and overall test cost for each sample, factoring in duplicate testing for the PCR-inhibited samples. For disease control/containment purposes, it is also important to opt for a highly sensitive assay that can detect samples with low viral loads, especially for outbreak surveillance testing for norovirus because the viral shedding period is long for nonsymptomatic patients who could still cause disease transmission.

ACKNOWLEDGMENTS

We thank Chia Wei Lim, Christopher Wai-Siong Ng, Lily Chiu, and Madeline Pei-Chin Ng for assistance in performing the norovirus PCR diagnosis work at the NUH between 2011 and 2015. The assay design work was supported by National Healthcare Group Small Innovative Grant SIG/08001 awarded to E.S.K.

REFERENCES

Ambert-Balay, K., Pothier, P., 2013. Evaluation of 4 immunochromatographic tests for rapid detection of norovirus in faecal samples. J. Clin. Virol. 56, 194–198.

Bert, F., Scaioli, G., Gualano, M.R., Passi, S., Specchia, M.L., Cadeddu, C., et al., 2014. Norovirus outbreaks on commercial cruise ships: a systematic review and new targets for the public health agenda. Food Environ. Virol. 6, 67–74.

Bharuthram, A., Paximadis, M., Picton, A.C., Tiemessen, C.T., 2014. Comparison of a quantitative real-time PCR assay and droplet digital PCR for copy number analysis of the CCL4L genes. Infect. Genet. Evol. 25, 28–35.

Bitler, E.J., Matthews, J.E., Dickey, B.W., Eisenberg, J.N., Leon, J.S., 2013. Norovirus outbreaks: a systematic review of commonly implicated transmission routes and vehicles. Epidemiol. Infect. 141, 1563–1571.

Buss, S.N., Leber, A., Chapin, K., Fey, P.D., Bankowski, M.J., Jones, M.K., et al., 2015. Multicenter evaluation of the BioFire FilmArray gastrointestinal panel for etiologic diagnosis of infectious gastroenteritis. J. Clin. Microbiol. 53, 915–925.

Chan, M.C., Sung, J.J., Lam, R.K., Chan, P.K., Lee, N.L., Lai, R.W., et al., 2006. Fecal viral load and norovirus-associated gastroenteritis. Emerg. Infect. Dis. 12, 1278–1280.

Costantini, V., Grenz, L., Fritzinger, A., Lewis, D., Biggs, C., Hale, A., et al., 2010. Diagnostic accuracy and analytical sensitivity of IDEIA Norovirus assay for routine screening of human norovirus. J. Clin. Microbiol. 48, 2770–2778.

Dong, L., Meng, Y., Sui, Z., Wang, J., Wu, L., Fu, B., 2015. Comparison of four digital PCR platforms for accurate quantification of DNA copy number of a certified plasmid DNA reference material. Sci. Rep. 5, 13174.

Duizer, E., Schwab, K.J., Neill, F.H., Atmar, R.L., Koopmans, M.P., Estes, M.K., 2004. Laboratory efforts to cultivate noroviruses. J. Gen. Virol. 85, 79–87.

Edgar, R.C., 2004. MUSCLE: multiple sequence alignment with high accuracy and high throughput. Nucleic Acids Res. 32, 1792–1797.

Frickmann, H., Hinz, R., Hagen, R.M., 2015. Comparison of an automated nucleic acid extraction system with the column-based procedure. Eur. J. Microbiol. Immunol. (Bp) 5, 94–102.

Gu, Z., Zhu, H., Rodriguez, A., Mhaissen, M., Schultz-Cherry, S., Adderson, E., et al., 2015. Comparative evaluation of broad-panel PCR assays for the detection of gastrointestinal pathogens in pediatric oncology patients. J. Mol. Diagn. 17, 715–721.

Herbst-Kralovetz, M.M., Radtke, A.L., Lay, M.K., Hjelm, B.E., Bolick, A.N., Sarker, S.S., et al., 2013. Lack of norovirus replication and histo-blood group antigen expression in 3-dimensional intestinal epithelial cells. Emerg. Infect. Dis. 19, 431–438.

Jones, M.K., Grau, K.R., Costantini, V., Kolawole, A.O., De Graaf, M., Freiden, P., et al., 2015. Human norovirus culture in B cells. Nat. Protoc. 10, 1939–1947.

Khare, R., Espy, M.J., Cebelinski, E., Boxrud, D., Sloan, L.M., Cunningham, S.A., et al., 2014. Comparative evaluation of two commercial multiplex panels for detection of gastrointestinal pathogens by use of clinical stool specimens. J. Clin. Microbiol. 52, 3667–3673.

Miura, T., Parnaudeau, S., Grodzki, M., Okabe, S., Atmar, R.L., LE Guyader, F.S., 2013. Environmental detection of genogroup I, II, and IV noroviruses by using a generic real-time reverse transcription-PCR assay. Appl. Environ. Microbiol. 79, 6585–6592.

Navidad, J.F., Griswold, D.J., Gradus, M.S., Bhattacharyya, S., 2013. Evaluation of Luminex xTAG gastrointestinal pathogen analyte-specific reagents for high-throughput, simultaneous detection of bacteria, viruses, and parasites of clinical and public health importance. J. Clin. Microbiol. 51, 3018–3024.

Papafragkou, E., Hewitt, J., Park, G.W., Greening, G., Vinje, J., 2014. Challenges of culturing human norovirus in three-dimensional organoid intestinal cell culture models. PLoS ONE 8, e63485.

Phillips, G., Lopman, B., Tam, C.C., Iturriza-Gomara, M., Brown, D., Gray, J., 2009. Diagnosing norovirus-associated infectious intestinal disease using viral load. BMC Infect. Dis. 9, 63.

Rolfe, K.J., Parmar, S., Mururi, D., Wreghitt, T.G., Jalal, H., Zhang, H., et al., 2007. An internally controlled, one-step, real-time RT-PCR assay for norovirus detection and genogrouping. J. Clin. Virol. 39, 318–321.

Scipioni, A., Bourgot, I., Mauroy, A., Ziant, D., Saegerman, C., Daube, G., et al., 2008. Detection and quantification of human and bovine noroviruses by a TaqMan RT-PCR assay with a control for inhibition. Mol. Cell. Probes. 22, 215–222.

Stals, A., Mathijs, E., Baert, L., Botteldoorn, N., Denayer, S., Mauroy, A., et al., 2012. Molecular detection and genotyping of noroviruses. Food Environ. Virol. 4, 153–167.

Trujillo, A.A., Mccaustland, K.A., Zheng, D.P., Hadley, L.A., Vaughn, G., Adams, S.M., et al., 2006. Use of TaqMan real-time reverse transcription-PCR for rapid detection, quantification, and typing of norovirus. J. Clin. Microbiol. 44, 1405–1412.

Vega, E., Barclay, L., Gregoricus, N., Williams, K., Lee, D., Vinje, J., 2011. Novel surveillance network for norovirus gastroenteritis outbreaks, United States. Emerg. Infect. Dis. 17, 1389–1395.

Vega, E., Barclay, L., Gregoricus, N., Shirley, S.H., Lee, D., Vinje, J., 2014. Genotypic and epidemiologic trends of norovirus outbreaks in the United States, 2009 to 2013. J. Clin. Microbiol. 52, 147–155.

Vinje, J., 2015. Advances in laboratory methods for detection and typing of norovirus. J. Clin. Microbiol. 53, 373–381.

"PANᴛʀᴀᴘ": A NOVEL DETECTION METHOD FOR GENERAL FOOD SAMPLES

10

Hiroyuki Saito[1], Miho Toho[2], Tomoyuki Tanaka[3] and Mamoru Noda[4]

[1]Akita Prefectural Research Center for Public Health and Environment, Akita, Japan [2]Fukui Prefectural Institute of Public Health and Environmental Science, Fukui, Japan [3]Hidaka General Hospital, Gobo, Japan [4]National Institute of Health Sciences, Tokyo, Japan

10.1 BACKGROUND

Norovirus (NoV) infection is a major cause of diarrhea, responsible for 20% of diarrhea cases worldwide and 50,000−100,000 deaths among children in developing countries each year. It has been reported that NoV affects approximately 1 in 15 people in the United States, causing 56,000−71,000 hospitalizations and 570−800 deaths annually; that more than 50% of cases of NoV infection are foodborne; and that NoV infection is associated with an annual health care cost of $5.5 billion.

In Japan, numerous cases of NoV-related illness, including food poisoning, are reported during the seasonal outbreak between late autumn and early spring. According to 2015 food poisoning statistics by the Ministry of Health, Labour and Welfare Japan, 65.5% of food poisoning cases were caused by NoV, and approximately 70% of the reported incidents of NoV infection were attributable to food prepared in restaurants.

NoV has been characterized as the major causative agent of viral food poisoning. However, there are only a few cases in which NoV was successfully detected from common food items, except for oysters, resulting in difficulties in identifying the sources and routes of contamination as well as in establishing effective strategies for the prevention of food poisoning.

In Japan, the concept of viral food poisoning was first established in the Food Sanitation Act of Japan in 1997. Since then, the detection of NoV genes from stool samples has become an essential component of epidemiological investigations of food poisoning outbreaks and, thus, marked technical progress has been made in recent years. In contrast, NoV detection from food samples has been a difficult pursuit for more than 10 years, creating an urgent need to develop detection methods for viruses in food.

We have explored practical procedures to detect NoV in food items and developed a novel method, termed the PANtrap method, that allows the detection of NoV from various types of food, including solid, liquid, paste, and fried items (Saito et al., 2015). This chapter discusses the advantages of the PANtrap method and prospects for its future applications.

The Norovirus. DOI: http://dx.doi.org/10.1016/B978-0-12-804177-2.00010-5

10.2 REASONS FOR DIFFICULTIES IN DETECTING NOVs IN FOOD

The lack of an established culture system for NoV has hampered the isolation and identification of NoV from food samples. Although direct detection by polymerase chain reaction (PCR) or other techniques is recognized as the only available assay for NoV, this approach involves greater procedural difficulties for the following reasons:

1. *Sample numbers*: Virological analysis of food must be performed on all samples collected; therefore, a large number of samples are required. The use of pooled food samples is associated with the problem of sample volume, as described next.
2. *Sample volume*: The volume of an emulsion of a food sample suspended in a buffer solution is at least approximately 50 mL, in marked contrast to a 10% stool suspension, of which the initial volume for extraction is 1 mL. For PCR assays, such a food emulsion must be concentrated nearly 1000-fold to obtain approximately 50 μL of RNA extract.
3. *Material properties of samples*: It may be possible to collect NoV from a smooth-surfaced, solid food item by rinsing it in a buffer, and the resulting sample solution may have relatively low turbidity. However, an emulsion of a paste-type or oily item remains turbid after multiple centrifugation steps. Filtration is not successful due to particulate materials clogging the filters, and a commonly used polyethylene glycol (PEG) concentration method often gives rise to a large amount of the pellet that is not related to NoV.
4. *Equipment, time, and cost*: The PEG concentration method generally involves overnight treatment followed by centrifugation at approximately 9500g to collect the precipitate. High-speed refrigerated centrifuges often require the use of proprietary centrifuge tubes. Such special equipment is not only costly but also poses the potential risk of cross-contamination due to its nondisposable nature.

10.3 PRINCIPLE OF THE PANtrap METHOD

In the PANtrap method, a food-emulsion sample is incubated with a specific antibody against NoV, and the resulting antigen−antibody complex is precipitated by adsorption to *Staphylococcus aureus* surface protein A. Following this process, NoV particles captured in the immune complex can be detected by PCR. The most important advantage of this method is that turbid food emulsions can be analyzed directly without any pretreatment. Fig. 10.1 shows the basic protocol of the PANtrap method. In brief, a food sample is suspended in 50 mL of homogenizing buffer (0.1 M Tris−HCl, 0.5 M NaCl, 0.1% Tween 20; pH 8.4) and centrifuged at 1870g for 30 minutes. The turbidity of the supernatant does not affect the assay. The supernatant is then incubated with anti-NoV antibody and heat-treated, formalin-fixed *S. aureus* (PANSORBIN Cells, Merk, Darmstadt, Germany) for 15 minutes to form complexes of NoV−IgG−bacterial cells. After centrifugation at 1870g for 20 minutes, the pellet of *S. aureus*-adsorbed complexes containing NoV is collected, resuspended in a small volume of buffer, and subjected to RNA extraction followed by real-time reverse transcription (RT)-PCR, as described previously. This method allows the efficient extraction and concentration of 50 mL of a food-emulsion sample into 50 μL of RNA solution for PCR assays.

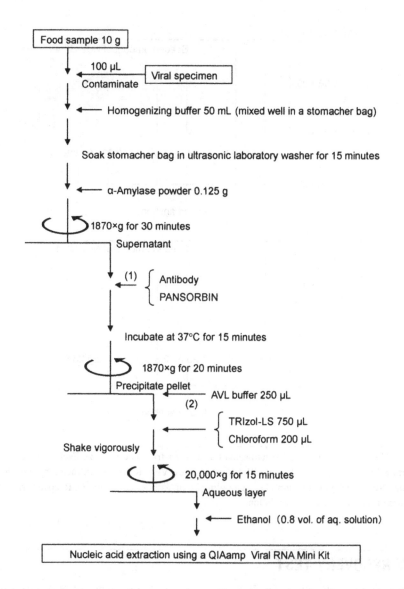

FIGURE 10.1

General protocol of the PANtrap method. (1) In order to construct the virus-IgG-*Staphylococcus aureus* (protein A) complex, 5 μL of virus-specific rabbit antiserum and 0.3 mL of PANSORBIN Cells or 0.15 mL of gamma globulin and 1.0 mL of PANSORBIN Cells were added. (2) The pellet was resuspended in AVL buffer (QIAamp Viral RNA Mini Kit).

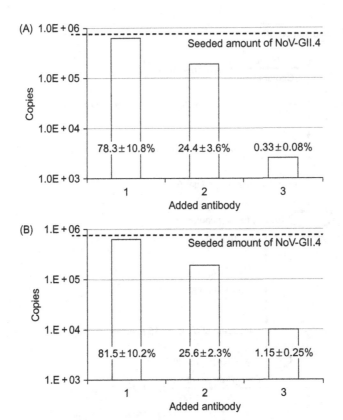

FIGURE 10.2

Recovery test of NoV GII.4 from spiked potato salad (A) and stir-fried noodles (B). Each 10 g of food sample was seeded with 8.18×10^5 copies of NoV GII.4 (dashed line). Viral RNA was extracted by the PANtrap method with anti-NoV GII.4 rabbit serum (1), γ-globulin (2), or without antibody (3). Recovery rate (%) is shown as a mean of three trials with standard deviation.

10.4 NOV RECOVERY TEST

Using the basic protocol shown in Fig. 10.1, we evaluated the recovery of NoV GII.4 from spiked food samples (Fig. 10.2). Rabbit antiserum against NoV GII.4 prepared by immunization with virus-like particles (VLPs) (Hansman et al., 2006) or a 5% γ-globulin preparation (Gammagard, Baxter, Deerfield, IL) was used as the antibody source. Reasons for the use of the γ-globulin preparation are described in Section 10.6. Real-time PCR for NoV was performed as described previously (Kageyama et al., 2003). cDNA was synthesized with the same primer as used in the PCR. Potato salad (a carbohydrate-rich food) and stir-fried noodles (oily food) were selected as sample items. As shown in Fig. 10.2, the assay with anti-NoV GII.4 rabbit serum achieved a recovery rate of approximately 80% in both samples, demonstrating a marked difference compared with

Table 10.1 Recovery Rates of NoV GII.4 From Various Foods Using the PANtrap Method and the PEG Concentration Method

Food[a]	Recovery Rate With the PANtrap Method (%)[b]	Recovery Rate With the PEG Concentration Method (%)	Relative Ratio (PANtrap: PEG)
Burdock salad	19.7	0.0197	1000
Fried lotus root	69.0	0.0820	841
Chicken boiled with vegetables	18.3	0.451	40.6
Spaghetti Napolitana	35.2	2.11	16.7
Sliced raw tuna	85.9	25.4	3.38
Mushroom mixed with mushed tofu	43.7	21.1	2. 07

[a]Food samples were spiked with NoV GII.4 at approximately 10^6 copies/g.
[b]NoVs were recovered with the PANtrap method using antirabbit serum against NoV GII.4.

the control assay without antibody addition (nonspecific adsorption). The use of the γ-globulin preparation led to a recovery rate of approximately 25%, resulting in a difference of three cycles or less in the PCR compared with the assay with specific antiserum.

We compared the PANtrap with PEG concentration methods in terms of the recovery of NoV GII.4 from spiked samples using food items with different mechanical/physical properties. The relative ratio (PANtrap:PEG) in Table 10.1 indicates the recovery rates for the PANtrap method relative to those for the PEG concentration method. There was no marked difference in the recovery rates between the two methods for smooth-surfaced foods, such as sliced raw tuna or mushrooms mixed with mashed tofu. The PANtrap method was particularly superior for certain types of food items, such as a mayonnaise-dressed burdock salad and stir-fried (oil-coated) lotus root, whose physical/mechanical properties readily allow the spread of viral contamination from the surface to the inside. Indeed, as mentioned previously, the turbid nature of their suspensions interfered with the procedures of the PEG concentration method. In contrast, the PANtrap method was successfully applied to all food items tested by following the same protocol, irrespective of the external form or physical/mechanical properties of the food items.

10.5 DETECTION LIMIT

In the recovery test described previously, we prepared test samples containing approximately 10^5 copies of NoV per 1 g of food. Because food poisoning incidents are considered to occur with a much lower level of viral contamination, we evaluated the detection limit of the PANtrap method using food samples spiked at different contamination levels with serially diluted NoV GII.4 (Table 10.2). Generally, a more sensitive technique, such as nested PCR, is employed to analyze a trace amount of virus. If currently available primers for NoV are to be used in nested PCR, the assay consists of a conventional PCR with the primers COG2F (Kageyama et al., 2003) and G2SKR (Kojima et al., 2002) and reamplification of the first-round PCR products by real-time PCR using inner primers. Although the results from this reaction system, irrespective of the use of real-time

Table 10.2 Detection of NoV GII.4 in Spiked Food Samples With Different Contamination Levels Using Seminested RT-PCR

Food[a]	Added Antibody	Contamination Level (copies/g)						
		3.5×10^4	3.5×10^3	3.5×10^2	1.0×10^2	3.5×10	1.0×10	3
Potato salad seeded with NoV GII.4	Anti-NoV GII.4 rabbit serum	3/3[b]	3/3	3/3	3/3	3/3	1/3	0/3
	γ-Globulin	3/3	3/3	3/3	3/3	3/3	0/3	0/3
Stir-fried noodles seeded with NoV GII.4	Anti-NoV GII.4 rabbit serum	3/3	3/3	3/3	3/3	3/3	2/3	0/3
	γ-Globulin	3/3	3/3	3/3	3/3	3/3	0/3	0/3

[a]*Food samples were spiked with different amounts of NoV GII.4.*
[b]*After the first PCR using primers COG2F (Kageyama et al., 2003) and G2SKR (Kojima et al., 2002), products of 387 bp were reamplified by real-time PCR. Detection was determined by the amplification curve raising. The experiments were repeated three times. The numerator indicates the number of the rising of the amplification curve (positive reactions/performed reactions).*

PCR, are qualitative in nature, they are comparable in terms of the predictive confirmatory value to those obtained by hybridization following gel electrophoresis and, thus, are useful in a time-constrained setting. When performed in conjunction with this nested PCR assay, the PANtrap method demonstrated a detection limit of 10 copies with the specific anti-NoV GII.4 rabbit serum and 35 copies per 1 g of food with the γ-globulin preparation. Note that these estimates of the detection limit reflect not only the effectiveness of the PANtrap method but also PCR reaction efficiency and that the final detection limit of this assay may vary due to a number of factors, including viral genotypes, genetic mutations in pandemic viruses, and the development of novel primers.

10.6 PANᴛʀᴀᴘ METHOD AS A GENERAL PROTOCOL

In the protocol development stage, we needed to simplify components of the assay system to optimize various reaction conditions, and we used food samples prepared by inoculating commercial food items with NoV GII.4 and antiserum raised by immunizing rabbits with GII.4 VLPs as a precipitating antibody. Laboratory-prepared antiserum is theoretically supported, but it is available only in a limited number of research facilities, requiring a steady supply of antibody to address numerous food poisoning cases. At the time of sample arrival in practical settings, it is difficult to select an appropriate capture antibody for NoV of an unknown genotype. In addition, the presence of other food poisoning viruses, such as sapovirus (SaV), should be taken into account.

Humans have antibodies against a variety of viruses, including (according to antibody prevalence studies) NoV, to which they are exposed in childhood. Therefore, commercial human serum can be effectively used as an antibody source against various types of NoV and other food

Table 10.3 Reactivity of Antibodies Against Foodborne Viruses Based on Recovery Rate

Virus[a]		Added Antibody and Recovery (%)	
		γ-Globulin	Rabbit Antiserum
NoV	GI.3	12.6	50.4
	GI.4	12.7	14.3
	GI.5	7.0	N.T.
	GI.6	2.7	13.0
	GII.2	45.1	93.4
	GII.3	12.4	14.8
	GII.4	45.7	77.3
	GII.5	22.4	36.4
	GII.6	11.9	18.4
	GII.12	43.0	65.8
	GII.13	17.1	N.T.
	GII.14	55.5	N.T.
	GII.22	9.4	N.T.
SaV	GI.1	8.0	N.T.
	GII.3	30.2	N.T.
	GIV.1	16.9	N.T.
	GV.1	35.3	N.T.
HAV		13.7	N.T.
AdV41		38.4	N.T.

[a]Approximately 10^5 copies of each foodborne virus suspended in 50 mL of homogenizing buffer were recovered by the PANtrap method. N.T., not tested.

poisoning viruses without quantity constraints. Although these advantages are beneficial, there is the problem of how to correct or minimize differences in antibody prevalence or titers between individuals. To overcome this drawback, we used a commercial γ-globulin preparation derived from pooled plasma from more than 10,000 donors. The γ-globulin preparation was effective against 13 NoV genotypes (GI.3, GI.4, GI.5, GI.6, GII.2, GII.3, GII.4, GII.5, GII.6, GII.12, GII.13, GII.14, and GII.22), 4 human-infective SaV genotypes (GI.1, GII.3, GIV.1, and GV.1), hepatitis A virus (HAV), and adenovirus type 41 (AdV41) (Table 10.3). Due to its content of high-titer antibodies to various food poisoning viruses, such as HAV and SaV, the use of γ-globulin in the PANtrap method allows the detection of a wide range of food poisoning viruses. The volume of antibody indicated in Fig. 10.1 is for a 5% γ-globulin preparation and should be optimized when using other γ-globulin preparations with different concentrations (75 and 50 μL for 10% and 15% preparations, respectively). An extremely large amount of antibody exceeding the antibody-binding capacity of PANSORBIN Cells results in a lower recovery rate.

Virus extraction with convalescent-phase serum samples from patients may serve as an effective initial approach to dealing with outbreaks of unknown viruses in the future. With its theoretical advantages, a virus-specific rabbit antiserum can be efficiently used to monitor assay performance, thereby circumventing the problem of quantity.

10.7 OTHER APPLICATION CONSIDERATIONS

We have extensively investigated the PANtrap method and note three major points that need to be discussed. First, carbohydrates are the major components interfering with the detection of viruses in food. Fats in food have a minimal impact on PCR reactions, as long as virus particles are efficiently recovered by rinsing (this is why the emulsification process using ultrasonic waves is incorporated into our protocol), whereas carbohydrates remain even after various separation procedures because their physical and chemical behavior is similar to that of nucleic acids. In our protocol (Fig. 10.1), this problem was overcome by employing Stomacher filter bags and α-amylase hydrolysis.

Second, it is recommended to perform cDNA synthesis with a virus-specific reverse transcription primer. Reverse transcription reactions with commonly used random primers or oligo-dT primers result in nonspecific amplification because RNA solution extracted using the PANtrap method contains a large amount of *S. aureus* RNA. DNA and RNA from *S. aureus* exert positive effects on some steps of the assay process by functioning as a carrier to stabilize a trace amount of viral RNA. Contaminated *S. aureus* DNA is removed by DNase treatment, which is commonly performed immediately before cDNA synthesis, and contamination with *S. aureus* RNA is ruled out using a virus-specific RT primer.

Third, PANSORBIN Cells, which form the basis of this method, are the commercially available product of only one company. Considering the possible unavailability of this product due to a supply shortage, depleted stocks, or future production cessation, a strategy to deal with this limitation needs be developed. An alternative reagent with similar properties can be prepared from laboratory-grown protein A-producing *S. aureus* Cowan I (cultured in liquid medium) with formalin fixation and heat treatment (Kessler, 1975). We have confirmed that this laboratory-prepared reagent is comparable in performance, such as recovery, to the commercial product, and it can be stored for approximately 1 year after preparation to facilitate a large stock.

10.8 CONCLUSIONS AND PERSPECTIVES

The detection of viruses in food has been a worldwide focus of investigation for more than 10 years, and various procedures have been developed based on different principles. The PANtrap method, which was designed with the original intention of applying it in routine examinations, has been perfected with regard to some aspects. The lack of the need for large laboratory instruments, such as high-speed refrigerated centrifuges, and the availability of the reagents from commercial sources allow ease of adaptability. From an operational perspective, due to its flexibility, the PANtrap method serves as a "backbone protocol," in which the antibody and reagents can be varied and tailored according to the circumstances. There has been one reported case of NoV detection from a food item using this method with a γ-globulin preparation (Tsuchiya et al., 2015). The PANtrap method will be further improved by its practical and widespread use in a large number of laboratories.

ACKNOWLEDGMENT

This study was partially supported by grants for research on food safety from the Ministry of Health, Labour, and Welfare of Japan.

REFERENCES

Hansman, G.S., Natori, K., Shirato-Horikoshi, H., Ogawa, S., Oka, T., Katayama, K., et al., 2006. Genetic and antigenic diversity among noroviruses. J. Gen. Virol. 87, 909−919.

Kageyama, T., Kojima, S., Shinohara, M., Uchida, K., Fukushi, S., Hoshino, F.B., et al., 2003. Broadly reactive and highly sensitive assay for Norwalk-like viruses based on real-time quantitative reverse transcription-PCR. J. Clin. Microbiol. 41, 1548−1577.

Kessler, S.W., 1975. Rapid isolation of antigens from cells with a staphylococcal protein A-antibody absorbent: parameters of the interaction of antibody−antigen complexes with protein A. J. Immunol. 115, 1617−1624.

Kojima, S., Kageyama, T., Fukushi, S., Hoshino, F.B., Shinohara, M., Uchida, K., et al., 2002. Genogroup-specific PCR primers for detection of Norwalk-like viruses. J. Virol. Methods 100, 107−114.

Saito, H., Toho, M., Tanaka, T., Noda, M., 2015. Development of a practical method to detect noroviruses contamination in composite meals. Food Environ. Virol 7, 239−248.

Tsuchiya, Y., Sahara, A., Jinbo, T., Nakano, T., Kato, K., Ogai, T., et al., 2015. A foodborne outbreak of norovirus caused by bread. Jpn. J. Food Microbiol. 32, 153−158 (in Japanese).

IMMUNOCHROMATOGRAPHIC TESTS FOR RAPID DIAGNOSIS OF NOROVIRUSES

11

Hiroshi Ushijima[1,2], Aksara Thongprachum[1,2], Shoko Okitsu[1,2] and Pattara Khamrin[1,3]

[1]Nihon University School of Medicine, Tokyo, Japan [2]The University of Tokyo, Tokyo, Japan
[3]Chiang Mai University, Chiang Mai, Thailand

11.1 BACKGROUND

Acute gastroenteritis or diarrhea is one of the most common diseases in children and adults and continues to be a significant cause of morbidity and mortality worldwide. Viruses are the major etiologic agents that cause diarrhea in both developed and developing countries (Liu and Black, 2015). More than 10 viruses have been reported to associate with diarrhea, including rotavirus, norovirus, sapovirus, adenovirus, and astrovirus (Table 11.1). Among the various types of viruses that cause diarrhea, rotavirus and norovirus are considered to be the major etiologic agents that cause diarrhea worldwide. In developing countries, rotavirus and norovirus are estimated to cause more than 400,000 and 200,000 deaths annually, respectively, among children younger than 5 years of age (Parashar et al., 2003; Tate et al., 2011; Liu and Black, 2015).

Previously, gastroenteritis caused by rotavirus infection had been reported as the most severe disease in children. However, with the successful development of rotavirus vaccines, the mortality rate associated with rotavirus has declined substantially. Rotavirus vaccine induces cross-protective antibody against different rotavirus genotypes, and vaccinated children usually show much milder symptoms (World Health Organizations, 2013).

In contrast, norovirus is reported to be a cause of gastroenteritis in all age groups. Norovirus infection-related death is often reported in elderly due to complications such as pneumonia or suffocation. Norovirus infection also leads to complications such as encephalopathy, kidney disorder, and febrile convulsion, especially in children (Ushijima et al., 2014). Foodborne transmission is a major route of norovirus infection. Eating raw oysters and shellfish may increase the risk of norovirus infection. Noroviruses have been found in drinking water, vegetables, and other food supplies. Infected food handlers are also one of the sources of the spread of norovirus (Ushijima et al., 2014).

Norovirus was discovered in 1972 by using an electron microscope from archive stools collected from acute gastroenteritis children in Norwalk, Ohio, in 1968 (Kapikian et al., 1972). Several different types of noroviruses have been recognized by immune electron microscopy (EM) with different convalescent sera (Okada et al., 1990). Initially, "Norwalk-like virus" was used to denote the prototype strain. With the availability of molecular methods, more strains have been identified, which has markedly enhanced our understanding of norovirus epidemiology. Recently,

The Norovirus. DOI: http://dx.doi.org/10.1016/B978-0-12-804177-2.00011-7

Table 11.1 Viruses Associated With Acute Gastroenteritis

Virus	Family	Size (nm)	Genome	Base Pair
Rotavirus	*Reoviridae*	70	dsRNA (11 segments)	18.5
Adenovirus	*Adenoviridae*	80	dsDNA	35
Norovirus	*Caliciviridae*	30–35	ss(+)RNA	7.5–7.7
Sapovirus	*Caliciviridae*	30–35	ss(+)RNA	7.6
Astrovirus	*Astroviridae*	30–35	ss(+)RNA	7.2
Human parechovirus	*Picornaviridae*	22–30	ss(+)RNA	7.3
Enterovirus	*Picornaviridae*	22–30	ss(+)RNA	7.3
Aichi virus	*Picornaviridae*	22–30	ss(+)RNA	7.3
Human cosavirus	*Picornaviridae*	22–30	ss(+)RNA	7.8
Saffold virus	*Picornaviridae*	22–30	ss(+)RNA	7.8
Human bocavirus	*Parvoviridae*	25	ss(+ or −)DNA	5.5

noroviruses in human and several animal species have been classified into at least seven genogroups (GI–GVII) (Rohayem et al., 2010; Green 2013; Vinjé, 2015). The norovirus strains relevant to human disease belong mainly to GI and GII, whereas GIV is rarely detected. GIII and GV have been found in bovine and murine, respectively. GVI and GVII are detected in canine species (Vinjé, 2015). Among each genogroup, noroviruses are classified further into several genotypes. GI is currently divided into 9 genotypes (GI.1–GI.9); GII contains at least 22 genotypes (GII.1–GII.22); GIII has 3 genotypes (GIII.1–GIII.3); GIV, GV, and GVI each have 2 genotypes; and GVII has only 1 genotype. The full-length sequence of the prototype of norovirus, the Norwalk virus, was determined in 1990 and was later found to be GI.1 (Jiang et al., 1990). Currently, the norovirus surveillance data from several countries worldwide indicate that the predominant strain is GII.4 (accounting for ~80% of all infections), and a new GII.4 variant emerges every 1 or 2 years (Thongprachum et al., 2015).

Human norovirus cannot be cultivated in vitro; therefore, most pathogenesis of and immunity to norovirus are obtained from studies in volunteers. Norovirus infection in humans can induce specific IgG, IgA, and IgM responses, and most patients are resistant to reinfection with the same genotype for 4–6 months. However, reinfection with different genogroups or genotypes can occur (Wilhelmi et al., 2003).

During approximately the past decade, significant progress on norovirus virion structure has been made by X-ray crystallography using norovirus-like particles. Recent studies of norovirus receptors have shown that different noroviruses bind to different histo-blood group antigens (HBGAs). All three major HBGA families—ABH, Lewis, and secretor families—have been shown to be involved in norovirus binding (Tan and Jiang, 2011). Norovirus GII.4, as the most common genotype, can bind to a wider range of HBGAs than other genotypes and is able to infect a larger susceptible population. The combination of strain-specific binding and variable expression on the HBGA receptors may explain the variation in host susceptibility for norovirus infection.

11.2 **DEVELOPMENT OF DIAGNOSTIC METHODS**

Because of the inability to cultivate noroviruses, diagnosis of norovirus infection in the past was based on viral particle visualization using EM (Kapikian et al., 1972). However, the EM technique is only useful for stool specimens that are collected during first few days of symptoms where a large amount of viruses are present. This method is costly, insensitive, and requires well-trained microscopists; thus, it is not widely used in general diagnostic laboratories (Lewis, 1990).

In 1980, methods based on the antigen−antibody reaction, such as immune adherence hemagglutination assay (IAHA), radioimmuno assay (RIA), and enzyme immunoassay (EIA), were developed for diagnosis of norovirus infection (Madore et al., 1986). IAHA detects norovirus antibodies in patients' sera using viral particles purified from the stool of infected individuals as antigens, and antigen−antibody complexes are detected by agglutination of group O human red blood cells (Kapikian et al., 1978). This method has limitations for routine clinical use because of the shortage of norovirus antigen preparation.

The success of molecular cloning of the Norwalk virus genome in 1990 led to dramatic progress in understanding the molecular epidemiology of noroviruses (Jiang et al., 1992a). Several complete genomes of different norovirus strains have been characterized, and numerous partial sequences of noroviruses have been deposited in the GenBank database. These allowed the development of the first-generation broadly reactive primers for norovirus-specific reverse transcriptase−polymerase chain reaction (RT-PCR) (Kageyama et al., 2003). Application of RT-PCR and DNA sequencing to detect and characterize noroviruses has markedly enhanced our understanding of the epidemiology of norovirus.

At the same time, the baculovirus expression system was exploited to produce norovirus-like particles (VLPs) (Jiang et al., 1992b). These VLPs were subsequently shown to be morphologically and antigenically similar to native virus particles. Instead of using native norovirus antigen from stools, the VLPs have been used for immunization in animals (mice and rabbits) to produce norovirus-specific antibodies that can be utilized to establish antigen−antibody-based diagnostic assays such as enzyme-linked immunosorbent assays (ELISA) and immunochromatographic (IC) assays (Shiota et al., 2007; Khamrin et al., 2015).

11.3 **DEVELOPMENT OF IC ASSAY**

For rapid detection of diarrheal viruses, an IC test is one of the most convenient and accessible diagnostic tools commonly used in primary care units and private clinics (Khamrin et al., 2014). When an outbreak of diarrhea occurs in a community, rapid identification of the virus causing the outbreak is required to ensure the administration of appropriate control measures. For this reason, several rapid test kits for the detection of diarrheal viruses have been developed. The tests do not require sophisticated laboratory equipment, and the process of testing takes only 5−15 minutes (Table 11.2). Several IC kits for rapid detection of the viruses associated with diarrhea, such as rotavirus, norovirus, adenovirus, and astrovirus, have been developed (Khamrin et al., 2010, 2011, 2015).

Table 11.2 Characteristics of IC Kits[a]

				Product Name		
	GE Test Noro	**Quick Navi-Noro 2**	**Quick Chaser-Noro**	**Immuno Catch-Noro**	**Rapid SP-Noro**	**RIDA Quick Norovirus**
Purpose (detection)	Norovirus antigen from stool	Norovirus antigen from stool	Norovirus antigen from stool	Norovirus antigen from stool	Norovirus antigen from stool	Norovirus antigen from stool
Principle	IC of mouse MoAb–colloidal gold	IC of mouse MoAb–blue latex	IC of mouse MoAb–colloidal gold	IC of mouse MoAb–colloidal gold	IC of mouse MoAb–colloidal gold	IC of mouse MoAb–biotin and streptavidin
Target specimen	Stool	Stool, rectal enema	Stool, rectal enema	Stool	Stool	Stool
Amount of drops	3 drops	3 drops	3 drops	3 drops	5 drops	150 μL
Judgment time	15 min	15 min	5–10 min	15 min	10–15 min	15 min
Judgment indication	GI, GII lines	GI + GII line	GI + GII line	GI + GII line	GI + GII line	GI + GII line
Sample treatment	Filtration one buffer	Filtration one buffer	Filtration one buffer	Filtration one buffer	Filtration one buffer	Sedimentation two reagents

[a]IC kits of ImmunoCardSTAT!, NOROTOP, SD BIOLINE NOROVIRUS, Immunoquick, and Noroscreen are not shown.

11.4 HISTORY

The first norovirus IC kit was developed in 2003 by using rabbit polyclonal antibody against norovirus of GII.4 Loadsdale strain. The IC kit was compared with monoplex RT-PCR (first round) for the sensitivity and specificity of norovirus detection. The sensitivity and specificity of the IC kit were 73% and 91%, respectively (Okame et al., 2003). The next version of IC kit was produced by using rabbit polyclonal antibodies against strains of GII.4 and GII.3. The sensitivity and specificity of this kit were 70% and 94%, respectively. The kit can also detect other genotypes of noroviruses. This IC kit has a lower limit of detection of 10^6-10^7 copy numbers/g of feces (Takanashi et al., 2008).

Following the successful development of monoclonal antibodies that are broadly reactive to GI and GII, IC kits that can be used for simultaneous detection and identification of GI and GII together in one line or separately in two lines have been developed (Khamrin et al., 2010, 2014). Currently, five norovirus IC kits are available in Japan. Five IC kits have been developed in Japan by using broadly reactive monoclonal antibodies: Quick Navi-Noro2 (Denka Seiken, Tokyo), ImmunoCatch-Noro (Eiken Chemical, Tokyo), Quick Chaser-Noro (Mizuho Medy, Tosu City, Japan), GE Test Noro (Nissui Pharmaceutical, Tokyo), and Rapid SP-Noro (DS Pharma Biomedical, Osaka, Japan). Other IC kits—RIDA Quick Norovirus (R-Biopharm, Darmstadt, Germany), ImmunoCard STAT! Norovirus (Meridian Bioscience, Paris), NOROTOP (ALL. DIAG S.A., Strasburg, France), SD BIOLINE NOROVIRUS (Standard Diagnostics, Yongin-si, Gyeonggi-do, Korea), Immunoquick norovirus (Biosynex S.A., Strasbourg, France), and Noroscreen (Microgen Bioproducts, Surrey, UK)—are used in foreign countries, especially in Europe.

11.5 PRINCIPLE

The principle of the IC test is based on antigen–antibody reaction similar to that of latex agglutination assay and EIA. The reaction is carried out through the chromatographic membrane by capillary action. The first norovirus-specific antibodies (mouse monoclonal antibodies against norovirus GI and GII are described here) are fixed on the chromatographic membrane (paper) while the second norovirus-specific antibodies, which are the same as the first ones, are conjugated with latex particle or colloidal gold and inserted into sample pad. The sample pad together with the conjugated particle or colloidal gold are fixed on top of chromatographic membrane at one end of the membrane strip while the other end of the membrane strip is fixed with the absorbent substance. When the test sample containing norovirus antigen is loaded onto the sample pad at the sample area, the norovirus antigen will form a complex with antinorovirus GI and GII conjugated latex particle or colloidal gold. The complexes will move along the membrane toward the absorbent end of the strip and form a sandwich complexed at the test line area where the mouse monoclonal antinorovirus GI and GII are fixed on the membrane. The excess conjugated latex particles or colloidal gold will move further to the control line area where antimouse rabbit polyclonal antibody is fixed on the membrane. If the test sample contains norovirus antigen, a colored line will appear at the test line area. The control line results from the reaction of mouse immunoglobulin conjugated latex particle or colloidal gold with antimouse antibodies (Fig. 11.1). It takes approximately 5–15 minutes before the result of the test can be read. The test sample is considered to be positive only when

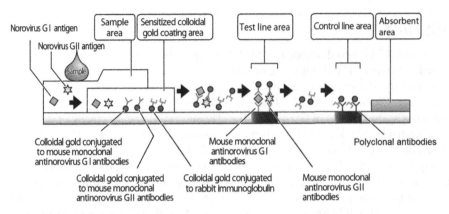

FIGURE 11.1

Principle of conventional IC assay.

both the test and control lines are observed. The test result is negative when no line is observed in the test line area with the appearance of control line. If both the test and control lines are not observed, the results are indeterminate.

11.6 IMPROVEMENT

Recently, rapid detection strips based on the IC principle have become commercially available for norovirus detection (Table 11.2). These IC kits have been proven to be more sensitive than ELISA tests. However, the limitation of the assay is that only a particular norovirus genotype that is reactive to the specific monoclonal antibodies can be detected. The development of broadly reactive antibodies for noroviruses is challenging, but it is needed due to the emergence of new variants. The advantage of IC lateral flow assays is that stool suspension can be applied directly to the test strip through the filter. Recently, IC kits have been developed by using broad reactive antibodies; therefore, they can be used to detect and identify both norovirus GI and norovirus GII.

11.7 EVALUATION

Recently, several IC kits have been developed from different manufacturers (Table 11.2). The sensitivity and specificity of these kits are variable. Therefore, validations of these kits by testing a panel of stool samples covering a wide variety of norovirus genogroups and genotypes is required to compare the sensitivity and specificity with the gold standard RT-PCR or real-time RT-PCR assays.

In general, the sensitivity and specificity of IC kits for norovirus detection are approximately 70% and 90%, respectively. A previous study demonstrated that the minimal detection limit of IC kits for norovirus GII.4 was approximately 10^6 virus copies/g of feces (Takanashi et al., 2008). However, it was observed that the sensitivity for the detection of norovirus variants was lower than that of GII.4. At least 10^8 virus copies/g of feces were required for the detection of GII.17 by each IC kit, which is approximately 1000-fold higher than that reported for the detection of GII.4 (Khamrin et al., 2015). Therefore, currently available norovirus IC kits must be redesigned and improved for the detection of novel norovirus variants. Laboratories and physicians should be aware of these findings, particularly when the novel norovirus variants emerge.

In addition to lack of sensitivity and the possibility of missing novel variants, false-positive results have been reported in stools taken from neonates (Takahashi et al., 2015). For these reasons, RT-PCR and real-time PCR methods are still the gold standard methods even though they are more technically demanding than IC assays.

11.8 CONCLUSIONS AND PERSPECTIVES

IC kits are useful tools for rapid diagnosis of norovirus infection. Although there is no specific therapy for norovirus infection, it is often important to reach a timely diagnosis to manage and control an outbreak. To make IC kits more clinically useful, further development to improve the analytical sensitivity and coverage of a broader spectrum of norovirus strains is needed.

REFERENCES

Green, K.Y., 2013. *Caliciviridae*: The noroviruses. In: Knipe, D.M., Howley, P.M., Griffin, D.E., Lamb, R.A., Martin, M.A., Roizman, B., Straus, S.E. (Eds.), Fields Virology, sixth ed. Lippincott Williams and Wilkins, Philadelphia, PA, pp. 582–608.

Jiang, X., Graham, D.Y., Wang, K.N., Estes, M.K., 1990. Norwalk virus genome cloning and characterization. Science 250, 1580–1583.

Jiang, X., Wang, J., Graham, D.Y., Estes, M.K., 1992a. Detection of Norwalk virus in stool by polymerase chain reaction. J. Clin. Microbiol. 30, 2529–2534.

Jiang, X., Wang, M., Graham, D.Y., Estes, M.K., 1992b. Expression, self-assembly, and antigenicity of the Norwalk virus capsid protein. J. Virol. 66, 6527–6532.

Kageyama, T., Kojima, S., Shinohara, M., Uchida, K., Fukushi, S., Hoshino, F.B., et al., 2003. Broadly reactive and highly sensitive assay for Norwalk-like viruses based on real-time quantitative reverse transcription-PCR. J. Clin. Microbiol. 41 (4), 1548–1557.

Kapikian, A.Z., Wyatt, R.G., Dolin, R., Thornhill, T.S., Kalica, A.R., Chanock, R.M., 1972. Visualization by immune electron microscopy of a 27-nm particle associated with acute infectious nonbacterial gastroenteritis. J. Virol. 10 (5), 1075–1081.

Kapikian, A.Z., Yolken, R.H., Wyatt, R.G., Kalica, A.R., Chanock, R.M., Kim, H.W., 1978. Viral diarrhea. Etiology and control. Am. J. Clin. Nutr. 31 (12), 2219–2236.

Khamrin, P., Chan-it, W., Satou, K., Nanba, Y., Yamashita, Y., Okitsu, S., et al., 2010. Evaluation of the newly developed immunochromatography test kit for rapid detection and differentiation of norovirus GI and GII. J. Trop. Pediatr. 56 (5), 368–369.

Khamrin, P., Tran, D.N., Chan-it, W., Thongprachum, A., Okitsu, S., Maneekarn, N., et al., 2011. Comparison of the rapid methods for screening of group a rotavirus in stool samples. J. Trop. Pediatr. 57 (5), 375–377.

Khamrin, P., Thongprachum, A., Okitsu, S., Maneekarn, N., Hayakawa, S., Ushijima, H., 2014. Comparison of three rapid tests for detection of norovirus in stool samples of acute gastroenteritis pediatric patients. J. Trop. Pediatr. 60 (6), 481–483.

Khamrin, P., Thongprachum, A., Takanashi, S., Okitsu, S., Maneekarn, N., Hayakawa, S., et al., 2015. Evaluation of immunochromatography tests for detection of novel GII.17 norovirus in stool samples. Eurosurveillance 20 (28), pii: 21185.

Lewis, D.C., 1990. Three serotypes of Norwalk-like virus demonstrated by solid-phase immune electron microscopy. J. Med. Virol. 30 (1), 77−81.

Liu, L., Black, R.E., 2015. Child survival in 2015: much accomplished, but more to do. Lancet. 386 (10010), 2234−2235.

Madore, H.P., Treanor, J.J., Pray, K.A., Dolin, R., 1986. Enzyme-linked immunosorbent assays for Snow Mountain and Norwalk agents of viral gastroenteritis. J. Clin. Microbiol. 24 (3), 456−459.

Okada, S., Sekine, S., Ando, T., Hayashi, Y., Murao, M., Yabuuchi, K., et al., 1990. Antigenic characterization of small, round-structured viruses by immune electron microscopy. J. Clin. Microbiol. 28 (6), 1244−1248.

Okame, M., Yan, H., Akihara, S., Okitsu, S., Tani, H., Matsuura, Y., et al., 2003. Evaluation of a newly developed immunochromatographic method for detection of norovirus. Kansenshogaku. Zasshi. 77 (8), 637−639.

Parashar, U.D., Hummelman, E.G., Bresee, J.S., Miller, M.A., Glass, R.I., 2003. Global illness and deaths caused by rotavirus disease in children. Emerg. Infect. Dis. J. 9 (5), 565−572.

Rohayem, J., Bergmann, M., Gebhardt, J., Gould, E., Tucker, P., Mattevi, A., et al., 2010. Antiviral strategies to control calicivirus infections. Antiviral. Res. 87, 162−178.

Shiota, T., Okame, M., Takanashi, S., Khamrin, P., Takagi, M., Satou, K., et al., 2007. Characterization of a broadly reactive monoclonal antibody against norovirus genogroups I and II: recognition of a novel conformational epitope. J. Virol. 81 (22), 12298−12306.

Takahashi, N., Nojima, I., Araki, T., Takasugi, M., Sakane, T., Kodera, A., et al., 2015. Evaluation of rapid immunochromatographic tests for norovirus in neonatal and infant faecal specimens. J. Int. Med. Res. 43, 648−652.

Takanashi, S., Okame, M., Shiota, T., Takagi, M., Yagyu, F., Tung, P.G., et al., 2008. Development of a rapid immunochromatographic test for noroviruses genogroups I and II. J. Virol. Methods 148 (1−2), 1−8.

Tan, M., Jiang, X., 2011. Norovirus−host interaction: multi-selections by human histo-blood group antigens. Trends. Microbiol. 19, 382−388.

Tate, J.E., Burton, A.H., Boschi-Pinto, C., Steele, A.D., Duque, J., Parashar, U.D., et al., 2011. 2008 estimate of worldwide rotavirus-associated mortality in children younger than 5 years before the introduction of universal rotavirus vaccination programmes: a systematic review and meta-analysis. Lancet. Infect. Dis. 12 (2), 136−141.

Thongprachum, A., Khamrin, P., Maneekarn, N., Hayakawa, S., Ushijima, H., 2015. Epidemiology of gastroenteritis viruses in Japan: prevalence, seasonality, and outbreak. J. Med. Virol. (Epub ahead of print).

Ushijima, H., Fujimoto, T., Müller, W.E.G., Hayakawa, S., 2014. Norovirus and foodborne disease: a review. Food Safety 2, 37−54.

Vinjé, J., 2015. Advances in laboratory methods for detection and typing of norovirus. J. Clin. Microbiol. 53 (2), 373−381.

Wilhelmi, I., Roman, E., Sánchez-Fauquier, A., 2003. Viruses causing gastroenteritis. Clin. Microbiol. Infect. 9 (4), 247−262.

World Health Organizations. (2013) Rotavirus vaccines WHO position paper: January 2013—recommendations. Vaccine. 31. p. 6170−6171.

CONTROL AND PREVENTION

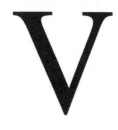

INFECTION CONTROL AND OUTBREAK MANAGEMENT

12

Bonita E. Lee

University of Alberta, Edmonton, Alberta, Canada

12.1 BACKGROUND

Understanding the characteristics that contribute to the high communicability of norovirus is an important first step to identifying critical areas in infection prevention and control for norovirus. Human norovirus, a member of the *Caliciviridae* family, is the etiological agent of at least six global epidemics of gastroenteritis outbreaks since 1996 (Siebenga et al., 2009). With the increasing use of molecular diagnostic assays in routine laboratory settings and the implementation of rotavirus vaccine worldwide, norovirus is also increasingly recognized as the leading cause of sporadic gastroenteritis in both adults and children (Ahmed et al., 2014; Lindsay et al., 2015; Platts-Mills et al., 2015). How does norovirus establish itself as a major etiological agent of gastroenteritis?

12.2 LEARNING ABOUT THE VIRUS

Until recently, there were no in vivo or in vitro culture models for human norovirus (Jones et al., 2015). Most of the studies on human norovirus have been limited to clinical and molecular epidemiological studies, genetic sequencing and cloning, the use of recombinant viral particles to study viral binding and serological response, and human challenged studies using classic norovirus strains. Norovirus is a small, nonenveloped, positive-strand RNA virus with three open reading frames (ORFs) (Glass et al., 2009; Robilotti et al., 2015). One of reasons why norovirus is a leading gastroenteritis pathogen is the genetic diversity residing in the viral capsid protein encoded in ORF2. Most norovirus infections in humans are caused by two genogroups: GI with 9 genotypes and GII with at least 22 genotypes. Although infections in infants and children are generally caused by a heterogeneous set of norovirus genotypes, norovirus epidemic outbreaks worldwide have been dominated by different variants of norovirus GII genotype 4 (GII.4 variants) that emerge every 2 or 3 years (Blazevic et al., 2015; Lee et al., 2008b; Siebenga et al., 2009; Yi et al., 2015). The understanding of immune response to norovirus infection is limited (Aliabadi et al., 2015b). Although norovirus GII infection provides some protection for subsequent GII infections, repeat norovirus infections by different genotypes and repeat infections by different GII.4 variants were observed in a prospective cohort study in Peruvian children (Saito et al., 2014). Experimental data on epitopes

The Norovirus. DOI: http://dx.doi.org/10.1016/B978-0-12-804177-2.00012-9

165

changes among the GII.4 variants supported the hypothesis that protective herd immunity drives the emergence of new GII.4 variants (Debbink et al., 2013; Lindesmith et al., 2013, 2008). Thus, the norovirus surveillance and scientific communities were quite excited about a novel GII. P17–GII.17 strain (GII.17 Kawasaki 2014) that had become dominant in various areas of China in the winter of 2014–15 (Fu et al., 2015; Han et al., 2015; Lu et al., 2015). Interestingly, only sporadic GII.17 Kawasaki 2014 outbreaks have been reported in North America and Europe (Lee and Pang, 2016). Proposed mechanisms for the dominance of GII.4 variants and the novel GII.17 stain over other norovirus strains include (1) a higher rate of mutations supporting the generation of variants (Bull et al., 2010; Chan et al., 2015) and (2) their affinity to a broad group of human histo-blood group antigens that have been shown to be important determinants of susceptibility to norovirus infections (Chan et al., 2015; Frenck et al., 2012; Zhang et al., 2015). Generation of norovirus variants that have escaped host immunity and are highly infectious to a large proportion of the population would result in a large human reservoir with reinfections over a lifetime. It has been postulated that immunocompromised and malnourished hosts who frequently present with chronic norovirus infections due to their suboptimal immune response are important reservoirs for evolutionary changes for norovirus (Karst and Baric, 2015).

12.3 MODE OF TRANSMISSION

Based on data from several human challenge studies with classic Norwalk virus (GI strain), norovirus has been shown to be highly infectious, with an estimated IC_{50} dose of 20–2800 virus depending on the type of human histo-blood group antigens of the study participants. (Atmar et al., 2014, 2015; Kirby et al., 2015; Teunis et al., 2008). There are various modes of transmission for norovirus. Norovirus-related waterborne outbreaks of different magnitudes have been reported in several countries (Cho et al., 2014; Giammanco et al., 2014; Kvitsand and Fiksdal, 2010; Poullis et al., 2002; Maunula et al., 2005; Zhou et al., 2015). A systematic review of waterborne outbreaks associated with small noncommunity drinking water systems in Canada and the United States identified norovirus as the etiological agent in 10% (29/293) of these outbreaks. In that study, norovirus and *Giardia intestinalis* were found to have caused the two largest proportions of human cases with illness (24% and 27%, respectively) (Pons et al., 2015). In the United States, norovirus was identified as the most common agent, causing 3444 (43%) of 7998 foodborne outbreaks that had a confirmed or suspected single etiology. These norovirus foodborne outbreaks resulted in 100,652 illnesses, 1028 hospitalizations, and five deaths from 1998 to 2008 (Gould et al., 2013). The most common reported settings for norovirus foodborne outbreaks in the United States were restaurant or deli ($n = 1885$), followed by a catering or banquet facility ($n = 318$); leafy vegetables were the most common single food item associated with norovirus ($n = 141$). Another analysis of foodborne outbreaks in the United States from 2001 to 2008 showed that most of these outbreaks were related to food worker health and hygiene, with contamination during preparation and service, except for mollusks and the occasional produce that were contaminated during production and processing (Hall et al., 2012). A study including data from systematic literature review as well as data from several surveillance systems including the Foodborne Viruses in Europe (FBVE) network and Noronet, CalicNet at the United States Centers for Disease Control and Prevention (CDC), and the Institute of environmental Science and Research (ESR) in New Zealand estimated that 14.5% of norovirus outbreaks from 2009 to 2012 could be attributed to food (Verhoef et al., 2015). On the other hand, it is recognized that the assignment of the mode of transmission for outbreaks (e.g., foodborne vs person-to-person) can be difficult and arbitrary (Hall et al., 2012; Imanishi et al., 2014).

Although important measures are needed to protect water and food safety to prevent and control norovirus infections and outbreaks, the remainder of this chapter focuses on norovirus infections in health care settings that are transmitted mainly by person-to-person or person-to-environmental contact. As mentioned previously, norovirus has a low infectious dose and can result in symptomatic or asymptomatic infections in both children and adults after a short incubation time of 24−48 hours (Atmar et al., 2008; Currier et al., 2015b; Graham et al., 1994; Lopman et al., 2015; O'Ryan et al., 2009; Ozawa et al., 2007; Phillips et al., 2010; Qi et al., 2015; Robilotti et al., 2015; Saito et al., 2014). Symptomatic norovirus infection generally is a short-lived illness for 24−48 hours. However, young infants and elderly infected with norovirus can be symptomatic up to 2 or 3 weeks (Costantini et al., 2016; Goller et al., 2004; Partridge et al., 2012; Miyoshi et al., 2015; Murata et al., 2007). Significant morbidity and mortality have been associated with norovirus outbreaks in health care settings, especially with GII.4 outbreaks (Desai et al., 2012). For immunocompromised patients, illness can be very severe and much prolonged with secondary complications (Bok and Green, 2012; Lee et al., 2008a; Roddie et al., 2009; Ye et al., 2015). Symptomatic norovirus infection often begins with nausea and vomiting, followed by abdominal cramps, fever (in $\sim$40% of cases), watery diarrhea, and other constitutional symptoms such as headache, chills, and myalgias (Glass et al., 2009; Robilotti et al., 2015). The term "winter vomiting illness" for norovirus infections describes a very effective mechanism for widespread dispersion of norovirus in the environment. A simulated vomiting system, "Vomiting Larry," was created to estimate the extent to which projected fluid can contaminate the environment (Makison, 2014). During an episode of projectile vomiting using this system, splashes and droplets were shown to travel great distances, with greater than 3-m forward spread and 2.6-m lateral spread. In a human challenge study using classic Norwalk virus, virus was detected in 56% of emesis samples with a median concentration of 41,000 (interquartile range, 3800−240,000) copies of virus per milliliter (Atmar et al., 2014). In addition to dispersing virus via emesis, $10^4–10^{13}$ copies of virus per milliliter are excreted in stool during infection (Atmar et al., 2014; Miyoshi et al., 2015; Costantini et al., 2016). Moreover, the duration of viral shedding in stool samples is longer than the symptomatic period and can be up to weeks after infection in pediatric patients and the elderly (>70 years). In immunocompromised patients, infections often result in a large volume of stool output at the acute stage and shedding of virus for months (Bok and Green, 2012; Lee et al., 2008a; Roddie et al., 2009; Ye et al., 2015). Sequence analysis and epidemiological data strongly suggested the transmission of norovirus from an immunocompromised patient at least 17 days after the initial diagnosis, but it was not clear whether the patient was still symptomatic at the time of transmission (Sukhrie et al., 2010). The relative role of symptomatic and asymptomatic patients and health care providers in norovirus transmission in three hospital-based outbreaks and two outbreaks in nursing homes was examined by estimating the onset of shedding of norovirus in various groups based on their shedding patterns using a nonlinear regression model (Sukhrie et al., 2012). The reproduction number (R_0) based on Monte Carol estimates for the probability of transmission showed that the contribution of transmission was symptomatic patients ($R_0 = 1.9$) > health care workers ($R_0 = 1.3$) > asymptomatic patients (R_0 not detected, with the contribution of asymptomatic patients being much lower than that of symptomatic patients in four of the five outbreaks). A later study by the same group showed that the peak norovirus genomic copies and duration of shedding in the stool samples in these symptomatic and asymptomatic patients were similar (Teunis et al., 2015). It is conceivable that asymptomatic adults who are continent and observing basic hygiene might not be an important infectious source for norovirus. On the other hand, the situation might be different in pediatric hospitals with infants and young children who need help with changes of diapers or in nursing homes, in which residents might need assistance with bowel routines. A previous review of norovirus outbreak reports from 1991 to 2004 identified patients as index case in 40% (25) of outbreaks, staff in 26% (16), and unknown index case in the remaining outbreaks (Mattner et al., 2005). Outbreaks started by patients were found to have a higher impact (more patients and individuals affected and twice the risk for patients to be affected) compared to the outbreaks started by staff. The risk of staff being affected was independent of the index source category group.

Why is norovirus in the environment a problem? Using reverse transcriptase–polymerase chain reaction (RT-PCR), human norovirus was recovered from fingers that touched moist tissue paper contaminated with fecal samples that tested positive for norovirus (Barker et al., 2004). The study then demonstrated consistent transfer of norovirus from dry contaminated fingers onto melamine surfaces. Moreover, norovirus was observed to be secondarily transferred from a melamine surface to telephone receiver, tap handle, and door handle approximately 50% of the time via clean hands. Norovirus is a nonenveloped virus, which is known to be more stable compared to enveloped virus. However, in the absence of an in vitro cell culture model, the stability and infectivity of human norovirus cannot be assessed, so most of these types of data were extrapolated from viral culture studies using animal caliciviruses such as feline calicivirus (FCV) and murine norovirus (MNV). Researchers demonstrated sequential transfer of infectious MNV from inoculated produce to kitchen utensils and then to produce cut by the same contaminated utensils (Wang et al., 2013). In a different study, infectious FCV was recovered on day 7 from lettuce, ham, and stainless-steel plates stored at 4°C and only from the ham and stainless steel stored at room temperature for the same period (Mattison et al., 2007). By measuring the infectivity of MNV inoculated in or placed on various surfaces after storage at room temperature for 42 days, it was estimated that a 1 log reduction in infectivity for MVN would occur in water after 42 days, after 15 days on stainless-steel disks, and after 4 days on lettuce (Fallahi and Mattison, 2011). On the other hand, different ways of preparing the inoculums of these animal calicivirus would affect their stability in these types of studies, thus explaining why the stability data might vary by different studies (Esseili et al., 2015).

Although the stability and infectivity of human norovirus still need to be studied, observations from various outbreak reports supported that human norovirus could remain infectious for days in the environment. An epidemiological investigation found that different contaminated areas in an auditorium from several vomiting episodes of an index case served as several point sources for a large norovirus outbreak in students attending a performance in the same auditorium on the following day. A higher attack rate was observed in students seated on the same level as the index case, suggesting that proximity to the environmental contamination is a factor (Evans et al., 2002). Similar observations and deductions were made for an outbreak in a hotel in which the index case vomited in two corridors, resulting in a higher risk of infection in cases exposed to the specific areas by history (Kimura et al., 2011). The best example demonstrating person-to-environmental contact transmission for norovirus is from an investigation of a long-haul flight. After a passenger vomited in the cabinet, different teams of flight attendants who had no other contact except for working on the same flight for successive flight sectors during the next 6 days developed norovirus gastroenteritis (Thornley et al., 2011). In that outbreak, molecular epidemiology provided additional evidence because the illness was associated with GI.6, an uncommon norovirus strain. Other studies have performed environmental sampling and testing for norovirus. A study used genetic sequence to characterize norovirus strains detected in patient samples and environmental samples (Nenonen et al., 2014). The environmental samples included swabs of various areas, dust samples, and ionized viral traps on seven wards that had had at least one norovirus outbreak during a 5-month period versus a control ward that had had no outbreaks. Norovirus were detected by RT-PCR in 48% of environmental samples on the outbreak wards versus 7% of environmental samples on the control ward, indicating a higher level of environmental contamination in the wards with outbreaks. This observation could also be related to the higher norovirus caseloads on the outbreak wards (58%) versus the control ward (12%), and a causal relationship could not be drawn. Sequence analyses identified 11 closely related GII.4 variants from patients from all eight wards and five clusters of GII.4 variants from the environmental samples. For outbreak periods in which both patient and environmental samples were sequenced, there was correlation with time and place for each outbreak. However, the GII.4 variants identified from a patient in the nonoutbreak control ward were also closely linked to a strain related to an outbreak on a different ward. Although only nucleic acids of norovirus were detected and infectivity was not assessed in the environmental samples, the importance of proper environmental cleaning procedures in rooms occupied by norovirus-infected patients is highlighted by the study.

Another interesting question is whether norovirus can withstand stress associated with aerosolization and result in airborne transmission through swallowing of airborne infectious virus. A research group in Quebec, Canada, detected nucleic acids of human norovirus in air samples collected by a two-stage cyclone aerosol sampler in six of eight health care facilities that had an active gastroenteritis outbreak. The concentration of virus was calculated to be 14–2350 genome copies/m^3 in 54% of air samples collected in patient rooms and 38% in the hallway outside the patient rooms (Bonifait et al., 2015). This group also used MNV as a surrogate virus to demonstrate that 76–86% of MNV that was nebulized as aerosols and desiccated remained infectious and that intact MNV was detected using a special molecular assay. However, airborne transmission of disease is complex and affected by many factors, including the droplet/aerosol generation process, the nature of the particle (e.g., viscosity), particle size, physical characteristics of the environment (e.g., temperature, humidity, and aerodynamics), pathogen load in particles, characteristics of the pathogen, and pathogen–host interaction (e.g., norovirus to be ingested) (Bunyan et al., 2013; Gralton et al., 2011; Robinson et al., 2012; Xie et al., 2007). Currently, measles, varicella, and *Mycobacterium tuberculosis* are the three pathogens well acknowledged to have airborne transmission—that is, transmission via droplet nucleic acids suspended in air containing infectious pathogens that can travel long distances (some defined as >1 m) and last a long time (World Health Organization, 2014).

According to the National Outbreak Reporting System in the United States, 5720 of 6223 confirmed norovirus outbreaks from 2009 to 2013 were classified as transmitted through person-to-person contact or environment (Wikswo et al., 2015). International guidelines for norovirus outbreak control recommend contact precautions with gowns and gloves for norovirus cases and additional droplet and contact precaution (i.e., including eyes and facial protection) when there is risk of aerosolization (e.g., with vomiting) (Table 12.1). Only the New Zealand norovirus outbreak

Table 12.1 Summary of Gastroenteritis/Norovirus Outbreak Control Guidelines[a]

	Definition of Outbreak and Laboratory Testing	Hand Hygiene	Point-of-Care Risk Assessment for PPE	Handling Patient Care Equipment	Environmental Cleaning	Patient Ambulation or Transfer	Visitors and New Admission	Waste and Sharps Handling
Routine practice for infection control (College and Association of Registered Nurses of Alberta, 2010; Siegel et al., 2007; World Health Organization, 2006)	Not applicable	MOST IMPORTANT • Perform hand hygiene before and after contact with patient and patient environment and appropriate donning and offing procedure if PPE is used • Clean hands before touching PPE supplies and clean hands in proper sequence with the removal of exposed PPE	Appropriate donning and offing procedure for risk-based assessment PPE: • Gloves: single use only; nonsterile gloves if contact with body fluids, mucous membranes or nonintact skin, contaminated items and environment • Gowns: single use only; protect exposed skin and clothing from body fluids or contact with contaminated environment • Mask and eye protection: single use only; protect from droplets in aerosols-generating process or procedure	• Bring minimal supplies into patient room • Discard single-use items • Clean and disinfect reusable equipment after and before use • Handle soiled or used linens with minimal agitation	• Cleaning and disinfection of frequently touched surfaces, from areas with lower likelihood of contamination to areas of higher likelihood • Regularly scheduled cleaning and perform discharge cleaning	Before leaving room, practice hand hygiene, put on clean clothing or hospital gown/ housecoat, and ensure body fluids or drainage are contained by dressing or appropriate apparatus	• Do not visit if ill • Practice hand hygiene • Observe additional precaution as applicable for the patient • In family-centered care, family not using PPE should not access hospital supplies or visit public areas designated for patient use in hospital	• Wear gloves to remove waste from patient rooms, treatment rooms, or if the outside of the bag is soiled • Double bag as needed; avoid contact with body
Caring for a patient with diarrhea and/or vomiting, unknown etiology extracted from routine practices (College and Association of Registered Nurses of Alberta, 2010; Siegel et al., 2007; World Health Organization, 2006)	Not applicable	Good hand hygiene, AS ALWAYS, and washing hands with soap and water is recommended for patients with gastroenteritis symptoms	IN ADDITION to above—clear signs to indicate contact precaution: gown and glove mask and eye protection if there is potential aerosolization (e.g., vomiting)	IN ADDITION to above—use appropriate agents or wipes that are sporicidal and virucidal	IN ADDITION to above—use appropriate agents or wipes that are sporicidal and virucidal	IN ADDITION to above—patient on contact precaution • Minimize patient movements except for essential care	Same as above NOTE—patient on contact precaution	Same as above
Guideline for norovirus outbreaks (Alberta Health Services, 2015)	*Start:* Two or more cases of GI illness with a common epidemiological	• Wash hands with soap and water when:	• In addition to Routine Practices, implement Contact	• Surfaces must first be cleaned prior to	• Surfaces must first be cleaned prior to	Consider • Minimizing patient	• Post outbreak signage at entrance	No specific instructions

	Hand hygiene	Precautions	Disinfection	Disinfection (two-step process)	Patient placement / movement	Visitor / admission restrictions
link (e.g., same location or same care giver, and evidence of health care–associated transmission within the facility), with initial onset within one 48-h period OR 96 h from onset of symptoms in the last case, whichever occurs first. *Lab test*: If one or more of outbreak samples are positive for an etiological agent, further specimens will not be tested unless there is specific request made to the laboratory. No more than six specimens from the same outbreak will be tested if the batch of specimens all tested negative for an etiological agent	• Hands are visibly soiled • After removal of gloves when caring for a patient who has diarrhea and/or vomiting • Alcohol-based hand rubs (≥70% alcohol) are an acceptable alternative to hand washing during gastroenteritis illness outbreaks, when used according to label directions	• Precautions (gown and gloves) when providing direct care for symptomatic patients • Implement Contact and Droplet Precautions (gown, glove, and face and eye protection) if patient is actively vomiting	disinfection (two-step process) • Hypochlorite at a concentration of 1000 ppm OR Surface disinfectant with a Drug Identification Number (DIN) issued by Health Canada with a specific label claim against norovirus, FCV, or MNV (e.g., 0.5% accelerated hydrogen peroxide)	disinfection (two-step process) • Hypochlorite at a concentration of 1000 ppm OR Surface disinfectant with a Drug Identification Number (DIN) issued by Health Canada with a specific label claim against norovirus, FCV, or MNV (e.g., 0.5% accelerated hydrogen peroxide) • Conduct a thorough enhanced cleaning in all affected areas at the end of the outbreak • Privacy curtains should be changed if visibly soiled and when isolation precautions for GI illness are lifted	movements and transfer • Suspending group activities	advising staff and visitors of necessary precautions • Discourage visit if ill • Visit only one patient and exit the facility immediately after the visit • Practice hand hygiene • Observe additional precaution as applicable for the patient • Consider restriction to admission No specific instructions
Guideline for norovirus outbreaks (Centers for Disease Control and Prevention, 2011) Definition of start and end of outbreak not specified. *Lab test*: Early collection of specimens; stool specimens from at least five ill persons are recommended	• Use soap and water for a minimum of 20 s • If available, ≥70% alcohol-based hand sanitizers can be used as an adjunct but should not be considered a substitute for soap-and-water hand washing	Reinforced effective preventive controls practices	Chlorine bleach solution 1000–5000 ppm OR EPA-registered cleaning products and disinfectants that have label claims for use in health care (https://www.epa.gov/sites/2016-06/documents/list_g_norovirus.pdf)	Chlorine bleach solution 1000–5000 ppm OR EPA-registered cleaning products and disinfectants that have label claims for use in health care (https://www.epa.gov/sites/2016-06/documents/list_g_norovirus.pdf)	• Isolation of patients • Cohort of ill patients with dedicated nursing staff • Minimize transfer	• Nonessential personnel, including visitors, may be screened for symptoms and excluded or, at a minimum, should be cautioned about the risks, with emphasis on hand hygiene • In certain situations, units in a health care facility may be closed to new admissions to prevent the introduction of new susceptible patients

Table 12.1 Summary of Gastroenteritis/Norovirus Outbreak Control Guidelines[a] *Continued*

	Definition of Outbreak and Laboratory Testing	Hand Hygiene	Point-of-Care Risk Assessment for PPE	Handling Patient Care Equipment	Environmental Cleaning	Patient Ambulation or Transfer	Visitors and New Admission	Waste and Sharps Handling
Guideline for norovirus outbreaks (MacCannell et al., 2011)	*Start:* If lab diagnosis is not available, use Kaplan criteria (vomiting in >50% of affected persons in the outbreak; a mean (or median) incubation period of 24–48 h; a mean (or median) duration of illness of 12–60 h; and lack of identification of a bacterial pathogen in culture of stool) (Turcios et al., 2006) *Lab test:* Using RT-PCR, sensitivity 84% for one positive among 2–4 specimens, sensitivity >92% for 2 positive among 5–11 specimens	• Use soap and water • For hand hygiene before contact with patients, consider ethanol-based hand sanitizers	Contact and routine precaution for at least 48 h after resolution of symptoms; may use longer periods for complex or immunocompromised patients and infants; face protection if vomiting	Use EPA-registered cleaning products and disinfectants that have label claims for use in health care (https://www.epa.gov/sites/production/files/2016-06/documents/list_g_norovirus.pdf)	• Increase frequency of cleaning to two or three times daily • Use EPA-registered cleaning products and disinfectants that have label claims for use in health care (https://www.epa.gov/sites/production/files/2016-06/documents/list_g_norovirus.pdf) • Consider steam clean of upholstered furniture upon discharge • Change privacy curtains if visibly soiled or upon discharge	Consider • Minimizing patient movements and transfer • Suspending group activities • Cohort staff • Allocate staff recovered from recent outbreak to care for symptomatic patients	• Exclude nonessential staff, students, and volunteers • Restrict nonessential visitors • Emphasize hand hygiene and PPE for visitors in extenuating circumstances • Consider closure of wards	No specific instructions
Guideline for norovirus outbreaks (Public Health England, 2012)	*Start:* Flexible definition with Infection Prevention and Control Team consultation *End:* Usually 48 h after resolution of vomiting/diarrhea in last known case or at least 72 h after initial onset of the last new case and usually related to completion of terminal cleaning *Lab test:* Isolate symptomatic patient pending testing; negative test will facilitate lifting of restriction more rapidly and support optimal use of isolation resource if limited	Use liquid soap and water	Use gloves and apron and only consider face protection if there is risk of droplets or aerosols	• Use single-use equipment if possible • Decontaminate all other equipment immediately after use	• Increase frequency of cleaning • After cleaning, disinfect with 1000 ppm available chlorine (0.1% sodium hypochlorite) • Use disposable mops/clothes or have robust laundry (71°C for at least 3 min or 65°C for at least 10 min) service for cloths • PPE for cleaning staff • Appropriate terminal cleaning on discharge • Prompt two-step process (cleaning and disinfection) for spillage or soiling by personnel with appropriate PPE	• Short-term norovirus isolation ward not recommended because of potential safety risk to patients and might not change progress of outbreak • Might need to decant ward to allow complete terminal clean	• Restricting visits to essential staff and essential social visitors only • Emphasize PPE for visitors in extenuating circumstances • Depending on the architecture of ward, use a risk-assessed approach for stepwise closure of areas with cohort nursing if possible (Public Health England, 2012)	No specific instructions

Guideline	Case definition / Lab test	Hand hygiene	Isolation / PPE	Disinfection	Environmental	Patient placement	Outbreak control / visitors	Other
Guideline for norovirus outbreaks (New Zealand Ministry of Health, 2009)	*Starr:* Two or more cases of illness linked to a common source. *Lab test:* Test in batches of three specimens until at least one positive has been identified. Subsequent testing is usually not necessary	• Wash hands with soap and water, with emphasis on protocol to dry hands effectively; use antiseptic hand wash; use antiseptic (waterless) hand rub or surgical hand antisepsis (reference to CDC). • Alcohol gel is recommended only after washing and drying hands in outbreaks; but alcohol hand sanitizers still recommended when access to adequate hand washing is limited	• Contact isolation. • Recommend airborne precautions when patient is vomiting	Disinfect with 1000 ppm available chlorine (0.1% sodium hypochlorite) or potassium peroxymonosulfate	• Discourage vacuuming of carpets. • Restrict access to contaminated area for at least 30 min	• Place patients on contact isolation until symptoms resolved for 48 h. • Consider cohorting patients if there are a number of cases. • Restrict patient movement out of isolation rooms except for essential activities. • Cohort staff to minimize exposure. • Exclude nonessential staff	• Post outbreak signage. • Minimize visits to symptomatic cases. • Prevent visitors of a suspected case from visiting other patients or residents. • Emphasize hand hygiene and PPE for visitors. • Tell visitors of a suspected case of norovirus infection that they must not visit patients or residents in other institutions for at least 3 days. • Closure of wards if there are ongoing cases despite implementation of outbreak control measures	No specific instruction.
Guideline for gastroenteritis outbreaks (Communicable Disease Network Australia, 2010)	*Starr:* Two or more associate cases of diarrhea and/or vomiting in a 24-h period or two or more associate cases of diarrhea and/or vomiting in a defined time frame in a setting that is prone to norovirus outbreak	Hands must be washed with soap and water whenever possible or decontaminated using an alcohol-based hand rub (70–80% alcohol) or gel when hand-washing facilities are not available	Gloves, gowns, masks, and eye protection if patient is vomiting or cleaning of areas contaminated by vomit or feces	Clean with detergent solution before disinfection using 1000 ppm bleach (0.1% sodium hypochlorite)	Increase frequency of cleaning (at least twice a day)	• Place patients on isolation until symptoms resolved for 72 h; restrict from common areas. • Cohorting of ill patients, especially in semiclosed environment	• Visiting affected areas should be restricted during the period of an outbreak. • Advise unwell visitors not to visit their relatives. • Emphasize PPE for visitors in extenuating circumstances. • Consider closure when there is significant ongoing risk of transmission	No specific instruction.

*Information specific for respiratory illness is not included in table.

management guideline recommends airborne precaution for norovirus when a patient is vomiting (New Zealand Ministry of Health, 2009). Further studies are needed to examine the true risk of airborne transmission for norovirus.

12.4 NOROVIRUS OUTBREAKS—GOING BACK TO THE BASICS

Several international guidelines on the management of norovirus outbreaks are summarized in Table 12.1. To be proactive, the following question should be asked: What can be done to prevent the transmission from a case of norovirus before widespread outbreak? Norovirus was first cloned and sequenced in 1990 so that molecular diagnostic assays could be developed (Jiang et al., 1990, 1992; Matsui et al., 1991). Until recently, the testing for norovirus was focused on outbreak settings with many norovirus cases being undiagnosed in patients of all ages presenting with sporadic gastroenteritis (Beersma et al., 2012; Borrows and Turner, 2014; Pang and Lee, 2015; Pang et al., 2014; Yen and Hall, 2013). In a study that performed retrospective norovirus testing of stool samples submitted only for bacterial investigations at four hospitals in the Netherlands, undiagnosed norovirus infections were associated with otherwise unrecognized nosocomial clusters of infection (Beersma et al., 2012).

On the other hand, even without laboratory diagnosis, striving for implementation of good routine infection control practice among all patients and early implementation of additional precautions for all patients presenting with symptoms of vomiting and diarrhea could still prevent the spread of infectious gastroenteritis pathogens. Routine practice in infection control is embedded with general principles and actions to prevent transmission of communicable disease in health care settings (College and Association of Registered Nurses of Alberta, 2010; Siegel et al., 2007; World Health Organization, 2006). It is important to always have point-of-care risk assessment in mind before providing care for any patient and carry out appropriate routine infection control practices. Applying additional precautions for patients with gastroenteritis symptoms by placing signs outside their rooms can enhance compliance of hand hygiene and use of personal protective equipment (PPE) for these patients. On the other hand, it is not easy to change human behavior, and achieving good hand hygiene and infection control practice is a well-recognized challenge in many health facilities (Allegranzi et al., 2013; Allegranzi and Pittet, 2009; Zingg et al., 2015). Much literature has been published on different ways to improve hand hygiene practice and use of PPE, and this is not reviewed here (Luangasanatip et al., 2015; Srigley et al., 2015). Another obstacle faced by many facilities is physical design. For example, many facilities have a small number of single rooms or have multi-bed rooms with beds that are less than 2 m apart or an open ward design, inconvenient or insufficient access to hand hygiene supplies, and limited space for placing clean versus used PPE to streamline workflow; all these issues are not conducive to good infection control practice. When the physical design of health facilities calls for cohorting of patients without physical barriers, it is important for health care providers to have an understanding and respect for the individual patient environment and perform appropriate hand hygiene and infection control practice at all times. Some facilities also have issues with regard to workload and insufficient staffing, both of which are important elements for a successful infection control program (Zingg et al., 2015).

Although it is important to implement routine practice and additional practices as appropriate for each patient's condition, it is still useful to have the diagnostics capabilities for norovirus. A study showed that 50% of patients diagnosed or undiagnosed with norovirus infection had vomiting, with a nonsignificant lower proportion of diarrhea in undiagnosed patients (80% vs 90%)—essentially nondifferentiable symptoms in the two groups (Beersma et al., 2012). Patients with undiagnosed norovirus infection underwent significantly more diagnostic imaging and had longer hospitalization. Moreover, having the diagnostic results would enhance the recognition of clusters of infections and support early implementation of outbreak control measurements. Mattner et al. (2015) emphasized the need for timely microbiological testing for the prevention of norovirus outbreaks because the number of cases in norovirus outbreaks was significantly lower when the norovirus test results were available before the start of the outbreak. In certain settings, molecular epidemiology can be helpful in tracing transmission and increases the ability to identify areas that need improvement to prevent future outbreaks (Sukhrie et al., 2011).

12.5 CONTROL AND MANAGEMENT MEASURES RECOMMENDED FOR NOROVIRUS OUTBREAKS

Table 12.1 summarizes and highlights some of the recommendations from several norovirus outbreak guidelines (Alberta Health Services, 2015; Centers for Disease Control and Prevention, 2011; Communicable Disease Network Australia, 2010; MacCannell et al., 2011; New Zealand Ministry of Health, 2009; Public Health England, 2012). Recent reviews of infection and outbreak control for norovirus by Barclay et al. (2014) and Kambhampati et al. (2015) also provide very useful information. One of the challenges in developing guidelines for the management of norovirus outbreaks as highlighted by a few authors is the absence of good-quality evidence for many of the recommended practices (Barclay et al., 2014; Donskey, 2013; Public Health England, 2012). However, it is important to recognize that these guidelines are developed and based on basic principles and best practice in infection control that make practical sense. Some of the elements that are keys to good infection control and outbreak management for norovirus are discussed next.

12.5.1 INITIATING AN OUTBREAK INVESTIGATION

Review of 27 norovirus outbreaks in the Netherlands found that early implementation of outbreak control measures, within 3 days of identifying the index case, was associated with outbreaks that had shorter durations (Friesema et al., 2009). The importance of having organization preparedness for outbreak management and effective communication pathways is emphasized in the guidelines for the management of norovirus outbreaks in the United Kingdom (Public Health England, 2012). In the United States, the Healthcare Infection Control Practices Advisory Committee (HICPAC) recommends having written policies that specify the chains of communication to manage and report norovirus outbreaks, but it indicates that more studies are needed to understand the benefits of having such policies in place (MacCannell et al., 2011). Definitions of the start and end of gastroenteritis or norovirus outbreaks and the recommendation for the numbers of samples to be submitted for norovirus testing vary among the guidelines (Table 12.1). Most guidelines state that no further testing is needed once norovirus has been identified as the etiological agent; however, the UK guidelines indicate that additional testing of suspected new cases can be useful in differentiating patients with nonspecific gastroenteritis and facilitating earlier lifting of restrictions when resources are limited.

12.5.2 HAND HYGIENE

The importance of hand hygiene in the reduction of transmission of infectious agents was recognized back in 1829 (Labarraque, 1829). Although it is difficult to quantify the isolated benefits of hand hygiene in disease transmission (McLaws, 2015), practicing correct hand hygiene techniques at all appropriate moments during provision of care is one of the most important elements of infection prevention and control (World Health Organization, 2009). An unanswered question with respect to hand hygiene for norovirus concerns the effectiveness of alcohol-based hand rubs in inactivating human norovirus. Disinfection studies conducted with FCV or MNV showed different susceptibilities to disinfection by alcohol and various products, and which animal virus is a better surrogate for human norovirus remains unknown (Cromeans et al., 2014; Park et al., 2010; Chiu et al., 2015). All guidelines recommend washing hands with soap and water during norovirus outbreak, and alcohol-based hand rubs (at least 70%) are recommended as an adjunct if a handwashing facility is not accessible (Table 12.1). Using RT-PCR, which tests for the presence of viral nucleic acids but not infectious viruses, hand washing with soap and water was found to be more effective in reducing viral contamination on an artificially inoculated finger pad (Tuladhar et al., 2015). Another point to consider is that patients with undiagnosed etiology for diarrhea could have *Clostridium difficile* infection, and hand washing with soap and water is necessary because *C. difficile* spores are resistant to alcohol (Dubberke et al., 2014). Except for dealing with pathogens resistant to alcohol products (mainly agents of gastroenteritis) and/or when hands are visibly soiled, alcohol hand rubs are still preferred over hand washing with soap because hand rubs have the following advantages: (1) short time required for action (20—30 seconds), (2) better skin tolerability, (3) no need for infrastructure (compared to the need for clean water supply, soap, and supplies to dry hands), (4) availability at point of care, and (5) broad activity against many pathogens (World Health Organization, 2009).

12.5.3 ISOLATION PRECAUTION, PERSONAL PROTECTION EQUIPMENT, AND POLICY REGARDING VISITORS

All guidelines recommend contact precaution with gown and gloves for patients with norovirus and recommend eye and facial protection against droplets when patients are vomiting or during cleaning of areas contaminated by vomit or feces because of aerosolization risks (Table 12.1). As mentioned previously, only New Zealand recommends airborne precaution when a patient is vomiting. Most guidelines recommend suspending nonessential group activities but vary in their strictness in implementing restrictions for visitors (Table 12.1). A cross-sectional online survey of all 15 Territorial Health Boards in Scotland found inconsistencies in the availability of policies and use of criteria regarding suspension of visitors during norovirus outbreaks (Currie et al., 2015a). Professional judgment, rather than protocol, was mainly used in these types of decisions. Some guidelines suggest cohorting of symptomatic patients to reduce transmission, which needs to be balanced with the recommendation of minimizing patient movements that might increase transmission. According to all guidelines, symptomatic staff are to be excluded from work; HICPAC and the United Kingdom recommend that symptomatic staff be excluded from work until symptom-free for 48 hours.

12.5.4 WARD CLOSURE AND RESTRICTION TO ADMISSION

All guidelines listed ward closure and restriction to admission as an outbreak management strategy to be considered (Table 12.1). The UK guideline recommends a risk-based assessment and provides an algorithm for stepwise closure of areas depending on the design of the ward. Several studies have examined the evidence and cost-effectiveness for ward closure to control outbreaks of norovirus. Illingworth et al. (2011) compared the median number of bed-days lost per norovirus outbreak between two winter seasons, 2007—08 and 2009—10, because a new strategy was introduced in 2008 whereby admissions to the outbreak ward were restricted for at least 72 hours after the onset of the last case. They found a significantly shorter median bed-days lost in the winter of 2009—10 compared to 2007—08 (5 vs 29 days, respectively). However, there were other confounding factors during the implementation of the new strategy, such as a larger infection control team and a faster turnaround time for norovirus diagnostics tests. A different study performed regression analysis of 3457 laboratory-confirmed norovirus outbreaks during a 3-year period in the United Kingdom and found that outbreaks with ward closure within 3 days of the first reported date of onset of illness had a shorter duration of outbreak with fewer patients and staff affected per day compared to the wards that took more than 3 days to be closed (Harris et al., 2014). On the other hand, no significant difference in the duration of outbreaks and the number of persons affected per day was found between the outbreak wards that were closed within 3 days and the outbreak wards that were never closed, illustrating the complexities of these matters. An economic analysis using an epidemic simulation model based on active surveillance data collected from 232 outbreaks during a 12-month period in the United Kingdom found that ward closure is unlikely to be a cost-effective measure using opportunity cost of losing a bed-day versus cost per new case of norovirus and per outbreak that could be averted by ward closure (Sadique et al., 2016). Another way of considering the risks versus benefits of ward closure is to balance the risk for a previously unexposed patient to acquire norovirus infection with admission to an outbreak ward against risks due to potential delay in clinical management (e.g., admission to hospital or surgical procedures required by the patient when resources are limited, a phenomenon frequently encountered in the winter with cocirculation of respiratory viruses and norovirus).

12.5.5 ENVIRONMENT CLEANING

Thorough cleaning is essential before disinfection because inorganic and organic materials that remain on the surfaces of instruments can interfere with the effectiveness of the disinfection process (Barker et al., 2004; Rutala et al., 2008). Moreover, cleaning can remove some of the pathogen load from the environment (Dancer, 2014). Similar to the question regarding alcohol hand rubs versus water and soap in terms of hand hygiene for norovirus, there are no data on the effectiveness of various disinfectants on norovirus (Chiu et al., 2015; Cromeans et al., 2014; Zonta et al., 2015). Quaternary ammonium compounds are not used as disinfectants for norovirus due to their low activity against animal calicivirus and nonenveloped virus in general. All the outbreak guidelines recommend the use of 0.1% sodium hypochlorite (1000 ppm), with the CDC recommending a range of 0.1−0.5% sodium hypochlorite for disinfection (Table 12.1). North America guidelines also recommend using US Environmental Protection Agency-registered cleaning products and disinfectants (EPA updates their guideline regularly. Search for "US Environmental Protection Agency-registered cleaning products and disinfectants" on the web. The 2016 URL for cleaning products and disinfectants for norovirus is: https://www.epa.gov/sites/production/files/2016-06/documents/list_g_norovirus.pdf) that have label claims for use against norovirus in health care. Some guidelines recommend increased frequency of cleaning and use of disposable cloths or mops; some emphasize adopting process to minimize aerosolization during cleaning of heavily contaminated areas. Appropriate PPE for environmental staff is mentioned by a few guidelines. Another critical step is to perform appropriate terminal or isolation clean after patients are discharged.

12.6 CONCLUSIONS AND PERSPECTIVES

Because norovirus is one of the leading pathogens in community gastroenteritis for patients of all ages and due to the propensity for a large amount of virus to be dispensed in the environment with vomiting and diarrhea, it is not surprising that norovirus is the leading pathogen in institutional gastroenteritis outbreaks (Lopman et al., 2011; Shioda et al., 2015). A major advancement in norovirus research was the publication of an in vitro cell model for culturing human norovirus in 2015 (Jones et al., 2015). The ability to propagate natural human norovirus revolutionizes our ability to study viral replication, pathogenicity, and immunogenicity, and it will enhance the development of norovirus vaccine and antivirals. Rotavirus vaccine changed the landscape of childhood gastroenteritis in areas where rotavirus vaccine was implemented (Aliabadi et al., 2015a; Dóró et al., 2014; Tate and Parashar, 2014). Time will tell if the same will happen to norovirus or whether it will follow the path of influenza virus and occasionally reinvent itself through genetic changes (Aliabadi et al., 2015b).

The ability to differentiate infectious human norovirus from viral nucleic acids will help in the study of the effects of various disinfection agents/processes and transmission pathways. New technologies are being developed to disinfect the environment—for example, using no-touch automated modality such as modules that emit hydrogen peroxide vapor/mist or ultraviolet wavelength light after the patient room has been cleaned (Canadian Agency for Drugs and Technologies in Health Ottawa, 2014). More studies need to be performed to provide more evidence for the benefits of various recommended steps to prevent norovirus transmission and outbreaks.

ACKNOWLEDGMENT

I thank Mr. Brian Wong for his help with formatting the references and the table.

REFERENCES

Ahmed, S.M., Hall, A.J., Robinson, A.E., Verhoef, L., Premkumar, P., Parashar, U.D., et al., 2014. Global prevalence of norovirus in cases of gastroenteritis: a systematic review and meta-analysis. Lancet Infect. Dis. 14, 725−730.

Alberta Health Services, 2015. Guidelines for outbreak prevention, control and management in acute care & facility living sites. Includes influenza and gastrointestinal illness. Available from: <http://www.alberta-healthservices.ca/assets/healthinfo/Diseases/hi-dis-flu-prov-hlsl.pdf> (accessed 10.01.16.).

Aliabadi, N., Tate, J.E., Haynes, A.K., Parashar, U.D., 2015a. Centers for Disease Control and Prevention (CDC). Sustained decrease in laboratory detection of rotavirus after implementation of routine vaccination—United States, 2000—2014. MMWR Morb. Mortal. Wkly. Rep. 64 (13), 337—342.

Aliabadi, N., Lopman, B.A., Parashar, U.D., Hall, A.J., 2015b. Progress toward norovirus vaccines: considerations for further development and implementation in potential target populations. Expert. Rev. Vaccines. 14 (9), 1241—1253.

Allegranzi, B., Pittet, D., 2009. Role of hand hygiene in healthcare-associated infection prevention. J. Hosp. Infect. 73 (4), 305—315.

Allegranzi, B., Sax, H., Pittet, D., 2013. Hand hygiene and healthcare system change within multi-modal promotion: a narrative review. J. Hosp. Infect. 83 (Suppl. 1), S3—S10.

Atmar, R.L., Opekun, A.R., Gilger, M.A., Estes, M.K., Crawford, S.E., Neill, F.H., et al., 2008. Norwalk virus shedding after experimental human infection. Emerg. Infect. Dis. 14 (10), 1553—1557.

Atmar, R.L., Opekun, A.R., Gilger, M.A., Estes, M.K., Crawford, S.E., Neill, F.H., et al., 2014. Determination of the 50% human infectious dose for Norwalk virus. J. Infect. Dis. 209 (7), 1016—1022.

Atmar, R.L., Opekun, A.R., Estes, M.K., Graham, D.Y., 2015. Reply to Kirby et al. J. Infect. Dis. 211 (1), 167.

Barclay, L., Park, G.W., Vega, E., Hall, A., Parashar, U., Vinjé, J., et al., 2014. Infection control for norovirus. Clin. Microbiol. Infect. 20 (8), 731—740.

Barker, J., Vipond, I.B., Bloomfield, S.F., 2004. Effects of cleaning and disinfection in reducing the spread of norovirus contamination via environmental surfaces. J. Hosp. Infect. 58 (1), 42—49.

Beersma, M.F., Sukhrie, F.H., Bogerman, J., Verhoef, L., Mde Melo, M., Vonk, A.G., et al., 2012. Unrecognized norovirus infections in health care institutions and their clinical impact. J. Clin. Microbiol. 50 (9), 3040—3045.

Blazevic, V., Malm, M., Salminen, M., Oikarinen, S., Hyöty, H., Veijola, R., et al., 2015. Multiple consecutive norovirus infections in the first 2 years of life. Eur. J. Pediatr. 174 (12), 1679—1683.

Bok, K., Green, K.Y., 2012. Norovirus gastroenteritis in immunocompromised patients. New Engl. J. Med. 367, 2126—2132.

Bonifait, L., Charlebois, R., Vimont, A., Turgeon, N., Veillette, M., Longtin, Y., et al., 2015. Detection and quantification of airborne norovirus during outbreaks in healthcare facilities. Clin. Infect. Dis. 61 (3), 299—304.

Borrows, C.L., Turner, P.C., 2014. Seasonal screening for viral gastroenteritis in young children and elderly hospitalized patients: is it worthwhile? J. Hosp. Infect. 87 (2), 98—102.

Bull, R.A., Eden, J.S., Rawlinson, W.D., White, P.A., 2010. Rapid evolution of pandemic noroviruses of the GII.4 lineage. PLoS. Pathog. 6, e1000831. Available from: <http://journals.plos.org/plospathogens/article?id = 10.1371/journal.ppat.1000831> (accessed 10.01.16.)

Bunyan, D., Ritchie, L., Jenkins, D., Coia, J.E., 2013. Respiratory and facial protection: a critical review of recent literature. J. Hosp. Infect. 85 (3), 165—169.

Canadian Agency for Drugs and Technologies in Health Ottawa, 2014. Non-manual techniques for room disinfection in healthcare facilities: a review of clinical effectiveness and guidelines. Available from: <http://www.ncbi.nlm.nih.gov/pubmedhealth/PMH0071555/> (accessed 20.01.16.).

Centers for Disease Control and Prevention, 2011. Updated norovirus outbreak management and disease prevention guidelines. MMWR Recomm. Rep. 60 (RR-3), 1—18.

Chan, M.C., Lee, N., Hung, T.N., Kwok, K., Cheung, K., Tin, E.K., et al., 2015. Rapid emergence and predominance of a broadly recognizing and fast-evolving norovirus GII.17 variant in late 2014. Nat. Commun. 6, 10061.

Chiu, S., Skura, B., Petric, M., McIntyre, L., Gamage, B., Isaac-Renton, J., 2015. Efficacy of common disinfectant/cleaning agents in inactivating murine norovirus and feline calicivirus as surrogate viruses for human norovirus. Am. J. Infect. Control. 43 (11), 1208—1212.

Cho, H.G., Lee, S.G., Kim, W.H., Lee, J.S., Park, P.H., Cheon, D.S., et al., 2014. Acute gastroenteritis outbreaks associated with ground-waterborne norovirus in South Korea during 2008–2012. Epidemiol. Infect. 142 (12), 2604–2609.

College and Association of Registered Nurses of Alberta, 2010. Routine practices to reduce the risk of infectious diseases. Alta. RN 66 (6), 7–9.

Communicable Disease Network Australia, 2010. Guidelines for the public health management of gastroenteritis outbreaks due to norovirus or suspected viral agents in Australia. Available from: <https://www.health.gov.au/internet/main/publishing.nsf/Content/cda-cdna-norovirus.htm/$File/norovirus-guidelines.pdf> (accessed 20.01.16.).

Costantini, V.P., Cooper, E.M., Hardaker, H.L., Lee, L.E., Bierhoff, M., Biggs, C., et al., 2016. Epidemiologic, virologic, and host genetic factors of norovirus outbreaks in long-term care facilities. Clin. Infect. Dis. 62 (1), 1–10.

Cromeans, T., Park, G.W., Costantini, V., Lee, D., Wang, Q., Farkas, T., et al., 2014. Comprehensive comparison of cultivable norovirus surrogates in response to different inactivation and disinfection treatments. Appl. Environ. Microbiol. 80 (18), 5743–5751.

Currie, K., Curran, E., Strachan, E., Bunyan, D., Price, L., 2015a. Temporary suspension of visiting during norovirus outbreaks in NHS Boards and the independent care home sector in Scotland: a cross-sectional survey of practice. J. Hosp. Infect. (Epub ahead of print). Available from: <http://www.journalofhospitalinfection.com/article/S0195-6701(15)00433-8/fulltext> (accessed 20.01.16).

Currier, R.L., Payne, D.C., Staat, M.A., Selvarangan, R., Shirley, S.H., Halasa, N., et al., 2015b. Innate susceptibility to norovirus infections influenced by FUT2 genotype in a United States pediatric population. Clin. Infect. Dis. 60 (11), 1631–1638.

Dancer, S.J., 2014. Controlling hospital-acquired infection: focus on the role of the environment and new technologies for decontamination. Clin. Microbiol. Rev. 27 (4), 665–690.

Debbink, K., Lindesmith, L.C., Donaldson, E.F., Costantini, V., Beltramello, M., Corti, D., et al., 2013. Emergence of new pandemic GII.4Sydney norovirus strain correlates with escape from herd immunity. J. Infect. Dis. 208 (11), 1877–1887.

Desai, R., Hembree, C.D., Handel, A., Matthews, J.E., Dickey, B.W., McDonald, S., et al., 2012. Severe outcomes are associated with genogroup 2 genotype 4 norovirus outbreaks: a systematic literature review. Clin. Infect. Dis. 55 (2), 189–193.

Donskey, C.J., 2013. Does improving surface cleaning and disinfection reduce health care-associated infections?. Am. J. Infect. Control. 41 (5 Suppl.), S12–S19.

Dóró, R., László, B., Martella, V., Leshem, E., Gentsch, J., Parashar, U., et al., 2014. Review of global rotavirus strain prevalence data from six years post vaccine licensure surveillance: is there evidence of strain selection from vaccine pressure? Infect. Genet. Evol. 28, 446–461.

Dubberke, E.R., Carling, P., Carrico, R., Donskey, C.J., Loo, V.G., McDonald, L.C., et al., 2014. Strategies to prevent *Clostridium difficile* infections in acute care hospitals: 2014 update. Infect. Control. Hosp. Epidemiol 35 (Suppl. 2), S48–S65.

Esseili, M.A., Saif, L.J., Farkas, T., Wang, Q., 2015. Feline calicivirus, murine norovirus, porcine sapovirus, and tulane virus survival on postharvest lettuce. Appl. Environ. Microbiol. 81 (15), 5085–5092.

Evans, M.R., Meldrum, R., Lane, W., Gardner, D., Ribeiro, C.D., Gallimore, C.I., et al., 2002. An outbreak of viral gastroenteritis following environmental contamination at a concert hall. Epidemiol. Infect. 129 (2), 355–360.

Fallahi, S., Mattison, K., 2011. Evaluation of murine norovirus persistence in environments relevant to food production and processing. J. Food. Prot. 74 (11), 1847–1851.

Frenck, R., Bernstein, D.I., Xia, M., Huang, P., Zhong, W., Parker, S., et al., 2012. Predicting susceptibility to norovirus GII.4 by use of a challenge model involving humans. J. Infect. Dis. 206, 1386–1393.

Friesema, I.H., Vennema, H., Heijne, J.C., de Jager, C.M., Morroy, G., van den Kerkhof, J.H., et al., 2009. Norovirus outbreaks in nursing homes: the evaluation of infection control measures. Epidemiol. Infect. 137 (12), 1722–1733.

Fu, J., Ai, J., Jin, M., Jiang, C., Zhang, J., Shi, C., et al., 2015. Emergence of a new GII.17 norovirus variant in patients with acute gastroenteritis in Jiangsu, China, September 2014 to March 2015. Euro. Surveill. 20, (24).

Giammanco, G.M., Di Bartolo, I., Purpari, G., Costantino, C., Rotolo, V., Spoto, V., et al., 2014. Investigation and control of a norovirus outbreak of probable waterborne transmission through a municipal groundwater system. J. Water Health 12 (3), 452−464.

Glass, R.I., Parashar, U.D., Estes, M.K., 2009. Norovirus gastroenteritis. New Engl. J. Med. 361 (18), 1776−1785.

Goller, J.L., Dimitriadis, A., Tan, A., Kelly, H., Marshall, J.A., 2004. Long-term features of norovirus gastroenteritis in the elderly. J. Hosp. Infect. 58 (4), 286−291.

Gould, L.H., Walsh, K.A., Vieira, A.R., Herman, K., Williams, I.T., Hall, A.J., et al., 2013. Centers for Disease Control and Prevention. Surveillance for foodborne disease outbreaks—United States, 1998−2008. MMWR Surveill. Summ. 62 (2), 1−34.

Graham, D.Y., Jiang, X., Tanaka, T., Opekun, A.R., Madore, H.P., Estes, M.K., 1994. Norwalk virus infection of volunteers: new insights based on improved assays. J. Infect. Dis. 170 (1), 34−43.

Gralton, J., Tovey, E., McLaws, M.L., Rawlinson, W.D., 2011. The role of particle size in aerosolised pathogen transmission: a review. J. Infect. 62 (1), 1−13.

Hall, A.J., Eisenbart, V.G., Etingüe, A.L., Gould, L.H., Lopman, B.A., Parashar, U.D., 2012. Epidemiology of foodborne norovirus outbreaks, United States, 2001−2008. Emerg. Infect. Dis. 18 (10), 1566−1573.

Han, J., Ji, L., Shen, Y., Wu, X., Xu, D., Chen, L., 2015. Emergence and predominance of norovirus GII.17 in Huzhou, China, 2014−2015. Virol. J. 12, 139.

Harris, J.P., Adak, G.K., O'Brien, S.J., 2014. To close or not to close? Analysis of 4 year's data from national surveillance of norovirus outbreaks in hospitals in England. BMJ Open. 4 (1), e003919.

Illingworth, E., Taborn, E., Fielding, D., Cheesbrough, J., Diggle, P.J., Orr, D., 2011. Is closure of entire wards necessary to control norovirus outbreaks in hospital? Comparing the effectiveness of two infection control strategies. J. Hosp. Infect. 79 (1), 32−37.

Imanishi, M., Manikonda, K., Murthy, B.P., Gould, L.H., 2014. Factors contributing to decline in foodborne disease outbreak reports, United States. Emerg. Infect. Dis. 20 (9), 1551−1553.

Jiang, X., Graham, D.Y., Wang, K., Estes, M.K., 1990. Norwalk virus genome: cloning and characterization. Science 250, 1580−1583.

Jiang, X., Wang, J., Graham, D.Y., Estes, M.K., 1992. Detection of Norwalk virus in stool by polymerase chain reaction. J. Clin. Microbiol. 30 (10), 2529−2534.

Jones, M.K., Grau, K.R., Costantini, V., Kolawole, A.O., de Graaf, M., Freiden, P., et al., 2015. Human norovirus culture in B cells. Nat Protoc. 10 (12), 1939−1947.

Kambhampati, A., Koopmans, M., Lopman, B.A., 2015. Burden of norovirus in healthcare facilities and strategies for outbreak control. J. Hosp. Infect. 89 (4), 296−301.

Karst, S.M., Baric, R.S., 2015. What is the reservoir of emergent human norovirus strains? J. Virol. 89 (11), 5756−5759.

Kimura, H., Nagano, K., Kimura, N., Shimizu, M., Ueno, Y., Morikane, K., et al., 2011. A norovirus outbreak associated with environmental contamination at a hotel. Epidemiol. Infect. 139 (2), 317−325.

Kirby, A.E., Teunis, P.F., Moe, C.L., 2015. Two human challenge studies confirm high infectivity of Norwalk virus. J. Infect. Dis. 211 (1), 166−167.

Kvitsand, H.M., Fiksdal, L., 2010. Waterborne disease in Norway: emphasizing outbreaks in groundwater systems. Water. Sci. Technol. 61 (3), 563−571.

Labarraque, A.G., 1829. In: Porter, J. (Ed.), Instructions and observations regarding the use of the chlorides of soda and lime. Baldwin and Treadway, New Haven, CT.

Lee, B.E., Pang, X.L., Robinson, J.L., Bigam, D., Monroe, S.S., Preiksaitis, J.K., 2008a. Chronic norovirus and adenovirus infection in a solid organ transplant recipient. Pediatr. Infect. Dis. J. 27 (4), 360−362.

Lee, B.E., Preiksaitis, J.K., Chui, N., Chui, L., Pang, X.L., 2008b. Genetic relatedness of noroviruses identified in sporadic gastroenteritis in children and gastroenteritis outbreaks in northern Alberta. J. Med. Virol. 80 (2), 330–337.

Lee, B.E., Pang, X.L., 2016. The amazing race of norovirus. Can. J. Infect. Dis Med Microbiol. (in press).

Lindesmith, L.C., Donaldson, E.F., Lobue, A.D., Cannon, J.L., Zheng, D.P., Vinje, J., et al., 2008. Mechanisms of GII.4 norovirus persistence in human populations. PLoS Med. 5, e31. Available from: <http://journals.plos.org/plosmedicine/article?id=10.1371/journal.pmed.0050031> (accessed 20.01.16.).

Lindesmith, L.C., Costantini, V., Swanstrom, J., Debbink, K., Donaldson, E.F., Vinjé, J., et al., 2013. Emergence of a norovirus GII.4 strain correlates with changes in evolving blockade epitopes. J. Virol. 87, 2803–2813.

Lindsay, L., Wolter, J., De Coster, I., Van Damme, P., Verstraeten, T., 2015. A decade of norovirus disease risk among older adults in upper-middle and high income countries: a systematic review. BMC Infect Dis. 15, 425. Available from: <http://bmcinfectdis.biomedcentral.com/articles/10.1186/s12879-015-1168-5> (accessed 20.01.16.).

Lopman, B.A., Hall, A.J., Curns, A.T., Parashar, U.D., 2011. Increasing rates of gastroenteritis hospital discharges in US adults and the contribution of norovirus, 1996–2007. Clin. Infect. Dis. 52 (4), 466–474.

Lopman, B.A., Trivedi, T., Vicuña, Y., Costantini, V., Collins, N., Gregoricus, N., et al., 2015. Norovirus infection and disease in an Ecuadorian Birth Cohort: association of certain norovirus genotypes with host FUT2 secretor status. J. Infect. Dis. 211 (11), 1813–1821.

Lu, J., Sun, L., Fang, L., Yang, F., Mo, Y., Lao, J., et al., 2015. Gastroenteritis outbreaks caused by norovirus GII.17, Guangdong Province, China, 2014–2015. Emerg. Infect. Dis. 21 (7), 1240–1242.

Luangasanatip, N., Hongsuwan, M., Limmathurotsakul, D., Lubell, Y., Lee, A.S., Harbarth, S., et al., 2015. Comparative efficacy of interventions to promote hand hygiene in hospital: systematic review and network meta-analysis. BMJ 351, h3728. Available from: <http://www.bmj.com/cgi/pmidlookup?view=long&pmid=26220070> (accessed 20.01.16.).

MacCannell, T., Umscheid, C.A., Agarwal, R.K., Lee, I., Kuntz, G., Stevenson, K.B., et al., 2011. Guideline for the prevention and control of norovirus gastroenteritis outbreaks in healthcare settings. Infect. Control. Hosp. Epidemiol. 32 (10), 939–969.

Makison Booth, C., 2014. Vomiting Larry: a simulated vomiting system for assessing environmental contamination from projectile vomiting related to norovirus infection. J. Infect. Prev 15 (5), 176–180.

Matsui, S.M., Kim, J.P., Greenberg, H.B., Su, W., Sun, Q., Johnson, P.C., et al., 1991. The isolation and characterization of a Norwalk virus-specific cDNA. J. Clin. Invest. 87, 1456–1461.

Mattison, K., Karthikeyan, K., Abebe, M., Malik, N., Sattar, S.A., Farber, J.M., et al., 2007. Survival of calicivirus in foods and on surfaces: experiments with feline calicivirus as a surrogate for norovirus. J. Food. Prot. 70 (2), 500–503.

Mattner, F., Mattner, L., Borck, H.U., Gastmeier, P., 2005. Evaluation of the impact of the source (patient versus staff) on nosocomial norovirus outbreak severity. Infect. Control. Hosp. Epidemiol. 26 (3), 268–272.

Mattner, F., Guyot, A., Henke-Gendo, C., 2015. Analysis of norovirus outbreaks reveals the need for timely and extended microbiological testing. J. Hosp. Infect. 91 (4), 332–337.

Maunula, L., Miettinen, I.T., von Bonsdorff, C.H., 2005. Norovirus outbreaks from drinking water. Emerg. Infect. Dis. 11 (11), 1716–1721.

McLaws, M.L., 2015. The relationship between hand hygiene and health care-associated infection: it's complicated. Infect. Drug. Resist 8, 7–18.

Miyoshi, T., Uchino, K., Yoshida, H., Motomura, K., Takeda, N., Matsuura, Y., et al., 2015. Long-term viral shedding and viral genome mutation in norovirus infection. J. Med. Virol. 87 (11), 1872–1880.

Murata, T., Katsushima, N., Mizuta, K., Muraki, Y., Hongo, S., Matsuzaki, Y., 2007. Prolonged norovirus shedding in infants < or = 6 months of age with gastroenteritis. Pediatr. Infect. Dis. J. 26 (1), 46–49.

Nenonen, N.P., Hannoun, C., Svensson, L., Torén, K., Andersson, L.M., Westin, J., et al., 2014. Norovirus GII.4 detection in environmental samples from patient rooms during nosocomial outbreaks. J. Clin. Microbiol. 52 (7), 2352–2358.

New Zealand Ministry of Health, 2009. Guidelines for the Management of Norovirus Outbreaks in Hospitals and Elderly Care Institutions. Available from: < https://www.health.govt.nz/system/files/documents/publications/guidelines-management-norovirus_0.pdf > (accessed 10.01.16).

O'Ryan, M.L., Lucero, Y., Prado, V., Santolaya, M.E., Rabello, M., Solis, Y., et al., 2009. Symptomatic and asymptomatic rotavirus and norovirus infections during infancy in a Chilean birth cohort. Pediatr. Infect. Dis. J. 28 (10), 879–884.

Pang, X., Lee, B.E., 2015. Laboratory diagnosis of noroviruses: present and future. Clin. Lab. Med. 35 (2), 345–362.

Pang, X.L., Preiksaitis, J.K., Lee, B.E., 2014. Enhanced enteric virus detection in sporadic gastroenteritis using a multi-target real-time PCR panel: a one-year study. J. Med. Virol. 86 (9), 1594–1601.

Park, G.W., Barclay, L., Macinga, D., Charbonneau, D., Pettigrew, C.A., Vinjé, J., 2010. Comparative efficacy of seven hand sanitizers against murine norovirus, feline calicivirus, and GII.4 norovirus. J. Food. Prot. 73 (12), 2232–2238.

Partridge, D.G., Evans, C.M., Raza, M., Kudesia, G., Parsons, H.K., 2012. Lessons from a large norovirus outbreak: impact of viral load, patient age and ward design on duration of symptoms and shedding and likelihood of transmission. J. Hosp. Infect. 81 (1), 25–30.

Phillips, G., Tam, C.C., Rodrigues, L.C., Lopman, B., 2010. Prevalence and characteristics of asymptomatic norovirus infection in the community in England. Epidemiol. Infect. 138 (10), 1454–1458.

Platts-Mills, J.A., Babji, S., Bodhidatta, L., Gratz, J., Haque, R., Havt, A., et al., 2015. MAL-ED Network Investigators, Pathogen-specific burdens of community diarrhoea in developing countries: a multisite birth cohort study (MAL-ED). Lancet Glob. Health 3 (9), e564–e575.

Pons, W., Young, I., Truong, J., Jones-Bitton, A., McEwen, S., Pintar, K., et al., 2015. A systematic review of waterborne disease outbreaks associated with small non-community drinking water systems in Canada and the United States. PLoS One 10 (10), e0141646. Available from: <http://journals.plos.org/plosone/article?id=10.1371/journal.pone.0141646> (accessed 16.01.16).

Poullis, D.A., Attwell, R.W., Powell, S.C., 2002. An evaluation of waterborne diseasesurveillance in the European Union. Rev. Environ. Health 17 (2), 149–161.

Public Health England, 2012. Norovirus: Managing Outbreaks in Acute and community Health and Social Care Settings. Available from: https://www.gov.uk/government/uploads/system/uploads/attachment_data/file/322943/Guidance_for_managing_norovirus_outbreaks_in_healthcare_settings.pdf (accessed 10.01.16).

Qi, R., Ye, C., Chen, C., Yao, P., Hu, F., Lin, Q., 2015. Norovirus prevention and the prevalence of asymptomatic norovirus infection in kindergartens and primary schools in Changzhou, China: Status of the knowledge, attitudes, behaviors, and requirements. Am. J. Infect. Control 43 (8), 833–838.

Robilotti, E., Deresinski, S., Pinsky, B.A., 2015. Norovirus. Clin. Microbiol. Rev. 28 (1), 134–164.

Robinson, M., Stilianakis, N.I., Drossinos, Y., 2012. Spatial dynamics of airborne infectious diseases. J. Theor. Biol. 297, 116–126.

Roddie, C., Paul, J.P., Benjamin, R., Gallimore, C.I., Xerry, J., Gray, J.J., et al., 2009. Allogeneic hematopoietic stem cell transplantation and norovirus gastroenteritis: a previously unrecognized cause of morbidity. Clin. Infect. Dis. 49 (7), 1061–1068.

Rutala, W.A., Weber, D.J., The Healthcare Infection Control Practices Advisory Committee (HICPAC), 2008. Guideline for Disinfection and Sterilization in Healthcare Facilities. Available from: http://www.cdc.gov/hicpac/pdf/guidelines/disinfection_nov_2008.pdf (accessed 20.01.16).

Sadique, Z., Lopman, B., Cooper, B.S., Edmunds, W.J., 2016. Cost-effectiveness of ward closure to control outbreaks of norovirus infection in United Kingdom National Health Service Hospitals. J. Infect. Dis. 213 (Suppl. 1), S19–S26.

Saito, M., Goel-Apaza, S., Espetia, S., Velasquez, D., Cabrera, L., Loli, S., et al., 2014. Multiple norovirus infections in a birth cohort in a Peruvian Periurban community. Clin. Infect. Dis. 58 (4), 483–491.

Shioda, K., Kambhampati, A., Hall, A.J., Lopman, B.A., 2015. Global age distribution of pediatric norovirus cases. Vaccine 33 (33), 4065–4068.

Siebenga, J.J., Vennema, H., Zheng, D.P., Vinjé, J., Lee, B.E., Pang, X.L., et al., 2009. Norovirus illness is a global problem: emergence and spread of norovirus GII.4 variants, 2001–2007. J. Infect. Dis. 200 (5), 802–812.

Siegel, J.D., Rhinehart, E., Jackson, M., Chiarello, L., Health Care Infection Control Practices Advisory Committee, 2007. Guideline for isolation precautions: preventing transmission of infectious agents in health care settings, 2007. Am. J. Infect. Control 35 (10 Suppl. 2), S65–S164

Srigley, J.A., Corace, K., Hargadon, D.P., Yu, D., MacDonald, T., Fabrigar, L., et al., 2015. Applying psychological frameworks of behaviour change to improve healthcare worker hand hygiene: a systematic review. J. Hosp. Infect. 91 (3), 202–210.

Sukhrie, F.H., Beersma, M.F., Wong, A., van der Veer, B., Vennema, H., Bogerman, J., et al., 2011. Using molecular epidemiology to trace transmission of nosocomial norovirus infection. J. Clin. Microbiol. 49 (2), 602–606.

Sukhrie, F.H., Siebenga, J.J., Beersma, M.F., Koopmans, M., 2010. Chronic shedders as reservoir for nosocomial transmission of norovirus. J. Clin. Microbiol. 48 (11), 4303–4305.

Sukhrie, F.H., Teunis, P., Vennema, H., Copra, C., Thijs Beersma, M.F., Bogerman, J., et al., 2012. Nosocomial transmission of norovirus is mainly caused by symptomatic cases. Clin. Infect. Dis. 54 (7), 931–937.

Tate, J.E., Parashar, U.D., 2014. Rotavirus vaccines in routine use. Clin. Infect. Dis. 59 (9), 1291–1301.

Teunis, P.F., Moe, C.L., Liu, P., Miller, S.E., Lindesmith, L., Baric, R.S., et al., 2008. Norwalk virus: how infectious is it? J. Med. Virol. 80 (8), 1468–1476.

Teunis, P.F., Sukhrie, F.H., Vennema, H., Bogerman, J., Beersma, M.F., Koopmans, M.P., 2015. Shedding of norovirus in symptomatic and asymptomatic infections. Epidemiol. Infect. 143 (8), 1710–1717.

Thornley, C.N., Emslie, N.A., Sprott, T.W., Greening, G.E., Rapana, J.P., 2011. Recurring norovirus transmission on an airplane. Clin. Infect. Dis. 53 (6), 515–520.

Tuladhar, E., Hazeleger, W.C., Koopmans, M., Zwietering, M.H., Duizer, E., Beumer, R.R., 2015. Reducing viral contamination from finger pads: handwashing is more effective than alcohol-based hand disinfectants. J. Hosp. Infect. 90 (3), 226–234.

Turcios, R.M., Widdowson, M.A., Sulka, A.C., Mead, P.S., Glass, R.I., 2006. Reevaluation of epidemiological criteria for identifying outbreaks of acute gastroenteritis due to norovirus: United States, 1998–2000. Clin. Infect. Dis 42 (7), 964–969.

Verhoef, L., Hewitt, J., Barclay, L., Ahmed, S.M., Lake, R., Hall, A.J., et al., 2015. Norovirus genotype profiles associated with foodborne transmission, 1999–2012. Emerg. Infect. Dis. 21 (4), 592–599.

Wang, Q., Erickson, M., Ortega, Y.R., Cannon, J.L., 2013. The fate of murine norovirus and hepatitis A virus during preparation of fresh produce by cutting and grating. Food. Environ. Virol 5 (1), 52–60.

Wikswo, M.E., Kambhampati, A., Shioda, K., Walsh, K.A., Bowen, A., Hall, A.J., 2015. Outbreaks of acute gastroenteritis transmitted by person-to-person contact, environmental contamination, and unknown modes of transmission—United States, 2009–2013. MMWR Surveill. Summ. 64 (12), 1–16.

World Health Organization, 2006. Epidemic and Pandemic Alert and Response. Aide-memoire -Infection Control Standard Precautions in Health Care. Available from: <http://www.who.int/csr/resources/publications/4EPR_AM2.pdf> (accessed 09.01.16).

World Health Organization, 2009. WHO Guidelines on Hand Hygiene in Health Care First Global Patient Safety Challenge. Clean Care is Safer Care. Available from: <http://apps.who.int/iris/bitstream/10665/44102/1/9789241597906_eng.pdf> (accessed 20.01.16).

World Health Organization, 2014. Infection Prevention and Control of Epidemic-and Pandemic-Prone Acute Respiratory Infections in Health Care. Available from: <http://apps.who.int/iris/bitstream/10665/112656/1/9789241507134_eng.pdf> (accessed 17.01.16).

Xie, X., Li, Y., Chwang, A.T., Ho, P.L., Seto, W.H., 2007. How far droplets can move in indoor environments–revisiting the Wells evaporation-falling curve. Indoor Air 17 (3), 211–225.

Ye, X., Van, J.N., Munoz, F.M., Revell, P.A., Kozinetz, C.A., Krance, R.A., et al., 2015. Noroviruses as a cause of diarrhea in immunocompromised pediatric hematopoietic stem cell and solid organ transplant recipients. Am. J. Transplant 15 (7), 1874–1881.

Yen, C., Hall, A.J., 2013. Editorial commentary: challenges to estimating norovirus disease burden. J. Pediatric. Infect. Dis. Soc. 2 (1), 61–62.

Yi, J., Wahl, K., Sederdahl, B.K., Jerris, R.R., Kraft, C.S., McCracken, C., et al., 2015. Molecular epidemiology of norovirus in children and the elderly in Atlanta, Georgia, United States. J. Med. Virol. Available from: <http://onlinelibrary.wiley.com/doi/10.1002/jmv.24436/abstract;jsessionid=CAC217DB6F1390664662B5610A36DFE5.f04t02> (last accessed 10.01.16)

Zhang, X.F., Huang, Q., Long, Y., Jiang, X., Zhang, T., Tan, M., et al., 2015. An outbreak caused by GII.17 norovirus with a wide spectrum of HBGA-associated susceptibility. Sci. Rep. 5, 17687.

Zhou, N., Zhang, H., Lin, X., Hou, P., Wang, S., Tao, Z., et al., 2015. A waterborne norovirus gastroenteritis outbreak in a school, Eastern China. Epidemiol. Infect. 20, 1–8.

Zingg, W., Holmes, A., Dettenkofer, M., Goetting, T., Secci, F., Clack, L., et al., 2015. Systematic review and evidence-based guidance on organization of hospital infection control programmes (SIGHT) study group. Hospital organisation, management, and structure for prevention of health-care-associated infection: a systematic review and expert consensus. Lancet Infect. Dis. 15 (2), 212–224.

Zonta, W., Mauroy, A., Farnir, F., Thiry, E., 2015. Comparative virucidal efficacy of seven disinfectants against murine norovirus and feline calicivirus, surrogates of human norovirus. Food. Environ. Virol. 2015 Oct 7. Available from: <http://link.springer.com/article/10.1007/s12560-015-9216-2> (accessed 20.01.16).

VACCINE DEVELOPMENT

13

Zhong Huang, Xiaoli Wang and Qingwei Liu

Institute Pasteur of Shanghai, Huangpu, Shanghai, China

13.1 THE UNMET NEED FOR NOROVIRUS VACCINE

Noroviruses (NoVs) are an important cause of gastroenteritis worldwide. The viruses are primarily transmitted via the fecal—oral route. Although the disease is often self-limited, a proportion of individuals, especially the young and the elderly, infected with NoVs may develop severe gastroenteritis and other complications, which in some cases may lead to death. In the United States alone, NoVs are responsible for up to 21 million cases of acute gastroenteritis, 1.9 million outpatient visits, 400,000 emergency department visits, 70,000 hospitalizations, and nearly 800 deaths annually (Hall et al., 2013). It is estimated that NoVs cause 218,000 deaths worldwide each year (Patel et al., 2008). Thus, NoVs pose a serious threat to public health, affecting people of all ages. Currently, there is no licensed vaccine to prevent NoV infection. A NoV vaccine, if available, would have a profound beneficial impact on public health and significantly reduce the economic burden. For example, it is estimated that a NoV vaccine with 50% efficacy within 12 months after administration would avert 1—2.2 million cases of NoV-caused acute gastroenteritis each year in the United States (Bartsch et al., 2012). Therefore, developing a NoV vaccine is now the top priority for prevention of viral gastroenteritis.

13.2 KNOWLEDGE REGARDING PROTECTIVE IMMUNITY AGAINST NoV INFECTIONS

Understanding the correlates of protection against a given viral infection is the key to its vaccine development. Due to the lack of a robust immune-competent small animal model for NoV, current knowledge regarding anti-NoV protective immunity has largely come from clinical studies of natural infections and experimental challenges in humans. Important correlates of protection against NoV infection have been identified, strongly suggesting that it is possible to develop a prophylactic vaccine for NoVs.

The Norovirus. DOI: http://dx.doi.org/10.1016/B978-0-12-804177-2.00013-0

13.2.1 **HOST FACTORS**

Several host factors have been found to be important for human NoV infection, including histo-blood group antigens (HBGAs), secretor status, age, and immune status (Kocher and Yuan, 2015). HBGAs are diverse carbohydrates present on red blood cells, mucosal epithelial cells, and as free antigens in biological fluids. NoVs can directly bind to HBGAs in a strain-specific manner. HBGAs are considered as a cellular receptor for NoVs (Ravn and Dabelsteen, 2000; Hutson et al., 2002; Harrington et al., 2002a; Marionneau et al., 2002), although other receptors or coreceptors may exist. The expression of HBGA is controlled by the $\alpha(1,2)$-fucosyltransferase (*FUT2*) gene. Individuals carrying functional mutations in the *FUT2* gene have been found to be resistant to infection with human NoVs (Thorven et al., 2005), suggesting that HBGAs may play an important role in NoV infections. Clinical studies have further demonstrated that the susceptibility to NoV infections is associated with HBGAs in a strain-specific manner (Hutson et al., 2002; Trang et al., 2014). It is now believed that HBGA is the most critical host factor that determines the susceptibility to NoVs in human.

13.2.2 **THE ROLE OF ANTIBODIES IN PROTECTION AGAINST NoV INFECTION AND DISEASE**

NoV infection stimulates the production of NoV-specific serum IgG antibodies and the generation of IgA-biased antibody-secreting cells (ASCs) and IgG-biased memory B cells (Ramani et al., 2015; Chachu et al., 2008). Serological studies showed the presence of NoV-specific IgG and IgA antibodies and increasing titers following NoV infection (Nurminen et al., 2011). The resulting NoV-specific antibodies appeared to be able to provide protection against a second NoV infection because it was reported that children with higher preexisting NoV-specific antibody titers were less likely to contract NoV infection compared to those with lower titers (Lew et al., 1994).

In the past, it was not possible to evaluate the inhibitory effect of NoV-specific antibodies by neutralization assay due to the lack of a NoV cell culture model. Recombinant virus-like particles (VLPs) can bind HBGA as efficiently as authentic virion. Therefore, a blockade enzyme-linked immunosorbent assay (ELISA) based on the VLP–HBGA interaction has been developed as a surrogate neutralization assay (Lobue et al., 2006; Harrington et al., 2002a). Antibodies from individuals previously infected with NoVs can block the binding of VLPs to HBGA to various degrees. Clinical studies showed that the titers of blocking antibodies inversely correlate with the incident rate and severity of NoV-induced gastroenteritis (Reeck et al., 2010; Czako et al., 2012). Hence, it is currently well-accepted that blocking antibodies are the most important correlate of protective immunity against NoV infection and disease.

NoV infection occurs at mucosal sites. As a consequence, mucosal responses, as measured by salivary and fecal antibodies, are elicited. These antibodies may also play a role in the protection against NoV infection. A recent study showed that levels of preexisting NoV-specific salivary IgA antibodies were greater in infected subjects who did not develop gastroenteritis compared to those who did develop gastroenteritis (Ramani et al., 2015). Thus, NoV-specific salivary IgA antibody is also considered as a correlate of protection.

13.2.3 DURATION OF PROTECTIVE IMMUNITY

Duration of acquired protection after human NoV infection remains inadequately defined. A recent mathematical model predicted the duration of NoV immunity to be between 4.1 and 8.7 years (Simmons et al., 2013), which is longer than the results from human NoV challenge studies. One early human volunteer study suggested that immunity of up to 34 weeks could be developed following challenge with a GI.1 NoV strain (Parrino et al., 1977). A human multiple-challenge study indicated that the duration of protective immunity against GI.1 NoV lasted up to 6 months, and the protection was associated with high titers of preexisting antibodies (Johnson et al., 1990). A chimpanzee challenge study showed that protective immunity against homologous NoV infection sustained up to 10 months (Bok et al., 2011). These in vivo challenge data implicate that it is possible to induce at least short-term (6 months) protective immunity by vaccination.

Short-term protective immunity observed in human challenge studies is likely contributed partially by NoV-specific memory B cells. For example, resistance to GI.1 NoV challenge was found to correlate with an early increase in mucosal IgA in volunteers who had previous exposure to the same strain (Lindesmith et al., 2003). A study suggested that NoV-specific circulating memory B cells were associated with the protection against gastroenteritis, and these cells could be traced 180 days after infection (Johnson et al., 1990). This study identified NoV-specific memory IgG cells as a new correlate of protection against NoV gastroenteritis and also suggested that immune memory should be taken into consideration in the development and evaluation of NoV vaccines.

13.3 PRECLINICAL DEVELOPMENT OF NoV VACCINE

Culturing NoVs in vitro had not been successful until recently (Jones et al., 2014). Thus, in the past it was not possible to employ traditional live attenuated or inactivated vaccine approaches to develop NoV vaccines. Instead, previous efforts at NoV vaccine development focused on utilizing genetic engineering technologies to generate recombinant subunit vaccines targeting the NoV capsid (Table 13.1).

13.3.1 SUBUNIT VACCINE MODALITIES

13.3.1.1 NoV VLPs

Human NoVs are nonenveloped viruses. Their genome is a linear positive-sense RNA, approximately 7.6 kb (Jiang et al., 1993), which contains three open reading frames (ORFs). ORF1 encodes nonstructural proteins, including the NoV protease and RNA-dependent RNA polymerase (Thorne and Goodfellow, 2014). ORF3 encodes a minor capsid protein VP2. The exact biological function of VP2 remains unknown; however, the presence of VP2 could stabilize the secondary structure of recombinant VLPs in alkaline condition (Lin et al., 2014). ORF2 encodes a major capsid protein VP1.

Expression of VP1 capsid protein in recombinant systems results in the formation of VLPs that are morphologically similar to the infective virion but lack NoV viral genetic material (Jiang et al., 1992). Each VLP is approximately 38 nm in diameter (Fig. 13.1). Structural studies revealed that each VLP consists of 180 mers of VP1 assembled in a $T = 3$ icosahedra symmetry (Prasad et al., 1999).

Table 13.1 Representative Preclinical Studies of NoV Vaccine Candidates

Study/Reference	Vaccine Candidate	Genotype	Dose	Adjuvant	Route	Immunogenicity
Ball et al. (1998)	VLPs derived from insect cells	GI.1	5, 25, 50, 75, 100, 200, 300, 400, or 500 μg	CT	Oral	Specific serum IgG and intestinal IgA were detected; CT increased the levels of serum IgG but not the number of responders.
Nicollier-Jamot et al. (2004)	VLPs derived from insect cells	GII	10 μg	LT or mutant LT	Intranasal Oral	Specific serum IgG and intestinal IgA were induced; enhancing effects were observed with both adjuvants; local T-cell responses were induced for both routes with either adjuvant.
Parra et al. (2012)	VLPs derived from insect cells	GI.1 and consensus GII.4	50/50 μg; 150/150 μg	Alhydrogel Chitosan MPL	Intramuscular Intranasal	GII.4 consensus VLP induced broadly cross-reactive antibodies against GII.4 but not GI strains; intramuscular administration of the bivalent GI.1/GII.4 vaccine with Alhydrogel elicited the highest homologous and heterologous serum antibody titers.
Zhang et al. (2006)	Transgenic tomato expressing VLPs	GI.1	0.4 g and 0.8 g tomato powder containing 40 μg and 80 μg VLPs, respectively	None	Oral	Robust systemic and mucosal antibody responses were induced.
Fang et al. (2013)	P particle derived from *E. coli*	GII.4	30 μg	None	Intranasal	High-level antibody and T-cell responses were induced; innate immune cells were activated.
Guo et al. (2008)	Adenovirus expressing VP1 protein	GII.4	10^6 infectious units	None	Intranasal	Systemic and mucosal IgG and IgA antibodies were induced; antigen-specific cellular Th1/Th2 responses were stimulated.
Harrington et al. (2002b)	Venezuelan equine encephalitis virus replicon expressing VLPs	GI.1	10^7 infectious units	None	Subcutaneous Oral	Systemic and mucosal antibodies against homotypic and heterotypic VLPs were induced by subcutaneous inoculation with the vaccine.

LT, heat-labile E. coli toxin.

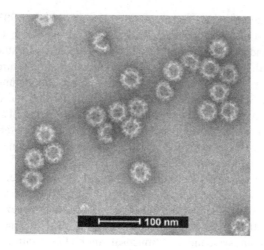

FIGURE 13.1

Electron microscope image of GII.4 VLPs.

VLPs derived from a variety of NoV genotypes have been successfully generated and tested, including GI.1 (Xi et al., 1992), GI.3 (Malm et al., 2015), GI.7 (Czako et al., 2015), GII.2 (Swanstrom et al., 2014), GII.3 (Boon et al., 2011), and GII.4 (Okame et al., 2003). Immunization studies indicated that these VLPs were in general highly immunogenic in animal models. For instance, mice immunized intramuscularly with GI.1 or GI.3 VLPs developed robust genotype-specific IgG antibodies against each VLPs with end point titer greater than 51,200; the titers of virus-specific IgG2a and IgG1 subclass antibodies were greater than 25,600 and 51,200, respectively; the blocking antibody titers ranged from 1:200 to 1:400, as defined by a 90% or greater reduction of GI.1 or GI.3 VLPs binding to saliva or synthetic HBGAs (Malm et al., 2015). The potent immunogenicity of NoV VLPs is likely attributed to the particulate nature and ordered repetitive presentation of epitopes on VLPs. These characteristic features inherent in the VLP structure can enhance immune activation by effector cells and uptake by antigen-presenting cells (Jennings and Bachmann, 2008). Indeed, it was reported that NoV VLPs could be efficiently presented by dendritic cells (DCs) to induce or activate several cellular immunity factors, including central memory $CD4^+$ T-cell phenotypes ($CD4^+CD44^+CD62L^+CCR7^+$), polyclonal $CD4^+$ T cells, an antigen-specific $CD4^+$ T cell, bone marrow-derived DC maturation, and mature DCs. Hence, NoV VLPs immunization resulted in strong innate, humoral, and cellular immune responses (Fang et al., 2013).

In addition to VLPs of clinical NoV strains, a consensus GII.4 VLP derived from three genetically distinct GII.4 NoV strains was designed and generated (Parra et al., 2012). Immunization with the consensus GII.4 VLP resulted in high antibody titers against a panel of GII.4 VLPs representing distinct variants that circulated over a period of 30 years.

Some previous human NoV challenges and epidemiologic studies suggested that NoVs could elicit antibodies with intragenogroup cross-reactivity (Wyatt et al., 1974; Swanstrom et al., 2014; Noel et al., 1997; Lobue et al., 2006; Lindesmith et al., 2010; Lindesmith et al., 2005; Iritani et al., 2007; Jiang et al., 1995), whereas evidence for the existence of intergenogroup cross-reactive serum antibody has also been described in some studies (Treanor et al., 1993; Rockx et al., 2005a; Madore et al., 1990; Higo-Moriguchi et al., 2014; Farkas et al., 2003; Green et al., 1993). The cross-reactivity of VLP-induced antibodies has been examined. One study (Malm et al., 2015) showed that each of the GI.1, GI.3, and GII.4 VLPs could elicit strong intragenogroup-specific IgG responses; however, only limited and significantly lower intergenogroup-specific antibody responses were observed. Specifically, antiserum of GI.1 VLPs did not show any cross-blocking activity, whereas antiserum of GI.3 VLPs blocked binding of GI.1 VLPs but not binding of GII VLPs; antiserum of GII.4 VLPs blocked the binding of GII.12 VLPs and GII.4 variants VLPs. These data indicate that VLPs derived from distinct genotypes have remarkably varied abilities to induce cross-reactive IgG and cross-blocking antibodies.

In addition to the form of purified protein, VLPs have also been delivered using a variety of viral vectors, including vesicular stomatitis virus (Ma et al., 2014; Ma and Li, 2011), Newcastle disease virus (Kim et al., 2014), adenovirus (Guo et al., 2008), and Venezuelan equine encephalitis virus (Harrington et al., 2002b). In general, these vectored VLP vaccine candidates were highly immunogenic, inducing both systemic and mucosal antibodies against VLP. However, further development of these vaccines was discouraged due to biosafety concerns and/or preexisting immunity against the vectors.

13.3.1.2 P particles

VP1 capsid protein can be virtually separated into a shell (S) domain and a protruding (P) domain, both of which are structurally and functionally independent. The P domain can be further divided into a P1 subdomain comprising residues 226–278 and 406–520 and a P2 subdomain consisting of residues 279–405 (Prasad et al., 1999). The P2 subdomain, which is located on the surface of the capsid, contains the most hypervariable sequence and determines interaction with both HBGAs and blocking antibodies (Chen et al., 2006; Cao et al., 2007; Lindesmith et al., 2008; Lochridge et al., 2005).

Expression of the S domain alone in insect cells results in the formation of spherical particles (termed S particles) with a smooth surface and a diameter smaller than 30 nm (Bertolotti-Ciarlet et al., 2002; Tan et al., 2004). The S particle is similar to the interior shell of NoV capsid in structure and does not bind to HBGAs (Bertolotti-Ciarlet et al., 2002; Tan et al., 2004).

Expression of the P domain in *Escherichia coli* leads to the formation of different P domain complexes including P domain dimer (Tan et al., 2004; Cao et al., 2007; Chen et al., 2011; Hansman et al., 2011; Bu et al., 2008; Choi et al., 2008), 24-mer P particle (Tan et al., 2008a; Tan and Jiang, 2005; Tan et al., 2008b, 2009), 12-mer small P particle (Tan et al., 2011), and polyvalent P domain complexes containing many P dimers (Wang et al., 2013). Among these P domain complexes, the P particle has been extensively studied for its potential as a vaccine candidate. P particles of GI.1 (Rubio-Del-Campo et al., 2014), GII.4 (Su et al., 2015; Jin et al., 2010; Bereszczak et al., 2012), GII.10 (Jin et al., 2015b) and GII.12 NoVs (Jin et al., 2015a) have been successfully produced. Mechanistic studies showed that P particles can be efficiently presented by DCs to induce humoral and cellular immune responses (Fang et al., 2013). Immunization with P particles of GII.4 NoV resulted in the production of GII.4-specific IgG1 and IgG2a response with titers of 51,200 and 1600, respectively (Tamminen et al., 2012). The study also demonstrated that P particle antiserum could block VLPs binding with four to eight folds lower efficiency as compared to anti-VLP sera. However, antisera against GII.4 P particles did not exhibit cross reactivity to heterologous antigens including GII.12 and GI.3 VLPs. A challenge study demonstrated that P particles derived from a GII.4 strain could induce homologous protection against viral shedding and diarrhea in gnotobiotic pigs (Kocher et al., 2014). These data suggested P particles as a viable NoV vaccine modality.

13.3.2 PRODUCTION SYSTEMS

13.3.2.1 Production systems for NoV VLPs

NoV VLPs could be generated by the expression of the major capsid protein VP1 in eukaryotic cells, including insect cells via recombinant baculoviruses (Xi et al., 1992; Jiang et al., 1995), mammalian cells (Harrington et al., 2002b; Taube et al., 2005), transformed yeast (Xia et al., 2007), and transgenic plants (Tacket et al., 2000; Mason et al., 1996) (Table 13.2).

Assembly of NoV VLPs was first achieved in insect cells infected with baculoviruses expressing the VP1 gene from a GI.1 strain previously named Norwalk virus (Xi et al., 1992). The resulting insect cell-produced VLPs were morphologically similar to the authentic viral particles purified from human stools but lacked viral nucleic acid. The yields of Norwalk VLPs from 1 L baculovirus-infected insect cell cultures ranged from 65 to 125 mg after purification (Xi et al., 1992). The purified VLPs were stable for at least 6 months when stored at both 4°C and −20°C and they were also stable after lyophilization (Xi et al., 1992). The high immunogenicity of insect cell-produced NoV VLPs has been repeatedly demonstrated by many groups. A number of insect cell-produced GI.1 and/or GII.4 VLPs have advanced into clinical trials.

Alternatively, NoV VLPs could be generated in mammalian cells by infecting baby hamster kidney cell with Venezuelan equine encephalitis virus replicon particles (VRP) (Baric et al., 2002, Harrington et al., 2002b) or transfecting human endothelial kidney cells with a plasmid encoding VP1 (Taube et al., 2005). The resulting VLPs were morphologically and antigenically indistinguishable to the ones produced in insect cells. In addition to the utility in the NoV VLP production, the VLP-expressing VRP vectors could induce strong immune responses toward NoV and therefore has the potential for serving as a NoV vaccine modality.

Table 13.2 Production Systems for VLP and P Particle

Antigen	Expression System	Yield	Reference
VLP (GI.1)	Insect cell/baculovirus	65–125 mg/L	Xi et al. (1992)
VLP (GII.4)	Insect cell/baculovirus	35 mg/L	Huo et al. (2015)
VLP (GI)	Baby hamster kidney cell/Venezuelan equine encephalitis virus replicon	10^{10} particles/mL	Baric et al. (2002)
VLP (GII.4)	Human endothelial kidney cell/plasmid	10^9 particles/10^7 cells	Taube et al. (2005)
VLP (GI.1)	Transgenic tobacco	0.23% TSP	Mason et al. (1996)
VLP (GI.1)	Transgenic tomato	0.4% TSP	Zhang et al. (2006)
VLP (GI.1)	Transgenic potato	8% TSP	Zhang et al. (2006)
VLP (GII.4)	*P. pastoris*	5–10 mg/L	Xia et al. (2007)
P particle (GII.4)	*P. pastoris*	~7.5 mg/L	Tan et al. (2008a)
P particle (GI.1/GII.4)	*E. coli*	~5 mg/L	Tan et al. (2008a)

Compared to other eukaryotic expression system, yeast is easy to maintain and handle, and it has economic advantage in large scale production of biopharmaceutical proteins. The capsid of a GII.4 strain (VA387) was expressed in *Pichia pastoris* and spontaneously formed VLPs yielded 5–10 mg per 1 L yeast culture after purification (Xia et al., 2007). Oral administration of raw material from VLP-expressing yeast without adjuvant could induce virus-specific systemic and mucosal immune response in mice (Xia et al., 2007).

Plant-based production systems, including stable transgenic plants (Mason et al., 1996) and transient expression with viral vectors (Huang et al., 2005), have been tested for NoV VLPs production with the aim to develop edible vaccines at a lower cost. Early studies showed that transgenic tobacco and potato could produce VLPs of GI.1 NoV, however, the yield of recombinant protein was low (Mason et al., 1996). The maximum level of VLPs accumulation in the leaves of tobacco transformants was only 0.23% of the total soluble protein (TSP) which was similar to the accumulation level in the tubers of transgenic potato. Subsequently, tomato as a vehicle for expression and delivery of full-length, truncated, and plant-optimized versions of VLPs was evaluated (Zhang et al., 2006; Huang et al., 2005). The maximum level of VLPs was up to 8% of the TSP in tomato fruit and 0.4% in potato tubers with the plant-optimized gene. In general, plant-based NoV vaccines were immunogenic in animal models and in clinical trials.

13.3.2.2 Production systems for P particles

P particles can be expressed and assembled in *E. coli* with yields of approximately 5 mg/L culture (Tan et al., 2008a). The formation of P particles is P protein concentration-dependent, with more than 90% of P protein forming particles at 2.5 mg/mL (Tan and Jiang, 2005). The antigenic and HBGA-binding profiles of P particles were similar to those of the corresponding VLPs (Tan et al., 2008a).

Yeast has also been tested for P particle production, yielding approximately 7.5 mg of P particles per liter of yeast culture (Tan et al., 2008a).

13.3.3 DELIVERY ROUTES

13.3.3.1 Systemic injection

The immunogenicity of NoV vaccine candidates administered systemically via intramuscular, intradermal, or intraperitoneal injection has been extensively evaluated in preclinical studies. For example, mice that received a single dose (10 μg) of GII.4 VLPs by either intramuscular or intradermal injection developed strong antigen-specific IgG response (Tamminen et al., 2012). A recent study indicated that two doses of 5 μg of GII.4 VLPs with aluminum adjuvant could induce high-titer, long-lasting GII.4-specific IgG antibodies in mice (Wang et al., 2015). Compared to intranasal immunization, intramuscular injection of a bivalent (GI.1/GII.4) VLP formulation elicited higher titers of serum IgG antibodies in mice (Parra et al., 2012). More significantly, chimpanzees vaccinated intramuscularly with GI.1 VLPs were protected from viral challenge 2 and 18 months after vaccination (Bok et al., 2011).

13.3.3.2 Mucosal immunization

Vaccine would be more effective against viruses that establish infection at mucosal sites if it could induce immune responses at the site of infection (Van Ginkel et al., 2000). Hence, a number of preclinical studies of NoV vaccines have evaluated the immunogenic potential of oral and nasal routes of vaccine administration. Specifically, oral immunization with purified NoV VLPs or VLP-containing materials, such as raw yeast extracts and transgenic plants, was found to induce the production of antigen-specific serum IgG and fecal IgA antibodies (Xia et al., 2007; Van Ginkel et al., 2000; Mason et al., 1996; Ball et al., 1998; Zhang et al., 2006). The presence of cholera toxin (CT) as a mucosal adjuvant significantly boosted the antibody response, resulting in higher serum IgG and fecal IgA antibody titers compared to those induced by the formulation without an adjuvant (Ball et al., 1998). A comparative study demonstrated that the intranasal delivery of NoV VLPs was more effective than the oral route at inducing serum IgG and fecal IgA response to a low dose of the antigen (Guerrero et al., 2001). The choice of adjuvant is critical for mucosal immunization with VLPs, influencing the antibody subtype and titer. One study compared a variety of TLR agonists for their mucosal adjuvanticity for GI.1 VLPs (Hjelm et al., 2014). The results demonstrated that intranasal codelivery of VLPs with GARD (a TLR7 agonist) or CpG (a TLR9 agonist) induced greater production of antibodies systemically and at distal mucosal sites. Importantly, the serum and vaginal, intranasal, bronchoalveolar, salivary, and gastrointestinal samples from the mice immunized with VLPs plus GARD were able to block binding of VLPs to HBGA by 82.0%, 61.7%, 58.5%, 85.1%, 48.2%, and 34.6%, respectively, indicating that the serum and mucosal antibodies were functional.

13.4 CLINICAL TRIALS WITH VLP VACCINES

Among all NoV vaccine candidates, only VLPs have entered into clinical trials due to their robust immunogenicity and efficacy demonstrated in preclinical studies. Thus far, the completed clinical trials have shown that VLPs in a variety of formulations are safe and immunogenic in humans (Table 13.3). Protection against NoV disease to different extents was observed in VLP-vaccinated healthy volunteers following virus challenge.

13.4.1 ORAL VACCINE TRIALS

Because NoVs transmit primarily via the oral—fecal route, the initial clinical studies with VLP vaccines used oral delivery with the goal to induce local immune responses at the sites of infection. The first NoV VLP clinical trial evaluated the safety and immunogenicity of orally administered GI.1 (Norwalk) VLP in the absence of adjuvant (Ball et al., 1999). Two doses of 100 or 250 μg of GI.1 VLPs were orally administered without adjuvant at 3-week intervals to prescreened adult volunteers. Vaccine-induced antibody responses were measured by ELISA with homologous VLPs as the coating antigen. IgG seroconversion rates (as defined by fourfold or greater increase in antibody titer) were 60% for the 100-μg vaccine dosage group and 100% for the 250-μg group. An IgA seroresponse was observed in 40% and 50% of the 100- and 250-μg dosage groups, respectively. Subsequently, a similar trial with higher, escalating dosages of insect cell-produced GI.1 VLPs was conducted (Tacket et al., 2003). Healthy adult volunteers were administered orally with 250, 500, or 2000 μg of VLPs on day 1 and day 21. The vaccine was well tolerated, with no reports of severe illness within 3 days after vaccination. There was no significant difference in seroconversion or

Table 13.3 Clinical Trials With VLP Vaccines

Clinical Trial	Vaccination Route	Vaccine Formulation	Dose	Results/Conclusions	Reference
Ball et al. (1999)	Oral	GI.1 VLP	100 µg; 250 µg	No side effects were observed or reported; orally administered VLPs were immunogenic without adjuvant; serum IgG responses to VLPs were dose-dependent.	Ball et al. (1999)
Tacket et al. (2003)	Oral	GI.1 VLP	250 µg; 500 µg; 2000 µg	The vaccine was safe; the vaccinees showed significant increase in IgA ASCs; increased dosages did not enhance immune response.	Tacket et al. (2003)
Tacket et al. (2000)	Oral	GI.1 VLP	215−751 µg	The vaccine was safe; 95% of vaccinees showed significant increase in IgA ASCs; the levels of serum antibody increase were modest.	Tacket et al. (2000)
NCT00806962	Intranasal	GI.1 VLP Chitosan MPL	5 µg; 15 µg; 50 µg; 100 µg	No vaccine-related serious adverse events occurred and the vaccine was well tolerated and highly immunogenic.	El-Kamary et al. (2010)
NCT00973284	Intranasal	GI.1 VLP Chitosan MPL	100 µg	Adverse events occurred with similar frequency among vaccine and placebo recipients; vaccination significantly reduced the frequencies of Norwalk virus gastroenteritis and Norwalk virus infection.	Atmar et al. (2011)
NCT01168401	Intramuscular	GI.1/GII.4 VLPs MPL Alum	5/5 µg;15/ 15 µg; 50/ 50 µg;150/ 150 µg	The vaccine was well tolerated and immunogenic; broadly blocking antibodies were induced.	Treanor et al. (2014), Lindesmith et al. (2015)
NCT01609257	Intramuscular	GI.1/GII.4 VLPs MPL Alum	50/50 µg	The vaccine was well tolerated and immunogenic, and reduced acute gastroenteritis (vomiting and/or diarrhea) following challenge with GII.4 NoV.	Bernstein et al. (2015)

geometric mean titer (GMT) of anti-VLP IgG or IgA among the three dosage groups. All vaccinees developed significant increases in serum IgA ASCs following vaccination, whereas mucosal anti-VLP IgA was detected in only 30–40% vaccinees. A phase I clinical trial was launched to evaluate human immune responses to a plant-based NoV oral vaccine (Tacket et al., 2000). Healthy adult volunteers were fed two or three times with transgenetic potato expressing GI.1 Norwalk VLPs. Each vaccine dose was composed of 150 g of raw, peeled, diced potato that contained 215–751 μg of viral capsid protein. Among 20 volunteers who ingested transgenic potatoes, 19 (95%) developed significant increases in the numbers of specific IgA ASCs, 4 (20%) developed specific serum IgG, and 6 (30%) developed specific fecal IgA, although the level of serum antibody increase was modest.

13.4.2 NASAL VACCINE TRIALS

Intranasal delivery of GI.1 VLPs was tested as an alternative mucosal route administration in two phase I clinical studies (El-Kamary et al., 2010). A dry powder formulation of GI.1 Norwalk VLPs containing chitosan as a mucoadhesive and monophosphoryl lipid (MPL) as an adjuvant was developed and administered intranasally to healthy adult volunteers aged 18–49 years. Study 1 was a stepwise, dosage escalation study in which the safety and immunogenicity of increasing dosages (5, 15, or 50 μg) of the intranasal vaccine given on day 0 and day 21 were evaluated. Study 2 compared 50- and 100-μg dosages of the intranasal vaccine for their safety and immunogenicity. Vaccine-induced systemic and mucosal immune responses were evaluated by analyzing antibody profile, ASC, and ASC homing receptors. Results showed that this intranasal adjuvanted GI.1 VLP vaccine was well tolerated, and no vaccine-related adverse events were observed or reported by volunteers. The most common symptoms were nasal stuffiness, discharge, and sneezing. In study 1, VLP-specific circulating IgA ASC was detected in 39% and 53% of all vaccine-inoculated volunteers on days 7 and 28, respectively; VLP-specific IgG and IgA seroconversion rates (four-fold increases) showed a dose-dependent response; and VLP-specific IgG and IgA titers increased as the dosage of vaccine antigen increased. In study 2, all subjects who received 50 or 100 μg of the intranasal vaccine generated IgA ASCs that were detectable on days 7 and 28, respectively; the 100-μg group developed higher IgG and IgA titers than those in the 50-μg group, but the differences were not statistically significant; in the 100-μg dosage group, VLP-specific IgG and IgA antibodies increased 4.8- and 9.1-fold, respectively. The majority of the vaccine-specific IgA ASCs expressed molecules that are associated with homing to mucosal and peripheral lymphoid tissues (El-Kamary et al., 2010). Further analysis of the peripheral blood mononuclear cells from the subjects enrolled in the previously mentioned clinical studies showed that all subjects immunized with 100 μg of the vaccine and 90% of those who received 50 μg had significant specific IgA or IgG memory B-cell responses; a correlation of the memory B-cell frequencies with serum antibody levels and mucosally primed ASC responses was observed (Ramirez et al., 2012).

The intranasal GI.1 VLP vaccine was further evaluated for safety, immunogenicity, and efficacy in a randomized, double-blind, placebo-controlled trial in which vaccinees were challenged with the homologous GI.1 (Norwalk) virus (Atmar et al., 2011). Healthy volunteers aged 18–50 years were administered intranasally with two doses of either placebo or the vaccine containing 100 μg of GI.1 VLPs formulated with chitosan and MPL as the adjuvant at 3-week interval. No vaccine-related severe adverse events occurred. The most common symptoms after vaccination were nasal stuffiness, nasal discharge, and sneezing. Serum samples were collected prior to vaccine administration and 3 weeks after each vaccination, and they were analyzed for antibody titers. GI.1-specific IgA seroconversion (defined as an increase by a factor of 4 in serum antibody levels) was detected in 70% of the VLP vaccine recipients prior to virus challenge. Participants who completed the 3-week follow-up period after the second vaccination were eligible to participate in the NoV challenge. Per protocol analysis showed that vaccination significantly reduced the frequencies of gastroenteritis (occurring in 69% of placebo recipients vs 37% of vaccine recipients; $p = 0.006$) and NoV infection (82% of placebo recipients vs 61% of vaccine recipients; $p = 0.05$).

Collectively, these clinical studies demonstrated that intranasal monovalent VLP vaccination can induce both systemic and mucosal antibody responses and confer protection against homologous NoV challenge in human.

13.4.3 PARENTERAL VACCINE TRIALS

A randomized, double-blind, placebo-controlled study was conducted to evaluate an intramuscular bivalent VLP vaccine for its reactogenicity, safety, and immunogenicity as an injectable bivalent NoV vaccine (Treanor et al., 2014). The bivalent vaccine contained GI.1 VLP and a consensus GII.4 VLP as the immunogens and MPL and aluminum hydroxide as adjuvants. In the first stage of the study, healthy adults aged 18−49 years were injected intramuscularly with escalating doses (5, 15, 50, or 150 μg of each VLP) of the bivalent VLP vaccine or placebo twice 4 weeks apart. In the second stage, healthy adults of different age groups (18−49, 50−64, and 65−85 years old) received two doses of the bivalent vaccine containing 50 μg of each VLP. Total and class-specific antibody responses, as well as HBGA-blocking antibody responses, were measured before and after each dose. Results showed that the vaccine was well tolerated and no serious adverse events related to vaccination occurred during the 1-year safety surveillance for the entire study. One dose of the vaccine containing 50 μg of each VLP increased GI.1 GMTs by 118-, 83-, and 24-fold and increased GII.4 GMTs by 49-, 25-, and 9-fold in subjects aged 18−49, 50−64, and 65−83 years, respectively. Serum antibody responses peaked on day 7 after the first dose for both GI.1 and GII.4 VLPs. There was no evidence of antibody level increase following a second dose. Notably, the majority of vaccinees in all three age groups developed HBGA-blocking antibody titers of 200 or more against both GI.1 and GII.4 VLPs after the first dose. In a follow-up study (Lindesmith et al., 2015), serum samples from 10 subjects injected with the bivalent VLP vaccine (50 μg of each VLP) were analyzed for potential cross-strain protection by an antibody-binding blockade assay. The results indicated that the bivalent VLP vaccine-induced antibodies exhibited blockade activities against both vaccine components as well as additional VLPs representing diverse strains and genotypes not included in the vaccine. Notably, the blocking antibodies were cross-reactive against two novel GII.4 strains not in circulation at the time of vaccination or sample collection. These results indicated the potential of a multivalent VLP vaccine to induce a broadly blocking antibody response to multiple epitopes within vaccine and nonvaccine NoV strains and to novel antigenic variants not yet circulating at the time of vaccination.

The efficacy of the bivalent VLP vaccine was evaluated in a human GII.4 virus challenge study (Bernstein et al., 2015). Healthy adults aged 18−50 years with a functional *FUT2* gene were given two intramuscular injections of placebo or the bivalent VLP vaccine (containing 50 μg each of GI.1 and consensus GII.4 VLPs plus 50 μg MPL and 0.5 mg alum per dose) at a 4-week interval.

After the first dose, 100% of vaccinees had GI.1 seroresponse, and 83.7% of vaccinees displayed GII.4 seroresponse. There was no significant increase in antibody titers against either GI.1 or GII.4 following the second vaccination. After the second dose, the vaccinees were challenged with 4.4×10^3 reverse transcriptase—polymerase chain reaction units of a GII.4 NoV strain (Farmington Hill variant) and monitored for illness and infection. The vaccine did not efficiently protect vaccinees against infection, but it appeared to reduce the occurrence of diarrhea and vomiting (68% reduction for moderate to severe and 47% for any severity) and to reduce the modified Vesikari score from 7.3 to 4.5. These results indicated that the intramuscular bivalent vaccine could protect against severe NoV illness.

13.5 MAJOR CHALLENGES IN NoV VACCINE DEVELOPMENT

The NoVs that infect humans belong mainly to genogroups I and II (GI and GII), which are composed of at least 9 and 22 distinct genotypes, respectively (Kroneman et al., 2013). GI strains cause approximately 10% of human disease, whereas GII strains account for almost all of the remaining 90% (Vega et al., 2014). The high genetic diversity and corresponding antigenic diversity represent a major challenge to the development of broadly protective NoV vaccines. Antibody cross-reactivity between GI and GII is less than 5% (Lobue et al., 2006), and no shared neutralization epitope has been identified between the two genogroups. Therefore, a NoV vaccine for broad protection against diverse NoV types must contain multiple-antigen components derived from GI and GII genogroups. In addition, the GII.4 genotype, which is responsible for more than 70% of all human outbreaks since the mid-1990s (Vega et al., 2014), evolves constantly and undergoes antigenic drift periodically, probably driven by the host herd immunity (Karst et al., 2014). Therefore, it is important to continuously monitor NoV epidemiology to allow acute prediction of future GII.4 variants for guiding vaccine strain selection.

Until recently, lack of robust cell culture models and animal models of human NoV infection has impeded NoV vaccine evaluation. A recent study showed that a BJAB B-cell line supported the complete life cycle of NoV in vitro; however, the levels of NoV replication were relatively low (Jones et al., 2014). This newly developed NoV culture system remains to be independently validated and improved. To develop an animal model for human NoVs, a number of animal species have been evaluated for supporting human NoV infection. Chimpanzees were first reported to be permissive to infection with NoV strain Norwalk virus in 1978; however, infected chimpanzees did not show clinical signs of gastroenteritis (Wyatt et al., 1978). The use of chimpanzees for this kind of invasive experimentation is no longer allowed due to ethical considerations. As nonhuman primates, both rhesus macaque and pigtail macaque can support human NoV replication (Subekti et al., 2002; Rockx et al., 2005b), but only newborn pigtail macaques develop clinical illness (Subekti et al., 2002). In 2013, a genetically modified mouse model for human NoV was reported (Taube et al., 2013). Limited viral replication was observed in humanized and nonhumanized $Rag^{-/-}\gamma c^{-/-}$ BALB/c mice upon intraperitoneal inoculation with a GII.4 NoV. Due to the immune-deficient status of the mice, the model can be used for the study of pathogenesis of NoV, but it may not be used for vaccine assessment. Studies showed that gnotobiotic (Gn) pigs and calves were susceptible to GII.4 NoV infection, resulting in diarrhea and virus shedding in feces

(Cheetham et al., 2006; Souza et al., 2008). The Gn pig model has been successfully used to demonstrate the protective potential of NoV P particles (Kocher et al., 2014) and NoV VLPs (Souza et al., 2007). However, limitations such as high cost, route of infection, short-term viral shedding, and variability in disease response of NoV infection are associated with this model. Collectively, development of robust cell culture models and affordable convenient animal models of human NoV infection remains a major challenge in NoV vaccine development.

13.6 CONCLUSIONS AND PERSPECTIVES

There is an unmet need for an effective NoV vaccine to prevent disease and death associated with NoV infections on a global scale. Based on current knowledge regarding the correlates of protection and epidemiology of NoV infection, an ideal NoV vaccine should be able to induce strong, long-lasting systemic and mucosal antibody responses capable of cross-protecting against both GI and GII strains as well as the newly emerging variants. Significant progress has been made in this regard. With constant effort from academic and industrial entities, a number of NoV vaccine modalities are now in different developmental stages. In particular, monovalent and bivalent VLP vaccines have completed phase II clinical trials with promising outcomes. Breakthroughs have been made in the development of NoV cell culture models and animal models, which may further facilitate evaluation of existing and new vaccine candidates. However, challenges remain in the development of a broadly protective NoV vaccine. Due to the high antigenic heterogeneity of NoVs and the antigenic drift of some genotypes, it is necessary to identify the major antigenic types for inclusion into a "cocktail" multivalent vaccine formulation for broad protection. Because some NoV genotypes (e.g., GII.4) evolve quickly in response to human herd immunity, the epidemiological study of NoVs should be strengthened in order to update vaccine strain selection. In addition, efforts should be made to improve the cell culture and animal models of NoV infection in order to better determine the efficacy of vaccine candidates before evaluation in clinical trials. Ultimately, the system of assessing NoV vaccine effectiveness should be unified. Nonetheless, it is reasonable to believe that an effective NoV vaccine for human use could be developed in the relatively near future.

REFERENCES

Atmar, R.L., Bernstein, D.I., Harro, C.D., Al-Ibrahim, M.S., Chen, W.H., Ferreira, J., et al., 2011. Norovirus vaccine against experimental human Norwalk Virus illness. New Engl. J. Med. 365, 2178–2187.

Ball, J.M., Hardy, M.E., Atmar, R.L., Conner, M.E., Estes, M.K., 1998. Oral immunization with recombinant Norwalk virus-like particles induces a systemic and mucosal immune response in mice. J. Virol. 72, 1345–1353.

Ball, J.M., Graham, D.Y., Opekun, A.R., Gilger, M.A., Guerrero, R.A., Estes, M.K., 1999. Recombinant Norwalk virus-like particles given orally to volunteers: phase I study. Gastroenterology. 117, 40–48.

Baric, R.S., Yount, B., Lindesmith, L., Harrington, P.R., Greene, S.R., Tseng, F.C., et al., 2002. Expression and self-assembly of Norwalk virus capsid protein from Venezuelan equine encephalitis virus replicons. J. Virol. 76, 3023–3030.

Bartsch, S.M., Lopman, B.A., Hall, A.J., Parashar, U.D., Lee, B.Y., 2012. The potential economic value of a human norovirus vaccine for the United States. Vaccine. 30, 7097–7104.

Bereszczak, J.Z., Barbu, I.M., Tan, M., Xia, M., Jiang, X., Van Duijn, E., et al., 2012. Structure, stability and dynamics of norovirus P domain derived protein complexes studied by native mass spectrometry. J. Struct. Biol. 177, 273–282.

Bernstein, D.I., Atmar, R.L., Lyon, G.M., Treanor, J.J., Chen, W.H., Jiang, X., et al., 2015. Norovirus vaccine against experimental human GII.4 virus illness: a challenge study in healthy adults. J. Infect. Dis. 211, 870–878.

Bertolotti-Ciarlet, A., White, L.J., Chen, R., Prasad, B.V., Estes, M.K., 2002. Structural requirements for the assembly of Norwalk virus-like particles. J. Virol. 76, 4044–4055.

Bok, K., Parra, G.I., Mitra, T., Abente, E., Shaver, C.K., Boon, D., et al., 2011. Chimpanzees as an animal model for human norovirus infection and vaccine development. Proc. Natl. Acad. Sci. USA 108, 325–330.

Boon, D., Mahar, J.E., Abente, E.J., Kirkwood, C.D., Purcell, R.H., Kapikian, A.Z., et al., 2011. Comparative evolution of GII.3 and GII.4 norovirus over a 31-year period. J. Virol. 85, 8656–8666.

Bu, W., Mamedova, A., Tan, M., Xia, M., Jiang, X., Hegde, R.S., 2008. Structural basis for the receptor binding specificity of Norwalk virus. J. Virol. 82, 5340–5347.

Cao, S., Lou, Z., Tan, M., Chen, Y., Liu, Y., Zhang, Z., et al., 2007. Structural basis for the recognition of blood group trisaccharides by norovirus. J. Virol. 81, 5949–5957.

Chachu, K.A., Strong, D.W., Lobue, A.D., Wobus, C.E., Baric, R.S., Virgin, H.W., 2008. Antibody is critical for the clearance of murine norovirus infection. J. Virol. 82, 6610–6617.

Cheetham, S., Souza, M., Meulia, T., Grimes, S., Han, M.G., Saif, L.J., 2006. Pathogenesis of a genogroup II human norovirus in gnotobiotic pigs. J. Virol. 80, 10372–10381.

Chen, R., Neill, J.D., Estes, M.K., Prasad, B.V., 2006. X-ray structure of a native calicivirus: structural insights into antigenic diversity and host specificity. Proc. Natl. Acad. Sci. USA 103, 8048–8053.

Chen, Y., Tan, M., Xia, M., Hao, N., Zhang, X.C., Huang, P., et al., 2011. Crystallography of a Lewis-binding norovirus, elucidation of strain-specificity to the polymorphic human histo-blood group antigens. PLoS. Pathog. 7, e1002152.

Choi, J.M., Hutson, A.M., Estes, M.K., Prasad, B.V., 2008. Atomic resolution structural characterization of recognition of histo-blood group antigens by Norwalk virus. Proc. Natl. Acad. Sci. USA. 105, 9175–9180.

Czako, R., Atmar, R.L., Opekun, A.R., Gilger, M.A., Graham, D.Y., Estes, M.K., 2012. Serum hemagglutination inhibition activity correlates with protection from gastroenteritis in persons infected with Norwalk virus. Clin. Vaccine. Immunol. 19, 284–287.

Czako, R., Atmar, R.L., Opekun, A.R., Gilger, M.A., Graham, D.Y., Estes, M.K., 2015. Experimental human infection with Norwalk virus elicits a surrogate neutralizing antibody response with cross-genogroup activity. Clin. Vaccine. Immunol. 22, 221–228.

El-Kamary, S.S., Pasetti, M.F., Mendelman, P.M., Frey, S.E., Bernstein, D.I., Treanor, J.J., et al., 2010. Adjuvanted intranasal Norwalk virus-like particle vaccine elicits antibodies and antibody-secreting cells that express homing receptors for mucosal and peripheral lymphoid tissues. J. Infect. Dis. 202, 1649–1658.

Fang, H., Tan, M., Xia, M., Wang, L., Jiang, X., 2013. Norovirus P particle efficiently elicits innate, humoral and cellular immunity. PLoS ONE. 8, e63269.

Farkas, T., Thornton, S.A., Wilton, N., Zhong, W., Altaye, M., Jiang, X., 2003. Homologous versus heterologous immune responses to Norwalk-like viruses among crew members after acute gastroenteritis outbreaks on 2 US Navy vessels. J. Infect. Dis. 187, 187–193.

Green, K.Y., Lew, J.F., Xi, J., Kapikian, A.Z., Estes, M.K., 1993. Comparison of the reactivities of baculovirus-expressed recombinant Norwalk virus capsid antigen with those of the native Norwalk virus antigen in serologic assays and some epidemiologic observations. J. Clin. Microbiol. 31, 2185–2191.

Guerrero, R.A., Ball, J.M., Krater, S.S., Pacheco, S.E., Clements, J.D., Estes, M.K., 2001. Recombinant Norwalk virus-like particles administered intranasally to mice induce systemic and mucosal (fecal and vaginal) immune responses. J. Virol. 75, 9713–9722.

Guo, L., Wang, J., Zhou, H., Si, H., Wang, M., Song, J., et al., 2008. Intranasal administration of a recombinant adenovirus expressing the norovirus capsid protein stimulates specific humoral, mucosal, and cellular immune responses in mice. Vaccine. 26, 460–468.

Hall, A.J., Lopman, B.A., Payne, D.C., Patel, M.M., Gastanaduy, P.A., Vinje, J., et al., 2013. Norovirus disease in the United States. Emerg. Infect. Dis. 19, 1198–1205.

Hansman, G.S., Biertumpfel, C., Georgiev, I., Mclellan, J.S., Chen, L., Zhou, T., et al., 2011. Crystal structures of GII.10 and GII.12 norovirus protruding domains in complex with histo-blood group antigens reveal details for a potential site of vulnerability. J. Virol. 85, 6687–6701.

Harrington, P.R., Lindesmith, L., Yount, B., Moe, C.L., Baric, R.S., 2002a. Binding of Norwalk virus-like particles to ABH histo-blood group antigens is blocked by antisera from infected human volunteers or experimentally vaccinated mice. J. Virol. 76, 12335–12343.

Harrington, P.R., Yount, B., Johnston, R.E., Davis, N., Moe, C., Baric, R.S., 2002b. Systemic, mucosal, and heterotypic immune induction in mice inoculated with Venezuelan equine encephalitis replicons expressing Norwalk virus-like particles. J. Virol. 76, 730–742.

Higo-Moriguchi, K., Shirato, H., Someya, Y., Kurosawa, Y., Takeda, N., Taniguchi, K., 2014. Isolation of cross-reactive human monoclonal antibodies that prevent binding of human noroviruses to histo-blood group antigens. J. Med. Virol. 86, 558–567.

Hjelm, B.E., Kilbourne, J., Herbst-Kralovetz, M.M., 2014. TLR7 and 9 agonists are highly effective mucosal adjuvants for norovirus virus-like particle vaccines. Hum. Vaccin. Immunother. 10, 410–416.

Huang, Z., Elkin, G., Maloney, B.J., Beuhner, N., Arntzen, C.J., Thanavala, Y., et al., 2005. Virus-like particle expression and assembly in plants: hepatitis B and Norwalk viruses. Vaccine. 23, 1851–1858.

Huo, Y., Wan, X., Ling, T., Wu, J., Wang, Z., Meng, S., et al., 2015. Prevailing Sydney like Norovirus GII.4 VLPs induce systemic and mucosal immune responses in mice. Mol. Immunol 68, 367–372.

Hutson, A.M., Atmar, R.L., Graham, D.Y., Estes, M.K., 2002. Norwalk virus infection and disease is associated with ABO histo-blood group type. J. Infect. Dis. 185, 1335–1337.

Iritani, N., Seto, T., Hattori, H., Natori, K., Takeda, N., Kubo, H., et al., 2007. Humoral immune responses against norovirus infections of children. J. Med. Virol. 79, 1187–1193.

Jennings, G.T., Bachmann, M.F., 2008. The coming of age of virus-like particle vaccines. Biol. Chem. 389, 521–536.

Jiang, X., Wang, M., Graham, D.Y., Estes, M.K., 1992. Expression, self-assembly, and antigenicity of the Norwalk virus capsid protein. J. Virol. 66, 6527–6532.

Jiang, X., Wang, M., Wang, K., Estes, M.K., 1993. Sequence and genomic organization of Norwalk virus. Virology. 195, 51–61.

Jiang, X., Matson, D.O., Ruiz-Palacios, G.M., Hu, J., Treanor, J., Pickering, L.K., 1995. Expression, self-assembly, and antigenicity of a snow mountain agent-like calicivirus capsid protein. J. Clin. Microbiol. 33, 1452–1455.

Jin, M., He, Y.Q., Li, H.Y., Yang, H., Zhang, H.L., Qi, R., et al., 2010. [The preparation of P particle of the norovirus strain SZ9711 from China and its affinity analysis with human histo-blood group antigens in saliva]. Zhonghua. Shi. Yan. He. Lin. Chuang. Bing. Du. Xue. Za. Zhi. 24, 5–7.

Jin, M., Chen, K., Song, J., Li, H., Zhang, Q., Kong, X., et al., 2015a. Analyses of binding profiles of the GII. 12 norovirus with human histo-blood group antigens. Bing. Du. Xue. Bao. 31, 164–169.

Jin, M., Tan, M., Xia, M., Wei, C., Huang, P., Wang, L., et al., 2015b. Strain-specific interaction of a GII.10 Norovirus with HBGAs. Virology. 476, 386–394.

Johnson, P.C., Mathewson, J.J., Dupont, H.L., Greenberg, H.B., 1990. Multiple-challenge study of host susceptibility to Norwalk gastroenteritis in US adults. J. Infect. Dis. 161, 18–21.

Jones, M.K., Watanabe, M., Zhu, S., Graves, C.L., Keyes, L.R., Grau, K.R., et al., 2014. Enteric bacteria promote human and mouse norovirus infection of B cells. Science 346, 755–759.

Karst, S.M., Wobus, C.E., Goodfellow, I.G., Green, K.Y., Virgin, H.W., 2014. Advances in norovirus biology. Cell. Host. Microbe. 15, 668–680.

Kim, S.H., Chen, S., Jiang, X., Green, K.Y., Samal, S.K., 2014. Newcastle disease virus vector producing human norovirus-like particles induces serum, cellular, and mucosal immune responses in mice. J. Virol. 88, 9718–9727.

Kocher, J., Yuan, L., 2015. Norovirus vaccines and potential antinorovirus drugs: recent advances and future perspectives. Future Virol 10, 899–913.

Kocher, J., Bui, T., Giri-Rachman, E., Wen, K., Li, G., Yang, X., et al., 2014. Intranasal P particle vaccine provided partial cross-variant protection against human GII.4 norovirus diarrhea in gnotobiotic pigs. J. Virol. 88, 9728–9743.

Kroneman, A., Vega, E., Vennema, H., Vinje, J., White, P.A., Hansman, G., et al., 2013. Proposal for a unified norovirus nomenclature and genotyping. Arch. Virol. 158, 2059–2068.

Lew, J.F., Valdesuso, J., Vesikari, T., Kapikian, A.Z., Jiang, X., Estes, M.K., et al., 1994. Detection of Norwalk virus or Norwalk-like virus infections in Finnish infants and young children. J. Infect. Dis. 169, 1364–1367.

Lin, Y., Fengling, L., Lianzhu, W., Yuxiu, Z., Yanhua, J., 2014. Function of VP2 protein in the stability of the secondary structure of virus-like particles of genogroup II norovirus at different pH levels: function of VP2 protein in the stability of NoV VLPs. J. Microbiol. 52, 970–975.

Lindesmith, L., Moe, C., Marionneau, S., Ruvoen, N., Jiang, X., Lindblad, L., et al., 2003. Human susceptibility and resistance to Norwalk virus infection. Nat. Med. 9, 548–553.

Lindesmith, L., Moe, C., Lependu, J., Frelinger, J.A., Treanor, J., Baric, R.S., 2005. Cellular and humoral immunity following Snow Mountain virus challenge. J. Virol. 79, 2900–2909.

Lindesmith, L.C., Donaldson, E.F., Lobue, A.D., Cannon, J.L., Zheng, D.P., Vinje, J., et al., 2008. Mechanisms of GII.4 norovirus persistence in human populations. PLoS Med. 5, e31.

Lindesmith, L.C., Donaldson, E., Leon, J., Moe, C.L., Frelinger, J.A., Johnston, R.E., et al., 2010. Heterotypic humoral and cellular immune responses following Norwalk virus infection. J. Virol. 84, 1800–1815.

Lindesmith, L.C., Ferris, M.T., Mullan, C.W., Ferreira, J., Debbink, K., Swanstrom, J., et al., 2015. Broad blockade antibody responses in human volunteers after immunization with a multivalent norovirus VLP candidate vaccine: immunological analyses from a phase I clinical trial. PLoS Med. 12, e1001807.

Lobue, A.D., Lindesmith, L., Yount, B., Harrington, P.R., Thompson, J.M., Johnston, R.E., et al., 2006. Multivalent norovirus vaccines induce strong mucosal and systemic blocking antibodies against multiple strains. Vaccine. 24, 5220–5234.

Lochridge, V.P., Jutila, K.L., Graff, J.W., Hardy, M.E., 2005. Epitopes in the P2 domain of norovirus VP1 recognized by monoclonal antibodies that block cell interactions. J. Gen. Virol. 86, 2799–2806.

Ma, Y., Duan, Y., Wei, Y., Liang, X., Niewiesk, S., Oglesbee, M., et al., 2014. Heat shock protein 70 enhances mucosal immunity against human norovirus when coexpressed from a vesicular stomatitis virus vector. J. Virol. 88, 5122–5137.

Ma, Y.M., Li, J.R., 2011. Vesicular stomatitis virus as a vector to deliver virus-like particles of human norovirus: a new vaccine candidate against an important noncultivable virus. J. Virol. 85, 2942–2952.

Madore, H.P., Treanor, J.J., Buja, R., Dolin, R., 1990. Antigenic relatedness among the Norwalk-like agents by serum antibody rises. J. Med. Virol. 32, 96–101.

Malm, M., Tamminen, K., Lappalainen, S., Uusi-Kerttula, H., Vesikari, T., Blazevic, V., 2015. Genotype considerations for virus-like particle-based bivalent norovirus vaccine composition. Clin. Vaccine. Immunol. 22, 656–663.

Marionneau, S., Ruvoen, N., Le Moullac-Vaidye, B., Clement, M., Cailleau-Thomas, A., Ruiz-Palacois, G., et al., 2002. Norwalk virus binds to histo-blood group antigens present on gastroduodenal epithelial cells of secretor individuals. Gastroenterology. 122, 1967—1977.

Mason, H.S., Ball, J.M., Shi, J.J., Jiang, X., Estes, M.K., Arntzen, C.J., 1996. Expression of Norwalk virus capsid protein in transgenic tobacco and potato and its oral immunogenicity in mice. Proc. Natl. Acad. Sci. USA. 93, 5335—5340.

Nicollier-Jamot, B., Ogier, A., Piroth, L., Pothier, P., Kohli, E., 2004. Recombinant virus-like particles of a norovirus (genogroup II strain) administered intranasally and orally with mucosal adjuvants LT and LT (R192G) in BALB/c mice induce specific humoral and cellular Th1/Th2-like immune responses. Vaccine 22, 1079—1086.

Noel, J.S., Ando, T., Leite, J.P., Green, K.Y., Dingle, K.E., Estes, M.K., et al., 1997. Correlation of patient immune responses with genetically characterized small round-structured viruses involved in outbreaks of nonbacterial acute gastroenteritis in the United States, 1990 to 1995. J. Med. Virol. 53, 372—383.

Nurminen, K., Blazevic, V., Huhti, L., Rasanen, S., Koho, T., Hytonen, V.P., et al., 2011. Prevalence of norovirus GII-4 antibodies in Finnish children. J. Med. Virol. 83, 525—531.

Okame, M., Yan, H., Akihara, S., Okitsu, S., Tani, H., Matsuura, Y., et al., 2003. Evaluation of a newly developed immunochromatographic method for detection of norovirus. Kansenshogaku. Zasshi. 77, 637—639.

Parra, G.I., Bok, K., Taylor, R., Haynes, J.R., Sosnovtsev, S.V., Richardson, C., et al., 2012. Immunogenicity and specificity of norovirus consensus GII.4 virus-like particles in monovalent and bivalent vaccine formulations. Vaccine. 30, 3580—3586.

Parrino, T.A., Schreiber, D.S., Trier, J.S., Kapikian, A.Z., Blacklow, N.R., 1977. Clinical immunity in acute gastroenteritis caused by Norwalk agent. New Engl. J. Med. 297, 86—89.

Patel, M.M., Widdowson, M.A., Glass, R.I., Akazawa, K., Vinje, J., Parashar, U.D., 2008. Systematic literature review of role of noroviruses in sporadic gastroenteritis. Emerg. Infect. Dis. 14, 1224—1231.

Prasad, B.V., Hardy, M.E., Dokland, T., Bella, J., Rossmann, M.G., Estes, M.K., 1999. X-ray crystallographic structure of the Norwalk virus capsid. Science 286, 287—290.

Ramani, S., Neill, F.H., Opekun, A.R., Gilger, M.A., Graham, D.Y., Estes, M.K., et al., 2015. Mucosal and cellular immune responses to Norwalk virus. J. Infect. Dis. 212, 397—405.

Ramirez, K., Wahid, R., Richardson, C., Bargatze, R.F., El-Kamary, S.S., Sztein, M.B., et al., 2012. Intranasal vaccination with an adjuvanted Norwalk virus-like particle vaccine elicits antigen-specific B memory responses in human adult volunteers. Clin. Immunol. 144, 98—108.

Ravn, V., Dabelsteen, E., 2000. Tissue distribution of histo-blood group antigens. APMIS. 108, 1—28.

Reeck, A., Kavanagh, O., Estes, M.K., Opekun, A.R., Gilger, M.A., Graham, D.Y., et al., 2010. Serological correlate of protection against norovirus-induced gastroenteritis. J. Infect. Dis. 202, 1212—1218.

Rockx, B., Baric, R.S., De Grijs, I., Duizer, E., Koopmans, M.P.G., 2005a. Characterization of the homo- and heterotypic immune responses after natural norovirus infection. J. Med. Virol. 77, 439—446.

Rockx, B.H., Bogers, W.M., Heeney, J.L., Van Amerongen, G., Koopmans, M.P., 2005b. Experimental norovirus infections in non-human primates. J. Med. Virol. 75, 313—320.

Rubio-Del-Campo, A., Coll-Marques, J.M., Yebra, M.J., Buesa, J., Perez-Martinez, G., Monedero, V., et al., 2014. Noroviral P-particles as an in vitro model to assess the interactions of noroviruses with probiotics. PLoS ONE. 9.

Simmons, K., Gambhir, M., Leon, J., Lopman, B., 2013. Duration of immunity to norovirus gastroenteritis. Emerg. Infect. Dis. 19, 1260—1267.

Souza, M., Costantini, V., Azevedo, M.S., Saif, L.J., 2007. A human norovirus-like particle vaccine adjuvanted with ISCOM or mLT induces cytokine and antibody responses and protection to the homologous GII.4 human norovirus in a gnotobiotic pig disease model. Vaccine. 25, 8448—8459.

Souza, M., Azevedo, M.S., Jung, K., Cheetham, S., Saif, L.J., 2008. Pathogenesis and immune responses in gnotobiotic calves after infection with the genogroup II.4-HS66 strain of human norovirus. J. Virol. 82, 1777–1786.

Su, W., Gao, J., Zang, Y., Wu, H., Wang, L., Hu, H., et al., 2015. Production, characterization and immunogenicity of P particles derived from norovirus GII.4 genotype 2004 variant. Acta Virol. 59, 33–39.

Subekti, D.S., Tjaniadi, P., Lesmana, M., Mcardle, J., Iskandriati, D., Budiarsa, I.N., et al., 2002. Experimental infection of *Macaca nemestrina* with a Toronto Norwalk-like virus of epidemic viral gastroenteritis. J. Med. Virol. 66, 400–406.

Swanstrom, J., Lindesmith, L.C., Donaldson, E.F., Yount, B., Baric, R.S., 2014. Characterization of blockade antibody responses in GII.2.1976 Snow Mountain virus-infected subjects. J. Virol. 88, 829–837.

Tacket, C.O., Mason, H.S., Losonsky, G., Estes, M.K., Levine, M.M., Arntzen, C.J., 2000. Human immune responses to a novel Norwalk virus vaccine delivered in transgenic potatoes. J. Infect. Dis. 182, 302–305.

Tacket, C.O., Sztein, M.B., Losonsky, G.A., Wasserman, S.S., Estes, M.K., 2003. Humoral, mucosal, and cellular immune responses to oral Norwalk virus-like particles in volunteers. Clin. Immunol. 108, 241–247.

Tamminen, K., Huhti, L., Koho, T., Lappalainen, S., Hytonen, V.P., Vesikari, T., et al., 2012. A comparison of immunogenicity of norovirus GII-4 virus-like particles and P-particles. Immunology. 135, 89–99.

Tan, M., Jiang, X., 2005. The p domain of norovirus capsid protein forms a subviral particle that binds to histo-blood group antigen receptors. J. Virol. 79, 14017–14030.

Tan, M., Hegde, R.S., Jiang, X., 2004. The P domain of norovirus capsid protein forms dimer and binds to histo-blood group antigen receptors. J. Virol. 78, 6233–6242.

Tan, M., Fang, P., Chachiyo, T., Xia, M., Huang, P., Fang, Z., et al., 2008a. Noroviral P particle: structure, function and applications in virus–host interaction. Virology. 382, 115–123.

Tan, M., Xia, M., Cao, S., Huang, P., Farkas, T., Meller, J., et al., 2008b. Elucidation of strain-specific interaction of a GII-4 norovirus with HBGA receptors by site-directed mutagenesis study. Virology. 379, 324–334.

Tan, M., Xia, M., Chen, Y., Bu, W., Hegde, R.S., Meller, J., et al., 2009. Conservation of carbohydrate binding interfaces: evidence of human HBGA selection in norovirus evolution. PLoS One. 4, e5058.

Tan, M., Fang, P.A., Xia, M., Chachiyo, T., Jiang, W., Jiang, X., 2011. Terminal modifications of norovirus P domain resulted in a new type of subviral particles, the small P particles. Virology. 410, 345–352.

Taube, S., Kurth, A., Schreier, E., 2005. Generation of recombinant norovirus-like particles (VLP) in the human endothelial kidney cell line 293T. Arch. Virol. 150, 1425–1431.

Taube, S., Kolawole, A.O., Hohne, M., Wilkinson, J.E., Handley, S.A., Perry, J.W., et al., 2013. A mouse model for human norovirus. MBio 4.

Thorne, L.G., Goodfellow, I.G., 2014. Norovirus gene expression and replication. J. Gen. Virol. 95, 278–291.

Thorven, M., Grahn, A., Hedlund, K.O., Johansson, H., Wahlfrid, C., Larson, G., et al., 2005. A homozygous nonsense mutation (428G → A) in the human secretor (FUT2) gene provides resistance to symptomatic norovirus (GGII) infections. J. Virol. 79, 15351–15355.

Trang, N.V., Vu, H.T., Le, N.T., Huang, P.W., Jiang, X., Anh, D.D., 2014. Association between norovirus and rotavirus infection and histo-blood group antigen types in Vietnamese children. J. Clin. Microbiol. 52, 1366–1374.

Treanor, J.J., Xi, J., Madore, H.P., Estes, M.K., 1993. Subclass-specific serum antibody-responses to recombinant Norwalk virus capsid antigen (Rnv) in adults infected with Norwalk, Snow Mountain, or Hawaii Virus. J. Clin. Microbiol. 31, 1630–1634.

Treanor, J.J., Atmar, R.L., Frey, S.E., Gormley, R., Chen, W.H., Ferreira, J., et al., 2014. A novel intramuscular bivalent norovirus virus-like particle vaccine candidate—reactogenicity, safety, and immunogenicity in a phase 1 trial in healthy adults. J. Infect. Dis. 210, 1763–1771.

Van Ginkel, F.W., Nguyen, H.H., Mcghee, J.R., 2000. Vaccines for mucosal immunity to combat emerging infectious diseases. Emerg. Infect. Dis. 6, 123–132.

Vega, E., Barclay, L., Gregoricus, N., Shirley, S.H., Lee, D., Vinje, J., 2014. Genotypic and epidemiologic trends of norovirus outbreaks in the United States, 2009 to 2013. J. Clin. Microbiol. 52, 147–155.

Wang, L., Huang, P., Fang, H., Xia, M., Zhong, W., Mcneal, M.M., et al., 2013. Polyvalent complexes for vaccine development. Biomaterials. 34, 4480–4492.

Wang, X., Ku, Z., Dai, W., Chen, T., Ye, X., Zhang, C., et al., 2015. A bivalent virus-like particle based vaccine induces a balanced antibody response against both enterovirus 71 and norovirus in mice. Vaccine. 33, 5779–5785.

Wyatt, R.G., Dolin, R., Blacklow, N.R., Dupont, H.L., Buscho, R.F., Thornhill, T.S., et al., 1974. Comparison of three agents of acute infectious nonbacterial gastroenteritis by cross-challenge in volunteers. J. Infect. Dis. 129, 709–714.

Wyatt, R.G., Greenberg, H.B., Dalgard, D.W., Allen, W.P., Sly, D.L., Thornhill, T.S., et al., 1978. Experimental infection of chimpanzees with the Norwalk agent of epidemic viral gastroenteritis. J. Med. Virol. 2, 89–96.

Xi, J.A., Min, W., Graham, D.Y., Estes, M.K., 1992. Expression, self-assembly, and antigenicity of the Norwalk virus capsid protein. J. Virol. 66, 6527–6532.

Xia, M., Farkas, T., Jiang, X., 2007. Norovirus capsid protein expressed in yeast forms virus-like particles and stimulates systemic and mucosal immunity in mice following an oral administration of raw yeast extracts. J. Med. Virol. 79, 74–83.

Zhang, X., Buehner, N.A., Hutson, A.M., Estes, M.K., Mason, H.S., 2006. Tomato is a highly effective vehicle for expression and oral immunization with Norwalk virus capsid protein. Plant. Biotechnol. J. 4, 419–432.

Index

Note: Page numbers followed by "*f*" and "*t*" refer to figures and tables, respectively.

Printed in the United States
By Bookmasters